T0293132

SYSTOLIC BLOOD PRESSURE

INFLUENCES, ASSOCIATIONS AND MANAGEMENT

PUBLIC HEALTH IN THE 21ST CENTURY

Additional books in this series can be found on Nova's website
under the Series tab.

Additional E-books in this series can be found on Nova's website
under the E-book tab.

SYSTOLIC BLOOD PRESSURE

INFLUENCES, ASSOCIATIONS AND MANAGEMENT

ROBERT A. ARFI
EDITOR

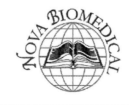

Nova Science Publishers, Inc.

New York

Library of Congress Cataloging-in-Publication Data

Systolic blood pressure : influences, associations, and management / editor,
Robert A. Arfi.
     p. ; cm.
  Includes bibliographical references and index.
  ISBN 978-1-61209-263-8 (hardcover)
  1. Hypertension. 2. Heart--Contraction. 3. Blood pressure--Regulation.
I. Arfi, Robert A.
  [DNLM: 1. Hypertension. 2. Angiotensin-Converting Enzyme
Inhibitors--therapeutic use. 3. Antihypertensive Agents--therapeutic use.
4. Blood Pressure. 5. Heart Diseases. WG 340]
  RC685.H8S97 2010
  616.1'32--dc22
                        2010047100

Published by Nova Science Publishers, Inc. † *New York*

Contents

Preface

This book presents topical research in the study of systolic blood pressure, including evidence that coping with psychological demands elicits an increase in systolic blood pressure; poor glucose control and stiff arteries; blood pressure changes in patients with migraines; transition from subclinical systolic dysfunction to heart failure and angiotensin converting enzyme inhibitors (ACE) in patients with hypertension.

Chapter I - Consistent empirical evidence suggests that active coping with psychological demands elicits large beta-adrenergically mediated increases in cardiac activity, with systolic blood pressure being most reliably affected. The myocardial effects of active coping are assumed to reflect energy mobilization or effort to facilitate coping with situational demands and they seem largely unrelated to affective arousal. Beginning with Obrist, blood pressure increases evoked by effortful coping have also been viewed as a primary biological pathway of hypertension development. This chapter tries to evaluate this traditional risk model in the framework of recent theories on adaptive versus maladaptive cardiovascular response patterns. A main aim is to demonstrate that disease risk is a complex construct that involves an interaction of cognitive-affective processes, dispositional attributes and environmental characteristics.

Chapter II - A strict control of the blood glucose level has been shown to be essential in order to prevent diabetic complications in patients with type 1 diabetes. However, the pathogenesis lying behind this complex cascade is far from clear. One pathway may lead via a toxic effect of glucose on the blood vessels resulting in a stiffening of the arteries and thus vascular complications. To date diabetes affects more than 240 million people worldwide and the number is rapidly increasing. The majority of cases have type 2 diabetes, but also type 1 diabetes shows a remarkable increase. The incidence of type 1 diabetes, was recently shown to have doubled from 1980 to 2005 in Finnish children. The reason is still largely unknown. The treatment of diabetes has markedly improved during recent years due to modern regimens. Despite better treatment it has not been able to eradicate the complications. Patients with type 1 diabetes are at increased risk of cardiovascular complications and diabetic nephropathy increases this risk markedly. As diabetic nephropathy influences one third of the patients, genetic predisposition seems evident. However, several studies have shown that diabetic kidney disease cannot exclusively be explained by genetic factors and a number of other players may be involved. Hyperglycemia causes extensive changes in the metabolic balance and has been shown to particularly influence the blood vessels. The track from a high blood glucose concentration to functional and structural arterial changes is long and various mechanisms seem to play their role. These include metabolic, hemodynamic and intracellular factors as well as growth factors and inflammatory components. Eventually, the function of the inner layer of the arteries, the endothelium, is disturbed. Endothelial dysfunction is believed to be tightly linked to arterial stiffness, a surrogate marker for cardiovascular disease. An increase in the arterial stiffness causes a premature return of reflected waves in the late systolic phase, increasing central pulse pressure (PP) and thus systolic blood pressure (SBP). SBP increases the load on the left ventricle, increasing the oxygen demand of the myocardium. The increase in central PP and the decrease in diastolic BP (DBP) may directly cause subendocardial ischemia. The measurement of aortic stiffness, which integrates the alterations of the arterial wall, may also reflect parallel lesions present at the site of the coronary arteries. Patients with type 1 diabetes have enhanced arterial stiffness even before clinically detectable diabetic complications compared to non-diabetic subjects. Arterial stiffness is further increased by micro- and macrovascular complications. Moreover, it has been shown in type 1 diabetes, that these patients suffer from premature arterial aging measured as increased PP, and the age – PP association was even steeper in the presence of diabetic nephropathy. Epidemiological studies have shown arterial stiffness to play an independent role in the prediction of cardiovascular disease in selected patients groups. The predictive value is especially high for patients with type 2 diabetes, end stage renal disease, and coronary heart disease but it is also shown in hypertensive patients as well as in the general population. Whether an attenuation of the arterial stiffness also reduces cardiovascular disease has to be determined. Only a few pharmacological studies have provided data regarding this subject. Two drugs that inhibit the renin-angiotensin-system (RAS), perindopril and losartan, have been shown to decrease arterial stiffness and alongside this effect also provide a protective effect against cardiovascular events. No interventional study has yet elucidated the role of strict glucose control on arterial stiffness in patients with type 1 diabetes. Tight metabolic and antihypertensive control are still the cornerstones in the prevention and treatment of diabetic complications. The specific role of tight glucose control cannot be emphasized enough. However, a need for a tool or surrogate marker to identify the patients at risk before clinically detectable complications is evident. One such marker may be arterial stiffness linking diabetes to increased cardiovascular risk. Future research will explore the mechanisms in more detail and hopefully provide the rationale for measures to retard the progression of arterial stiffness and thus diabetic complications.

Chapter III - Migraine and hypertension are common complaints and both have high prevalence worldwide.The comorbidity of migraine with hypertension is a common issue since 1913. Recent epidemiologic and population-based studies put some doubt regarding the association between migraine and hypertension, no association or even negative association was found by some authors. Authors who supported the positive association suggested that rennin-angiotensin system as a biological link between hypertension and CNS activities that are relevant for migraine pathogenesis. Authors who denied the association suggested a coincidental existence since any associationbetween two prevalent health conditions is likely to be detected in large series. Authors who supported the negative association suggested a central regulatory and homeostatic process resulting in reduction of sensitivity to pain(a phenomenon called hypertension-associated hypalgesia). Baroreflex stimulation, endogenous opioids, catecholamines and calcitonin peptide may influence blood pressure and pain sensitivity in patients with migraineand lowers the number of migraine attacks in hypertensives. Despite the uncertainty still present in this field, a unifying view among most recent studies suggests that migraine is positively correlated with diastolic blood pressure but negatively correlated with systolic blood pressure and pulse pressure. Similar vascular risk profile and the abnormal properties of systemic as well as cranial arterial vessels exist in subjects with migraine and hypertension. On the other hand poor control of blood pressure may exacerbate the frequency and severity of migraine and other headaches. These evidences may suggest that both conditions may coexist as part of a systemic disease. Thus establishing the blood pressure should be a routine task in the assessment of all headache patients and the control of hypertension in migraine patients is an important factor for the success of migraine treatment and to lower cardio- and cerebro-vascular risks.

Chapter IV - In the recent years, heart failure (HF) with relatively preserved ejection fraction (EF) has gained much attention owing to largely unproved pathogenesis, high morbidity and the lack of efficient therapeutic approach. Hypertension, a leading cause and threat of HF and cardiovascular co-morbidities in developed society, is currently becoming more and more widely recognized. Increasing arterial load of long duration, when coupled with elevated ventricular wall stress and after-load, has been observed to be associated with ventricular-arterial stiffening and subsequent heart failure (HF) development. Measure of ventricular contractility, such as end-systolic elastance, has been mentioned to be influenced by ventricular geometry. While myocardial contractility seemed to increase in asymptomatic hypertensive subjects in order to compensate for elevated arterial load, depressed contractility accompanied with increased passive myocardial stiffness was observed in the earlier stage HF patients. Indeed, it is well recognized that several systolic indices have actually declined in the earlier stage of HF though in this stage, conventional assessment of LV pumping in terms of ejection fraction (EF) may remain relatively unchanged. Altered cardiac structure and function such as concentric remodeling before over hypertrophy has been widely assessed and recognized in earlier stage of HTN though the exact clinical significance is unclear so far. A more severe form, ventricular hypertrophy, denotes a useful clinical marker of target organ damage and remained as robust cardiovascular prognosticator. However, diastolic dysfunction when utilizing tissue Doppler imaging (TDI) in detecting early myocardial damage in earlier stage hypertension (HTN) has been well-documented. More recently, emerging imaging technology and modality such as deformation imaging have allowed detection of early ventricular systolic dysfunction clinically feasible. Evidence of systolic dysfunction, in terms of the decline of deformation has also been proved in the recent studies. Even though, still there remained many issues unresolved regarding the interaction and mechanisms between ventricular remodeling and arterial adaptation in the transition from HTN to HF. A systemic approach and assessment to such link between ventricular remodeling, coupled ventricular-arterial stiffening and subclinical systolic dysfunction also remained to be established. More importantly, insights into the understanding of such transitional process may help identify subjects susceptible to HF development under increased arterial load and may warrant precise and earlier therapeutic intervention to prevent cascade of future unpleasant HF events.

Chapter V - It is well established that chronic, poorly controlled hypertension is an independent risk factor for cardiovascular morbidity and mortality, stroke and renal failure and in consequence controlling high blood pressure can reduce complications such as heart attack, heart failure, stroke, kidney failure and premature death. Confirming this statement, a prospective analysis of the 36-year follow-up data from the Framingham Heart Study demonstrated that hypertension (Systo-Diastolic blood pressure ≥ 140/90 mm Hg) is an important risk factor contributing to all major atherosclerotic CVD outcomes, including CHD, stroke, peripheral artery disease, and heart failure. Although a common and treatable risk factor for cardiovascular morbidity and mortality, hypertension is still highly prevalent, affecting approximately 1 billion individuals worldwide. Though awareness and treatment of hypertension has increased over the years, substantial improvements in blood pressure control rates are still lacking, despite availability of multiple antihypertensive agents with various pharmacological mechanisms of action and relatively few side effects. As a matter of facts because of the high prevalence of hypertension in the general population, approximately 35% of atherosclerotic CVD events may be attributable to hypertension. In addition to being a powerful risk factor for cardiovascular disease, hypertension in elderly patients increases the risk of decline in cognitive function. Due to the complex nature of hypertension, it is not surprising that single antihypertensive agents normalize blood pressure for less than a majority of hypertensive patients, and to lower the risk of complications from uncontrolled high blood pressure it is vital to treat patients early and aggressively. Given the just mentioned poor blood pressure control rates observed worldwide, it is important to carefully examine the numerous factors that influence blood pressure control. One important factor is the efficacy of the antihypertensive agent prescribed: it is important to choose an effective agent in order to maximize the chances of achieving goal blood pressure. Patient adherence is another critically important factor influencing blood pressure control. No matter how well an antihypertensive agent works in a short-term clinical trial, it will not be effective in the clinical setting if patients do not continue to take it over the long term. One of the most important factor that may impact control is convenience of dosing. The tolerability profile of an agent can have a major impact on patient adherence. Hypertension is generally asymptomatic for most patients; thus, a poorly tolerated drug with troublesome side effects may cause patients to feel worse while taking the drug than they did prior to the initiation of therapy; this fact will likely lead them to discontinue treatment, which, in turn, will lead to poor blood pressure control. An antihypertensive agent should, therefore, be effective and also have an excellent safety and tolerability profile and a simple, convenient dosing schedule. As we said, the lack of overt symptomatology in hypertension (until it progresses) makes side effects even more intolerable to patients; if the adverse events observed with many antihypertensive drugs occur too frequently or are too severe, patients often skip or completely discontinue their blood pressure medication altogether. If blood pressure medications are not taken as directed, drug efficacy is severely compromised, and a compromise in efficacy leads to uncontrolled blood pressure and, eventually, elevations above target range. There are many mechanisms involved in hypertension and it's now absolutely clear that one class of drug alone does not target all mechanisms at the same time; monotherapy is often insufficient to bring blood pressure down to a safe range. Actually several evidences coming from wide Clinical Studies confirm that the majority of hypertensive patients require two or more agents to reach blood pressure goal, and for those patients with stage 2 hypertension (or blood pressure > 20/10 mmHg above goal), it is recommended that treatment is initiated with a combination of two drugs from different classes; consequently most of the treatment guidelines for hypertension recommend that patients with baseline blood pressure ≥160/100 mmHg should be given a combination of two molecules from different drug classes as initial therapy. The renin-angiotensin-aldosterone system plays a crucial role in blood pressure regulation and hypertension-related complications. Angiotensin-converting enzyme inhibitors were the first to be used to block the RAAS and now have many compelling indications in the treatment of hypertension and its cardiovascular and renal complications. Angiotensin II receptor blockers, introduced 20 years later, have been shown to be equally as effective as antihypertensive treatment also in particular categories of patients and are also associated with a lower number of side effects. Furthermore, in clinical trials ARBs and ACEIs were associated with comparable benefits for their most typical indications. In addition, due to the development of direct renin inhibitors, blockade of the renin– angiotensin–aldosterone system at the level of theinteraction of renin with a substrate has become a clinical reality; the potential of renin inhibition must be viewed in the context of the remarkable efficacy of both angiotensin converting enzyme inhibition and angiotensin receptor blockers.There is an approximately linear relationship between relative risk of cardiovascular events and level of blood pressure, at least at levels between about 115/75 and 180/105 mmHg. Randomized clinical trials have demonstrated a 20% to 30% *relative* reduction in overall cardiovascular risk with antihypertensive treatment across this wide range of blood pressure levels. More importantly, the absolute cardiovascularrisk reduction is directly related to the pre-treatment blood pressure levels. Although specific clinical trial evidence only confirms the value of systolic blood pressure reduction to 140 mmHg, the totality of available evidence supports the benefit of blood pressure reduction to even lower levels in individuals at high risk. On the other hand, the benefits of lowering systolic blood pressure below that level in patients with mildly elevated blood pressure but at low absolute risk, are small. Multiple trials have addressed the question of whether more aggressive treatment of blood pressure improves outcomes. For instance, in the Hypertension Optimal Treatment (HOT) trial, the targeted blood pressure separations were not sufficient to determine whether "the lower" was "the better"; on the other hand in the United Kingdom Prospective Diabetes Study (UKPDS) a tighter control of blood pressure resulted in better cardiovascular disease outcome in individuals with diabetes. Although the available data are consistent with the notion that lower blood pressure levels, within the usual range seen in clinical settings, are beneficial, few clinical data currently support treatment to a level <140/90 mmHg in the overall population. The ESH/ESC 2007 Guidelines underlined that regardless of the drug employed, monotherapy allows to achieve blood pressure target in only a limited number of hypertensive patients and that the use of more than one agent is necessary to achieve target blood pressure in the majority of patients. A vast array of effective and well tolerated combinations is available; the ESH/ESC 2007 Guidelines also suggested that a combination of two drugs at low doses should be preferred as first step treatment when initial blood pressure is in the grade 2 or 3 range or if total cardiovascular risk is high or very high. Moreover, these Guidelines consider that in several patients blood pressure control is not achieved by two drugs, so introducing the concept that a combination of three or more drugs is sometimes required.

Chapter VI - Isolated systolic hypertension (ISH) is defined by the elevation of systolic blood pressure (SBP), with normal levels of diastolic blood pressure (DBP). The condition is recognized as a major cardiovascular risk factor, and current guidelines suggest values of SBP ≥ 140 mm Hg and DBP < 90 mm Hg for the diagnosis and treatment. Age-related changes in large arteries seem to have an important role in the pathogenesis and progression of SBP elevation. Ageing is associated with structural and functional alterations in the intima and media layers, characterized by thickening of large arteries, increased sympathetic activity and decreased sensitivity of beta-receptors, leading to deterioration in arterial compliance. These vessel modifications can determine differences in SBP levels for the same ejected volume. Even in apparently healthy individuals without known cardiovascular disease, SBP tends to increase throughout the life, whereas DBP increases up to 55-60, declining slowly thereafter.

In the elderly, ISH is considered the most common type of hypertension, particularly among very old subjects. For the correct diagnosis of ISH it is necessary to rule out the misdiagnosis of pseudo hypertension, white coat hypertension and to recognize the auscultatory hiatus.

The benefits of hypertension treatment have been fully demonstrated in controlled clinical trials, including those subjects with ISH. Beyond the reduction in major cardiovascular events, treatment of ISH also reduces the incidence of cognitive impairment and dementia.

The treatment goal for blood pressure levels should be below 140/90 mm Hg. Lifestyle changes have to be encouraged, are less expensive and have proven cardiovascular benefits. Elderly patients with ISH usually present other comorbidities and these conditions should guide the choice of anti-hypertensive agents, preferably with drugs that benefit other preexisting diseases and risk factors, even in borderline or stage I hypertension.

Thiazide diuretics are first-line agents for patients without comorbidities; indapamide, a sulfonamide derivative, seems to have the advantage of not interfering with glucose and lipid levels. When there is renal impairment with glomerular filtration rate < 30 mL/min loop diuretics should be chosen. Dihydropyridine calcium antagonists have been recognized as safe drugs with clear benefits among these patients, but some side effects can be more common in elderly patients. Angiotensin converting enzyme inhibitors are efficacious for treatment of ISH in the elderly, in spite of decreased renin levels. They reduce cardiovascular events, especially in high risk patients. Beta-blockers can be less effective in elderly patients but should be given for those with coronary heart disease or heart failure. Some beta-blockers such as metoprolol and bisoprolol are preferred due to lower risk of central nervous system side effects. Angiotensin receptor blockers (ARBs) are antihypertensives with excellent safety profile, and have proven benefits for ISH in the elderly. Central sympatholytic agents have limited use due to high risk of side effects.

Chapter VII - Hypertension, especially systolic hypertension, is the single most important modifiable risk factor for stroke. A number of recent studies have shown that for primary and secondary stroke prevention, beta blockers should no longer be considered first line agents because of a relatively higher risk of stroke recurrence, mortality (particularly in diabetics) and new onset diabetes compared to other drug classes. First-line choices should include calcium channel blockers, angiotensin converting enzyme inhibitors, angiotensin receptor blockers, and diuretics. Patients with diabetes and chronic kidney disease require specific treatment. Most patients require multiple agents for control. Initial polytherapy may be superior to monotherapy and graduated titration. Acute blood pressure management in stroke is less well defined. The available data suggest that excessive rises and declines in blood pressure may be associated with worse outcomes. Ongoing trials are designed to establish a scientific basis for acute stroke blood pressure management.

Chapter VIII - Atherosclerosis and aneurysm occur primarily near areas of disturbed flow such as bifurcations and large curvatures in the arterial tree. Changes to the geometry of these locations are believed to facilitate the development of atherosclerosis lesions and aneurysm ruptures. This fact has been observed*in vivo*, enforcing the importance of studying local hemodynamic conditions in these disease prone arterial sites. Three-dimensional angiographic non-invasive techniques, such as computerized axial tomography (CT) and magnetic resonance imaging (MRI), provide detailed anatomic information. Local hemodynamics can then be studied at patient-specific level using computational fluid-dynamics (CFD) applied to realistic geometric vasculature models. Therefore,it is important to reconstruct geometric models from CT or MR angiography images in order to gain accuracy in CFD computations and predictions. The aim of this chapter is to review the use of CFD methods in non-invasivediagnosis or screening of cardiovascular diseases.

Chapter IX - Beat-to-Beat R-R intervals and systolic blood pressure (SBP) variability signals were used for a quantitative study of coupling strength and synchronization in non linear interaction of heart rate and systolic blood pressure during spontaneous and controlled breathing. In addition to linear analysis that was based on spectral and cross-spectral analysis, we applied the independence of complexity test, the recurrence and the cross recurrence quantification analysis in order to estimate the values of coupling and synchronization in the two conditions of experimentation. The results indicate that the non linear R-R:SBP interaction is influenced at a high degree by the respiratory component because coupling strength and synchronization resulted strongly reduced during controlled respect to spontaneous respiration. In particular, the recurrence quantification analysis enabled us to confirm that a non deterministic dynamics, mathematically supported by the so called relaxation of Lipschitz conditions, is at the basis in cardiovascular control system.

Chapter X - Angiotensin converting enzyme inhibitors (ACEI) have been shown to be beneficial in patients with hypertension, recent myocardial infarction (MI), patients undergoing percutaneous coronary intervention (PCI) and/or left ventricular (LV) dysfunction. However, the evidence for routine administration of ACEI has been conflicting in patients with coronary artery disease (CAD) with preserved LV systolic function. In this chapter, the authors review the potential anti-atherosclerotic mechanisms of ACEI. In addition, they will summarize the randomized clinical trials supporting the potential benefitsof ACEI in patient with CAD and preserved LV function. The potential differences in the study design, patient population, individual ACEI pharmacokinetic and pharmacodynamic characteristics and therapeutic blood pressure differences between the trials will be addressed. In addition, the authors will also present an updated meta-analysis of the above trials. In summary, they believe that the current evidence supports that routine treatment with ACEI in patients with CAD who have preserved LV function.

In: Systolic Blood Pressure
Editor: Robert A. Arfi

ISBN: 978-1-61209-263-8
©2012 Nova Science Publishers, Inc.

Chapter I

Sympathetically-Mediated Blood Pressure Responses in Active Performance Situations: Cognitive Mediators, Dispositional Moderators and Cardiovascular Disease Risk

Margit Gramer
Department of Psychology, Karl-Franzens Universität, Graz, Austria

Abstract

Consistent empirical evidence suggests that active coping with psychological demands elicits large beta-adrenergically mediated increases in cardiac activity, with systolic blood pressure being most reliably affected. The myocardial effects of active coping are assumed to reflect energy mobilization or effort to facilitate coping with situational demands and they seem largely unrelated to affective arousal. Beginning with Obrist (1981), blood pressure increases evoked by effortful coping have also been viewed as a primary biological pathway of hypertension development. This chapter tries to evaluate this traditional risk model in the framework of recent theories on adaptive versus maladaptive cardiovascular response patterns. A main aim is to demonstrate that disease risk is a complex construct that involves an interaction of cognitive-affective processes, dispositional attributes and environmental characteristics.

Introduction

It is well established that the type of behavioral demand exerts a substantial influence on the intensity and patterning of cardiovascular responses. In particular, Obrist's (1981) task typology of *active vs. passive coping* has been found to elicit distinct cardiovascular adjustments. Active coping tasks provide the opportunity to exert control over outcomes in accordance with abilities and efforts. Consistent empirical evidence (Allen, Obrist, Sherwood, and Crowell, 1987; Bongard, 1995; Obrist, 1981; Sherwood, Dolan, and Light, 1990) demonstrates that the cardiovascular adjustments in active performance situations are characterized by large beta-adrenergically mediated increases in cardiac output (CO), indicated by elevations in systolic blood pressure (SBP) and heart rate (HR). Simultaneous effects on diastolic blood pressure (DBP) have also been observed but are considered less likely (Wright, 1996). In situations that require the passive tolerance or endurance of stressors cardiovascular responses appear to be primarily under alpha-adrenergic control, resulting in enhanced total peripheral resistance (TPR) and blood pressure (BP) reactivity, in particular, DBP reactivity (Hartley, Ginsburg, and Heffner, 1999; Lovallo et al., 1985; Sherwood et al., 1990). The myocardial effects of active coping have been observed in aversive (Lovallo et al., 1985) and appetitive (Gramer and Huber, 1996; Light and Obrist, 1983) conditions and are assumed to reflect effort, or task engagement, exerted to facilitate coping with situational demands. There seems to be no empirical basis to interpret the myocardial effects as indicative of affective arousal (Gendolla, 1999; Gendolla and Richter, 2005).

Research on the specific determinants of effort expenditure was greatly stimulated by Wright's (1996) integration of Obrist's (1981) active coping approach with Brehm's theory of motivational intensity (Brehm and Self, 1989). This *integrative analysis* or energization theory assumes that effort in active performance situations corresponds to experienced task demand as long as success is perceived as possible and worthwhile. In support of this view, several studies demonstrated that beta-adrenergically mediated cardiovascular activity increases with experienced task difficulty until active coping is impossible or maximal resources are exceeded (Eubanks, Wright and Williams, 2002; Gendolla, 1999; Richter, Friedrich and Gendolla, 2008; Wright and Kirby, 2001). Furthermore, cardiovascular effects were found to be minimal, irrespective of demand level, when success importance was low, e.g. in situations without evaluation potential (Wright, Dill, Geen and Anderson, 1998; Wright and Lockard, 2006). The difficulty/effort association may further be moderated by factors like ability perceptions (Annis, Wright and Williams, 2001; Gramer and Saria, 2007; Wright and Lockard, 2006), mood (Gendolla and Krüsken, 2001; 2002) and fatigue (Wright, Stewart, and Barnett, 2008). Individuals who view themselves as having low ability, who are in a negative mood or experience fatigue perceive tasks as more difficult and thus display enhanced effort and associated cardiovascular reactivity at low to moderate difficulty levels and abandon their efforts more readily at higher demand levels because they conclude earlier that success is too costly or impossible. These studies on the determinants of energy mobilization or *energization* have convincingly demonstrated that cardiovascular responses are a reliable indicator of effort in active coping situations and they have identified SBP as the most sensitive indicator of experienced task demand (e.g. Gendolla, 1999; Gendolla and Krüsken, 2001; Wright and Kirby, 2001). This is consistent with expectations. Cardiovascular responses in active performance situations are primarily of beta-adrenergic cardiac origin and there is reliable evidence that effort-related SBP effects are largely a function of cardiac sympathetic activity (Annis et al., 2001; Obrist, 1981; Richter et al., 2008). DBP was found to reflect both cardiac and vascular activity during active coping (Hartley et al., 1999; Obrist, 1981) and thus shows effort effects less reliably. HR is controlled by the sympathetic and parasympathetic branch of the autonomic system and may show effort effects only under strong sympathetic stimulation (Obrist, 1981; Wright, 1996).

The energization concept (Wright, 1996; Wright and Kirby, 2001) is a motivation theory. Its central focus is on the intensity of motivation or magnitude of effort. Wright and coworkers did not consider the potential etiological significance of effort-related cardiovascular activation. However, beginning with Obrist (1981), blood pressure increases evoked by effortful coping have also been viewed as a primary biological pathway of hypertension development. This chapter tries to evaluate this traditional risk model in the framework of recent theories on adaptive versus maladaptive cardiovascular response patterns. A main aim is to demonstrate that disease risk is a complex construct that involves an interaction of cognitive-affective processes, dispositional attributes and situational (environmental) characteristics.

The Reactivity Hypothesis

Theories that relate effortful coping to cardiovascular disease have mainly been based on the so-called "reactivity hypothesis". In its simplest form, this hypothesis assumes that exaggerated BP and HR responses to psychological stressors may serve as a marker or constitute a causal factor in the etiology of cardiovascular disease (Blascovich and Katkin, 1993; Gerin et al., 2000; Kamarck and Lovallo, 2003; Manuck, 1994; Schwartz et al., 2003). Initially, the etiological relevance of active coping was primarily derived from the observation that the elicited myocardial effects exceed metabolic demands by reference to the exercise cardiac output/oxygen consumption relationship (e.g. Carroll, Turner, and Hellawell, 1986; Langer et al., 1985). Obrist (1981), complementing Folkow (1978), hypothesized that the overperfusion of oxygen may result in blood vessel hypertrophy and an increase in total peripheral resistance, thereby leading to chronically elevated blood pressure. The potential relevance of structural changes is also considered in recent evaluations of pathogenic mechanisms (Larkin, 2005). A central implication of the reactivity hypothesis is frequent exposure to episodes of enhanced cardiovascular reactivity (CVR). Research on active coping and energization has mainly utilized cognitive stressors, such as mental arithmetic or memory tasks.

These non-social studies have been very informative about the determinants of enhanced CVR; however, they may lack ecological validity. However, Smith and coworkers (Brown and Smith, 1992; Smith, Allred, Morrison, and Carlson, 1989; Smith, Baldwin, and Christensen, 1990; Smith, Limon, Gallo, and Ngu, 1996; Smith, Ruiz, and Uchino, 2000) demonstrated in a series of studies that interpersonal equivalents of active coping, i.e. attempts to exert influence and control in dyadic discussions or persuasive speech tasks, elicit the same myocardial effects that occur in traditional, non-social studies of active coping. The effects were noted in men and women; they covaried with the difficulty of influence attempts and success importance. Furthermore, the intensity of cardiovascular effects elicited in a social context was found to surpass effects of cognitive stressors (Gramer and Huber, 1996). These studies suggest that effects of active coping might be sufficiently frequent to be involved in the development of hypertension.

Adaptive and Maladaptive Cardiovascular Responses

Although certain tasks allow for active coping, not all individuals may display a cardiovascular response pattern that indicates enhanced task engagement. Active tasks may also elicit vascular effects (i.e. enhanced peripheral resistance and DBP reactivity) or increases in both vascular and myocardial activity (Gregg, Matyas, and James, 2002; Llabre,Klein, Saab, McCalla, and Schneiderman, 1998). These response patterns are considered to characterize passive, inhibitory coping or vigilance (Sherwood et al., 1990; Smith et al., 2000). In search of potential mediators, there seems to be considerable evidence for an influence of cognitive-emotional processes. In particular, the *biopsychosocial model of challenge and threat* (BPS) developed by Tomaka and colleagues (Blascovich and Tomaka, 1996; Tomaka, Blascovich, Kelsey, and Leitten, 1993), which draws from the cognitive appraisal model of Lazarus and Folkman (1984) and the psychophysiological theories of Obrist (1981) and Dienstbier (1989), suggests that the predominance of cardiac versus vascular activity in active performance situations is partly determined by the cognitive evaluation of tasks as "challenges" or "threats". The BPS specifies cognitive appraisal as initial mediator of cardiovascular responses to active performance situations. Threat and challenge perceptions are based on a comparison of demand and resource/ability appraisals. An experience of threat occurs when demands are perceived to outweigh resources, challenge occurs when resources equal or exceed situational demands. Physiologically, challenge appraisals were found to be characterized by an increase in cardiac performance coupled with low peripheral resistance (cardiac pattern), whereas threat appraisals tend to elicit moderate cardiac effects and increased vascular resistance (vascular pattern). Furthermore, challenge appraisals may relate to lower distress emotions and better performance compared to threat appraisals (Tomaka et al., 1993; 1999). Drawing from Dienstbier's (1989) conceptualization of adaptiveness, these distinct psychophysiological response patterns are considered to reflect differences in coping efficiency, with challenge responses indicating greater efficiency in mobilization of resources for coping.

The mediating influence of cognitive appraisals has been confirmed in a series of studies (for reviews see Blascovich, Mendes, Tomaka, Salomon, and Seery, 2003; Blascovich and Tomaka, 1996), there are exceptions, though (e.g. Hartley et al., 1999; Kelsey et al., 2000). Furthermore, Wright and Kirby (2003) have suggested that the cardiovascular findings of the BPS might be interpreted in terms of effort or energization. It is difficult to maintain sharp distinctions between the energization concept and the BPS. As long as coping resources are considered sufficient both models predict a cardiac response pattern; beyond a certain difficulty level, the energization model predicts an abandonment of effort and low cardiac activity, whereas the BPS predicts a conversion from cardiac to vascular activity (i.e. a threat pattern). However, the BPS allows an evaluation of adaptiveness, at least partially, and it is one of the first concepts that challenge the notion that enhanced cardiac activity in active performance situations might be a pathway for hypertension development. It rather strengthens research suggesting vascular reactivity (i.e. threat responses) might relate to enhanced cardiovascular disease risk (Lovallo and al'Absi, 1998; Saab and Schneiderman, 1993; Steptoe, Willemsen, Kunz-Ebrecht, and Owen, 2003). In this respect, some words of caution have to be stated. Both the integrative analysis (Wright, 1996) and the BPS

(Blascovich and Tomaka, 1996; Tomaka et al., 1993) have mainly focused on physiological responses during initial stressor confrontation and have neglected some essential aspects of the stress process, that is, the speed of arousal decline after stressor ending (recovery), and the speed of decline across repeated stressor exposure (habituation). According to Dienstbier (1989), an adaptive response is characterized by fast and strong onset of sympathetic (cardiac) activity with stressor confrontation, fast arousal decline with stressor offset, and fast arousal decline across repeated similar episodes.

Empirical research on the recovery response suggests that myocardial activity shows fast decline with stressor offset, whereas vascular activity is sustained (Glynn, Christenfeld and Gerin, 2002; Gregg, James, Matyas, and Thorsteinsson, 1999; Steptoe et al., 2003) and distress emotions are considered a primary mediator of prolonged stress induced cardiovascular arousal (Glynn et al., 2002; Vitaliano, Russo, Paulsen, and Bailey, 1995). As regards adaptation to recurrent psychological stress, there is consistent evidence (Kelsey, 1993; Kelsey et al., 2000; Kelsey, Soderlund and Arthur, 2004; Quigley, Russo, Paulsen, and Bailey, 2002) that repeated exposure to active coping tasks results in attenuation of cardiac but not vascular activity. The decline in cardiac activity over tasks was found to be accompanied by a decline in primary (demand) appraisals of stress and improvements in performance and secondary (resources) appraisals. These findings suggest that the habituation of cardiac reactivity might reflect an active adaptation process resulting from reappraisals of prior experiences rather than a passive process involving fatigue (Kelsey et al., 2004). Overall, these differences in cardiovascular patterns over time are consistent with the view that vascular reactivity might be more pathologically relevant than transient cardiac activation in active performance situations (Blascovich and Katkin, 1993; Dienstbier, 1989; Steptoe et al., 2003). However, when occurring with great frequency and intensity, basic adaptive physiological patterns might be of etiological relevance (McEwen, 1998).

Dispositional Moderators of Cardiovascular Disease Risk

It might be perceived that cognitive processes and related physiological responses are moderated by personality factors. Research on the differential effects of active coping has considered the potential influence of trait characteristics. However, the majority of studies on dispositional moderators were based on negative constructions of sympathetic cardiac activity equating heightened cardiac reactivity with the experience of distress emotions and enhanced disease risk. Few studies in this field have attended to predictions of the BPS (Blascovich and Tomaka, 1996) and energization research (Wright, 1996) and/or have tried to evaluate the adaptiveness of cardiovascular responses (Dienstbier, 1989). Evidence from prospective epidemiological research has mainly implicated two independent personality traits with increased risk of coronary heart disease (CHD): hostility (Chida and Steptoe, 2009; Everson et al., 1997; Miller, Russo, Paulsen, and Bailey, 1996) and trait dominance (Houston, Chesney, Black, Cates, and Hecker, 1992; 1997; Siegman, et al., 2000a; Siegman, Townsend, Civelek, and Blumenthal, 2000b; Smith, Gallo and Ruiz, 2003). CVR is one proposed factor linking these traits and cardiovascular disease (Manuck, 1994).

Hostility

Presently, hostility represents one of the most widely studied psychosocial risk factors for CHD. It is regarded as a cognitive trait that involves the dislike and negative evaluation of others (Smith, 1994). Central features of the hostility construct involve cynicism (believing others are selfishly motivated), mistrust (an overgeneralization that others are intentionally provoking), and denigration (evaluating others as dishonest, mean and non-social) (Miller et al., 1996). Furthermore, there is some evidence that high-hostile individualstend to appraise interpersonal stressors as threats rather than as challenges (Kline, Fekete, and Sears, 2008) and they seem to prefer avoidant coping strategies to active control attempts (Piferi and Lawler, 2000). Viewing these characteristics within the framework of the BPS, it might be assumed that high hostile individuals are predisposed to exhibit enhanced vascular activity in active performance situations. According to the energization model and ability analysis high hostiles might withhold effort in demanding interpersonal situations and thus should exhibit reduced myocardial (SBP, HR) activity.

Available empirical evidence in this field appears more complex. In interpersonal situations that are *not deliberately anger provoking*, such as discussions or situations involving self-disclosure, cardiovascular findings are consistent with the view that hostile individuals might display passive inhibitory coping and disengagement in social/interpersonal situations. Several studies observed enhanced vascular activity, i.e. elevations in BP that resulted from increases in TPR (Christensen and Smith, 1993;Hardy and Smith, 1988; Smith and Allred, 1989). This tendency to vascular effects seems to be more pronounced in hostile individuals with a predisposition to anger inhibition (Vella and Friedman, 2009) or low emotional expressiveness (Kline et al., 2008). Other researchers observed attenuated cardiac activity in high hostile individuals, indicated by reductions in SBP and HR reactivity (Hernandez, Larkin, and Whited, 2009; Kline et al., 2008; Piferi and Lawler, 2000), or both elevations in vascular and reductions in cardiac activity (Davis, Matthews, and McGrath, 2000). Furthermore, there was some evidence that reduced task engagement might be more likely in men than in women (Chatkoff, Maier, Javaid, Hammouda, Munkrishna, 2009). In situations involving *explicit anger provocation* (e.g. harassment), a different response pattern has been observed. Several authors found high hostiles to display enhanced cardiac activity, indicated by marked elevations in SBP, HR and CO reactivity (Miller et al., 1996; Suarez et al., 1993; 1998). Anderson et al. (2005) noted a reduction of cardiac activity, though. Overall, these discrepant findings seem to suggest, that the cardiovascular response patterns of high hostile individuals may vary with the type of social situations. In situations without deliberate anger provocation, their suspicious and mistrustful nature may make them feel uncertain about actual demands and evoke a passive inhibitory response pattern and reduced effort mobilization. In situations with explicit anger provocation, demands are clear, and active defense behavior might be elicited as long as sufficient coping resources are experienced (Wright, 1996; Wright and Kirby, 2001). Alternatively, a reduction of task engagement in these situations might also be interpreted because of response habituation due to greater experience with anger provoking situations (Hernandez et al., 2009).

In this respect, it is also interesting that cardiovascular effects in situations without deliberate anger provocation were unrelated to affective arousal (Davis et al., 2000; Hernandez et al., 2009; Kline et al., 2008), whereas in situations with harassment cardiac activity of high hostile individuals was mediated by distress emotions, in particular, anger and irritation (Suarez,Harlan, Peoples, and Williams, 1993; 1998). This result contrasts with theories on active coping and energization (Gendolla, 1999; Obrist, 1981; Wright, 1996) which attribute cardiac activity to effort rather than affective arousal. However, a study by Harmon-Jones (2003) indicates that anger emotions are related to the behavioral approach system (BAS), and Tomaka and Palacios-Esquivel (1997) observed an association between the BAS and enhanced sympathetic myocardial activity. In light of this evidence, it might be concluded that myocardial activity in the presence of strong anger emotions might represent a "hot" active response that does not necessarily relate to the determinants of energy investment defined in energization research (i.e. difficulty, ability level). Considering that the majority of daily experiences among hostile individuals may not be explicitly anger provoking (Davis et al., 2000), enhanced vascular activity, or inhibited coping, might implicate greater cardiovascular disease risk. However, it is of note that anger provoking situations were consistently found to go along with impaired cardiac recovery in hostile individuals (Smith, Cranford, and Green, 2001; Suarez et al., 1993; 1998), even if there were no differential cardiovascular effects during task exposure (Neumann,Waldstein, Sollers, Thayer, and Sorkin, 2004). Studies without anger provocation either did not attend to recovery or found no evidence of prolonged vascular activity (Davis et al., 2000). Thus, sympathetically mediated SBP effects in anger provoking conditions do not show the characteristics of an adaptive response (Dienstbier, 1989). The anger induced blood pressure elevations may be sustained long after the interpersonal situation has ended and rumination over the anger-provoking situation may recreate the cardiovascular response even after return to resting levels (Glynn et al., 2002; Glynn, Christenfeld, and Gerin, 2007). Furthermore, there is some evidence that hostile individuals may show impaired nocturnal blood pressure dipping (Thomas, Nelesen, and Dimsdale, 2004). Thus, in an environment with high conflict potential, cardiac activity might be of greater etiological significance than vascular activity.

Dominance

Compared to hostility, there is a relative paucity of research on the cardiovascular effects of trait dominance. This psychosocial trait is characterized by motives to exert influence and control. Interpersonal circumplex accounts of personality consider dominance an aspect of agency, a metaconstruct that involves striving for mastery and power (Helgeson and Fritz, 1999). Converging evidence from human epidemiological and experimental animal research has identified dominance and social control as predictors of CHD. Several well-controlled prospective studies observed a significant relationship between behavioral indicators of dominance (Houston et al., 1992; 1997; Siegman et al., 2000b; Smith et al., 2003) or self-reported dominance (Siegman et al., 2000a) and increased incidence of CHD. The effect was independent of hostility. There is also some evidence that exposure to dominant others might contribute to coronary disease (Carmelli,Swan, and Rosenman, 1985). Experimental research on nonhuman primates (for reviews see Kaplan, Manuck, Williams, and Strawn, 1993; Shively,Adams, Kaplan, and Williams, 2000) suggests that environmental factors and gender may determine whether dominance status is related to cardiovascular disease. Cynomolgus macaque monkeys are considered an ideal animal model to study the effects of psychosocial factors on CHD risk. Macaques live in large social groups and form hierarchies of social status. They are susceptible to diet-induced atherogenesis and have a high frequency of myocardial infarction. In a series of studies, Kaplan and coworkers (Kaplan et al., 1993) demonstrated that male dominant monkeys display enhanced CHD risk in an unstable social environment, in which the constituency of the social group is changed at regular intervals and new status hierarchies have to be formed at each social reorganization. In stable environments, social status was unrelated to disease risk. The effects of social status and social instability were different in female monkeys. Social instability had no influence on atherogenesis. It was the subordinatesthat displayed enhanced atherosclerosis. Of interest, Kaplan,Manuck, Adams, Weingand, and Clarkson (1987) observed that treatment with a beta-adrenergic blocking agent could reduce atherosclerosis of dominant monkeys living in unstable groups. This result suggests atherogenic effects may result from enhanced sympathetic activity.

Experimental research on human beings was greatly influenced by studies on social equivalents of active coping. As indicated above, effortful attempts to exert social influence and control may elicit marked beta-adrenergic cardiac activity (Brown and Smith, 1992; Gramer and Huber, 1996; Smith et al., 1989; 2000). With its motives and tendencies, trait dominance might be conceived a dispositional marker of active coping and its cardiovascular manifestations (Gramer, 2003). In this respect, several studies have observed enhanced cardiac activity, indicated by elevations in SBP and/or HR (Gramer, 2003; Gramer and Berner, 2005; Hughes and Callinan, 2007; Newton and Bane, 2001; Newton, Bane, Flores and Greenfield, 1999; Rejeski, Parker, Gagne, and Koritnik, 1990) and attenuated vascular or DBP effects (Gramer, 2003; Gramer and Berner, 2005) in dominant compared to submissive individuals. Furthermore, there is some evidence that cardiovascular responses of dominant individuals might habituate over task exposure, whereas responses of low dominant individuals are sustained (Gramer and Huber, 1997; Rejeski,Gagne, Parker, and Koritnik, 1989). Low dominant individuals may also exhibit a delay of DBP recovery (Gramer, 2003). Cognitive task appraisals and affective processes indicate greater confidence of meeting situational demands (Gramer, 2003; Gramer and Berner, 2005) and less distress (Gramer, 2003; Gramer and Berner, 2005; Gramer and Huber, 1997; Hughes and Callinan, 2007; Newton, 2009) in high compared to low dominant individuals. In terms of the BPS (Blascovich and Tomaka, 1996) and energization research (Wright, 1996), the cardiovascular responses of dominant individuals might be interpreted as efficient energy mobilization to support coping with demands or "challenge" responses, whereas the vascular response pattern of submissive individuals might be described as a "threat pattern" or passive coping approach. The psychological and cardiovascular responses of dominant individuals are also consistent with Dienstbier's (1989) view of adaptiveness and seem to suggest a beneficial effect of trait dominance on stress-related responses.

This interpretation contradicts epidemiological evidence that relates trait dominance to CHD (e.g. Houston et al., 1992; 1997; Siegman et al., 2000a, b). In this respect, it has to be noted that theoretical contributions on trait dominance/agency do not necessarily suggest a relation to disease risk. Considerable evidence relates agency to greater psychological well-being, in particular, reduced anxiety, enhanced self-esteem, and fewer health complaints (for reviews see Helgeson, 1994; 2003). Negative health effects of agency are only expected for extreme expressions of an agentic orientation, that is, unmitigated agency (Helgeson, 1994; Helgeson and Fritz, 1999) or hostile dominance (Ghaed and Gallo, 2006). Research on nonhuman primates noted vulnerability for male dominants only in unstable environments and assigns disease risk in female animals to subordinates rather than dominants (Kaplan et al., 1993; Shively et al., 2000). Several studies with human beings also suggest a moderating influence of environmental characteristics. Interactions with dominant partners seem to provoke enhanced DBP reactivity (Brown, Smith and Benjamin, 1998; Newton et al., 1999; Newton, Watters, Philhower, and Weigel, 2005) or prolonged DBP recovery (Gramer and Berner, 2005), in both high and low dominant individuals. Furthermore, dominant interaction partners were found to provoke anger-related states (Gramer and Berner, 2005). Thus, situations that severely threaten dominant status may disrupt the effective coping pattern of dominant individuals. Due to their motive to maintain control, vascular activity in high dominant individuals should be accompanied by enhanced cardiac activation. This mixed cardiac/vascular response pattern represents a condition where the cardiovascular effects of effortful coping might be of pathological relevance (Blascovich and Katkin, 1993). Taken together, trait dominance might be related to disease risk if the motive to exert influence or maintain control is instigated very frequently and recovery periods are shortened, or environmental conditions interfere with controllability of demands. The vascular "threat" pattern of low dominant individuals might also be of importance if low dominant individuals are continually faced with environmental demands that do not fit their preferred response tendencies. Research on nonhuman primates assigns incongruous social positions pathogenic significance (Shively et al., 2000).

Conclusion

As a whole, this selective review revealed a complex picture of the potential etiological significance of enhanced sympathetic cardiac activity in active performance situations. The majority of studies seem to contradict the classical reactivity hypothesis, which assumes that heightened reactivity per se implicates disease risk. In agreement with Dienstbier's (1989) theory of physiological toughness and adaptive responses, findings rather suggest that transient elevations of SBP and/or HR in conditions with high-perceived control reflect an adaptive response indicative of successful coping. However, in interaction with specific psychosocial dispositions and environmental conditions involving a high degree of social conflict or threats to preferred response tendencies, this adaptive response pattern may gain pathological significance.

Taken together, the research findings suggest that the evaluation of disease risk requires an expanded research model that includes cognitive-emotional processes, potential dispositional moderators and measures of prolonged reactivity. Present concepts on cardiovascular reactivity in active performance situations cover only a portion of these aspects. The traditional reactivity hypothesis has held a "negative view of arousal" (Dienstbier, 1989) and equated heightened CVR with the experience of distress emotions. In light of research linking distress emotions to disease outcomes (e.g. Booth-Kewley and Friedman, 1987), cardiac reactivity was considered a maladaptive response. This view was greatly changed by the BPS (Blascovich and Tomaka, 1996) and energization theory (Wright, 1996). Research in the realm of these theoretical concepts has demonstrated that enhanced cardiac activity in active performance situations may result from energy mobilization in face of sufficient coping resources. This interpretation implicates adaptiveness and Blascovich and Tomaka (1996) have equated challenge responses with adaptive responses. However, as indicated above, they did not consider prolonged activation in their model, an essential aspect of adaptiveness. Research on hostility shows that enhanced cardiac activity in active coping situations need not always reflect effort and energy mobilization. It may also result from approach-related distress emotions. Thus, there are conditions where the predictions of traditional reactivity research might apply. A reliable differentiation of effort based cardiac reactivity and cardiac reactivity resulting from affective arousal requires an assessment of recovery responses. Effort based activity was found to go along with swift return to resting levels (Gramer, 2003; Steptoe et al., 2003), whereas distress-related cardiac arousal tends to be prolonged (Suarez et al., 1993; 1998) and may carry disease risk.

References

Allen, M.T., Obrist, P.A., Sherwood, A., and Crowell, M.D. (1987). Evaluation of myocardial and peripheral vascular responses during reaction time, mental arithmetic, and cold pressure tasks. *Psychophysiology, 24,* 648-656.

Anderson, J.C., Linden, W., and Habra, M.E. (2005). The importance of examining blood pressure reactivity and recovery in anger provocation research. *International Journal of Psychophysiology, 57,* 159-163.

Annis, S., Wright, R.A., and Williams, B.J. (2001). Interactional influence of ability perception and task demand on cardiovascular response: appetitive effects at three levels of challenge. *Journal of Applied Biobehavioral Research, 6,* 82-107.

Blascovich, J., Mendes, W.B., Tomaka, J., Salomon, K., and Seery, M. (2003). The robust nature of the biopsychosocial model of challenge and threat: A reply to Wright and Kirby. *Personality and Social Psychology Review, 7,* 234-243.

Blascovich, J., and Katkin, E.S. (Eds.) (1993). *Cardiovascular reactivity to psychological stress and disease.* Washington, DC: American Psychological Association.

Blascovich, J., and Tomaka, J. (1996). The biopsychosocial model of arousal regulation. *Advances in Experimental Social Psychology, 28,* 1-51.

Bongard, S. (1995). Mental effort during active and passive coping: a dual-task analysis. *Psychophysiology, 32,* 242-248.

Booth-Kewley, S., and Friedman, H.S. (1987). Psychological predictors of heart disease: A quantitative review. *Psychological Bulletin, 101,* 343-362.

Brehm, J.W., and Self, E.A. (1989). The intensity of motivation. *Annual Review of Psychology, 40,* 109-131.

Brosschot, J.F., Gerin, W., and Thayer, J.F. (2006). The perseverative cognition hypothesis: a review of worry, prolonged stress-related physiological activation, and health. *Journal of Psychosomatic Research, 60,* 113-124.

Brown, P.C., and Smith, T.W. (1992). Social influence, marriage and the heart: cardiovascular consequences of interpersonal control in husbands and wives. *Health Psychology, 11,* 88-96.

Brown, P.C., Smith, T.W., and Benjamin, L.S. (1998). Perceptions of spouse dominance predict blood pressure reactivity during marital interactions. *Annals of Behavioral Medicine, 20,* 294-301.

Carmelli, D., Swan, G.E., and Rosenman, R.H. (1985). The relationship between wives' social and psychologic status and their husbands' coronary heart disease. *American Journal of Epidemiology, 122*, 90-100.

Carroll, D., Turner, J.R., and Hellawell, J.C. (1986). Heart rate and oxygen consumption during active psychological challenge: The effects of level of difficulty. *Psychophysiology, 23*, 174-181.

Chatkoff, D.K., Maier, K. J., Javaid, J., Hammouda, M. K., and Munkrishna, P. (2009).Dispositional hostility and gender differentially relate to cognitive appraisal, engagement, and cardiovascular reactivity across cognitive and emotional laboratory tasks. *Personality and Individual Differences, 47*, 122-126.

Chida, Y., and Steptoe, A. (2009). The association of anger and hostility with future coronary heart disease. *Journal of the American College of Cardiology, 53*, 936-946.

Christensen, A.J., and Smith, T.W. (1993). Cynical hostility and cardiovascular reactivity during self-disclosure. *Psychosomatic Medicine, 55*, 193-202.

Davis, M.C., Matthews, K.A., and McGrath, C.E. (2000). Hostile attitudes predict elevated vascular resistance during interpersonal stress in men and women. *Psychosomatic Medicine, 62*, 17-25.

Dienstbier, R.A. (1989). Arousal and physiological toughness: implications for mental and physical health. *Psychological Review, 96*, 84-100.

Eubanks, L., Wright, R.A., and Williams, B.J. (2002). Reward influences on the heart: cardiovascular response as a function of incentive value at five levels of task demand. *Motivation and Emotion, 26*, 139-152.

Everson, S.A., Kauhanen, J., Kaplan, G.A., Goldberg, D.E., Julkunen, J., Tuomilehto, J., and Salonen, J.T. (1997). Hostility and increased risk of mortality and acute myocardial infarction: the mediating role of behavioral risk factors. *American Journal of Epidemiology, 146*, 142-152.

Folkow, B. (1978). Cardiovascular structural adaptation: Its role in the initiation and maintenance of primary hypertension. *Clinical Science and Molecular Medicine, 55*, 3s-22s.

Gendolla, G.H.E. (1999). Self-relevance of performance, task difficulty, and task engagement assessed as cardiovascular response. *Motivation and Emotion, 26*, 139-152.

Gendolla, G.H.E., and Krüsken, J. (2001). The joint impact of mood state and task difficulty on cardiovascular and electrodermal reactivity in active coping. *Psychophysiology, 38*, 548-556.

Gendolla, G.H.E., and Krüsken, J. (2002). Mood state, task demand, and effort-related cardiovascular response. *Cognition and Emotion, 16*, 577-603.

Gendolla, H.E., and Richter, M. (2005). Ego involvement and effort: cardiovascular, electrodermal, and performance effects. *Psychophysiology, 42*, 595-603.

Gerin, W., Pickering, T.G., Glynn, L., Christenfeld, N., Schwartz, A., Carroll, D., and Davidson, K. (2000). An historical context for behavioral models of hypertension. *Journal of Psychosomatic Research, 48*, 369-377.

Ghaed, S.G., and Gallo, L.C. (2006). Distinctions among agency, communion, and unmitigated agency and communion according to the interpersonal circumplex, five-factor model, and social emotional correlates. *Journal of Personality Assessment, 86*, 77-88.

Glynn, L.M., Christenfeld, N., and Gerin, W. (2002). The role of rumination in recovery from reactivity: cardiovascular consequences of emotional states. *Psychosomatic Medicine, 64*, 714-726.

Glynn, L.M., Christenfeld, N., and Gerin, W. (2007). Recreating cardiovascular responses with rumination: The effects of a delay between harassment and its recall. *International Journal of Psychophysiology, 66*, 135-140.

Gramer, M. (2003). Cognitive appraisals, emotional and cardiovascular responses of high and low dominant subjects in active performance situations. *Personality and Individual Differences, 34*, 1303-1318.

Gramer, M., and Berner, M. (2005). Effects of trait dominance on psychological and cardiovascular responses to social influence attempts: the role of gender and partner dominance. *International Journal of Psychophysiology, 55*, 279-289.

Gramer, M., and Huber, H.P. (1996). Kardiovaskuläre Effekte aktiven Bewältigungsverhaltens in mentalen und sozialen Belastungssituationen unter verschiedenen Anreizbedingungen. *Zeitschrift für Experimentelle Psychologie, 43*, 256-278.

Gramer, M., and Huber, H.P. (1997). Cardiovascular reactivity to active and passive task engagement: the role of dominance. *Psychologische Beiträge, 39*, 283-296.

Gramer, M., and Saria, K. (2007). Effects of social anxiety and evaluative threat on cardiovascular responses to active performance situations. *Biological Psychology, 74*, 67-74.

Gregg, M.E., Matyas, T.A., and James, J.E. (2002). A new model of individual differences in hemodynamic profile and blood pressure reactivity. *Psychophysiology, 39*, 64-72.

Gregg, M.E., James, J.E., Matyas, T.A., and Thorsteinsson, E.B. (1999). Hemodynamic profile of stress-induced anticipation and recovery. *International Journal of Psychophysiology, 34*, 147-162.

Hardy, J.D., and Smith, T.W. (1988). Cynical hostility and vulnerability to disease: Social support, life stress, and physiological response to conflict. *Health Psychology, 7*, 447-459.

Harmon-Jones, E. (2003). Anger and the behavioral approach system. *Personality and Individual Differences, 35*, 995-1005.

Hartley, T.R., Ginsburg, G.P., and Heffner, K. (1999). Self-presentation and cardiovascular reactivity. *International Journal of Psychophysiology, 32*, 75-88.

Helgeson, V.S. (1994). Relation of agency and communion to well-being: evidence and potential explanations. *Psychological Bulletin, 116*, 412-428.

Helgeson, V.S. (2003). Gender-related traits and health. In J. Suls and K.A. Wallston (Eds.), *Social psychological foundations of health and illness* (pp.367-394). Malden: Blackwell.

Helgeson, V.S., and Fritz, H.L. (1999). Unmitigated agency and unmitigated communion: distinctions from agency and communion. *Journal of Research in Personality, 33*, 131-154.

Hernandez, D.H., Larkin, K.T., and Whited, M. C. (2009). Cardiovascular response to interpersonal provocation and mental arithmetic among high and low hostile young adult males. *Applied Psychophysiology and Biofeedback, 34*, 27-35.

Houston, B.K., Chesney, M.A., Black, G.W., Cates, D.S., and Hecker, M.H.L. (1992). Behavioral clusters and coronary heart disease risk. *Psychosomatic Medicine, 54*, 447-461.

Houston, B.K., Babyak, M.A., Chesney, M.A., Black, G., and Ragland, D.R. (1997). Social dominance and 22-year all-cause mortality in men. *Psychosomatic Medicine, 59*, 5-12.

Hughes, B.M., and Callinan, S. (2007). Trait dominance and cardiovascular reactivity to social and nonsocial stressors: gender-specific implications. *Psychology and Health, 22*, 457-472.

Kaplan, J.R., Manuck, S.B., Williams, K.K., and Strawn, W. (1993). Psychosocial influences on atherosclerosis: evidence for effects and mechanisms in nonhuman primates. In J., Blascovich and E.S., Katkin (Eds.), *Cardiovascular reactivity to psychological stressand disease* (pp. 3-26). Washington, DC: APA.

Kaplan, J.R., Manuck, S.B., Adams, M.R., Weingand, K.W., and Clarkson, T.B. (1987). Inhibition of coronary atherosclerosis by propanolol in behaviorally predisposed monkeys fed an atherogenic diet. *Circulation, 76*, 1364-1372.

Kamarck, T.W., and Lovallo, W.R. (2003). Cardiovascular reactivity to psychological challenge: conceptual and measurement considerations. *Psychosomatic Medicine, 65*, 9-21.

Kelsey, R.M. (1993). Habituation of cardiovascular reactivity to psychological stress: evidence and implications. In J. Blascovich, and E.S. Katkin (Eds.), *Cardiovascular reactivity to psychological stress and disease* (pp. 135-153). Washington, DC: APA.

Kelsey, R.M., Blascovich, J., Leitten, C.L., Schneider, T.R., Tomaka, J., and Wiens, S. (2000). Cardiovascular reactivity and adaptation to recurrent psychological stress: the moderating effects of evaluative observation. *Psychophysiology, 37*, 748-756.

Kelsey, R.M., Soderlund, K., and Arthur, C.M. (2004). Cardiovascular reactivity and adaptation to recurrent psychological stress: Replication and extension. *Psychophysiology, 41*, 924-934.

Kline, K.A., Fekete, E.M., and Sears, C.M. (2008). Hostility, emotional expression, and hemodynamic responses to laboratory stressors: reactivity attenuating effects of a tendency to express emotions interpersonally. *International Journal of Psychophysiology, 68*, 177-185.

Langer, A.W., McCubbin, J.A., Stoney, C.M., Hutcheson, J.S., Charlton, J.D., and Obrist, P.A. (1985). Cardiopulmonary adjustments during exercise and an aversive reaction time task: effects of beta-adrenoceptor blockade. *Psychophysiology, 22*, 59-68.

Larkin, K.T. (2005). *Stress and hypertension. Examining the relation between psychological stress and high blood pressure*. New Haven: Yale University Press.

Lazarus, R.S., and Folkman, S. (1984). *Stress, Appraisal and Coping*. New York: Springer.

Light, K.C., and Obrist, P.A. (1983). Task difficulty, heart rate reactivity, and cardiovascular responses to an appetitive reaction time task. *Psychophysiology, 20*, 301-312.

Llabre, M.M., Klein, B.R., Saab, P.G., McCalla, J.B., and Schneiderman, N. (1998). Classification of individual differences in cardiovascular responsivity: the contribution of reactor type controlling for race and gender. *International Journal of Behavioral Medicine, 5*, 213-229.

Lovallo, W.R., and al'Absi, M. (1998). Hemodynamics during rest and behavioral stress in normotensive men at high risk for hypertension. *Psychophysiology, 35*, 47-53.

Lovallo, W.R., Wilson, M.F., Pincomb, G.A., Edwards, G.L., Tompkins, P., and Brackett, D.J. (1985). Activation patterns to aversive stimulation in man: passive exposure versus effort to control. *Psychophysiology, 22*, 283-291.

Manuck, S.B. (1994). Cardiovascular reactivity in cardiovascular disease: "once more unto the breach". *International Journal of Behavioral Medicine, 1*, 4-31.

McEwen, B.S. (1998). Protective and damaging effects of stress mediators. *New England Journal of Medicine, 338*, 171-179.

Miller, T.Q., Smith, T.W., Turner, C.W., Guijaro, M.L., Hallet, A.J. (1996). A meta-analytic review of research on hostility and physical health. *Psychological Bulletin, 119*, 332-348.

Neumann, S.A., Waldstein, S.R., Sollers III, J.J., Thayer, J.F., and Sorkin, J.D. (2004). Hostility and distraction have differential influences on cardiovascular recovery from anger recall in women. *Health Psychology, 23*, 631-640.

Newton, T.L. (2009). Cardiovascular functioning, personality, and the social world: The domain of hierarchical power. *Neuroscience and Biobehavioral Reviews, 33*, 145-159.

Newton, T.L., and Bane, C.M.H. (2001). Cardiovascular correlates of behavioral dominance and hostility during dyadic interaction. *International Journal of Psychophysiology, 40*, 33-46.

Newton, T.L., Bane, C.M.H, Flores, A., and Greenfield, J. (1999). Dominance, gender, and cardiovascular reactivity during social interaction. *Psychophysiology, 36*, 245-252.

Newton, T.L., Watters, C.A., Philhower, C.L., and Weigel, R.A. (2005). Cardiovascular reactivity during dyadic social interaction: the roles of gender and dominance. *International Journal of Psychophysiology, 57*, 219-228.

Obrist, P.A. (1981). *Cardiovascular psychophysiology: A perspective*. New York: Plenum.

Piferi, R.L., and Lawler, K.A. (2000). Hostility and the cardiovascular reactivity of women during interpersonal confrontation. *Women and Health, 30*, 111-129.

Quigley, K.S., Feldman Barrett, L., and Weinstein, S. (2002). Cardiovascular patterns associated with threat and challenge appraisals: a within-subject analysis. *Psychophysiology, 39*, 292-302.

Rejeski, W.J., Gagne, M., Parker, P.E., and Koritnik, D.R. (1989). Acute stress reactivity from contested dominance in dominant and submissive males. *Behavioral Medicine, 15*, 118-124.

Rejeski, W.J., Parker, P.E., Gagne, M., and Koritnik, D.R. (1990). Cardiovascular and testosterone responses to contested dominance in women. *Health Psychology, 9*, 35-47.

Richter, M., Friedrich, A., and Gendolla, G.H.E. (2008). Task difficulty effects on cardiac activity. *Psychophysiology, 45*, 869-875.

Saab, P.G., and Schneiderman, N. (1993). Biobehavioral stressors, laboratory investigation, and the risk of hypertension. In J. Blascovich, and E.S. Katkin (Eds.), *Cardiovascular reactivity to psychological stress and disease* (pp. 48-82). Washington, DC: APA.

Schwartz, A.R., Gerin, W., Davidson, K.W., Pickering, T.G., Brosschot, J.F., Thayer, J.F., Christenfeld, N., and Linden, W. (2003). Toward a causal model of cardiovascular responses to stress and the development of cardiovascular disease. *Psychosomatic Medicine, 65*, 22-35.

Sherwood, A., Dolan, C.A., and Light, K.C. (1990). Hemodynamics of blood pressure responses during active and passive coping. *Psychophysiology, 27*, 656-668.

Shively, C.A., Adams, M.R., Kaplan, J.R.,and Williams, J.K. (2000). Social stress, gender, and coronary heart disease risk in monkeys. In P.M. McCabe, N. Schneiderman, T. Field, and A.R. Wellens (Eds.), *Stress, coping, and cardiovascular disease* (pp. 71-84). New Jersey, Lawrence Erlbaum.

Siegman, A.W., Kubzansky, L.D., Kawachi, I., Boyle, S., Vokonas, P.S., and Sparrow, D. (2000a). A prospective study of dominance and coronary heart disease in the Normative Aging Study. *The American Journal of Cardiology, 86*, 145-149.

Siegman, A.W., Townsend, S.T., Civelek, A.C., and Blumenthal, R.S. (2000b). Antagonistic behavior, dominance, hostility and coronary heart disease. *Psychosomatic Medicine, 62*, 248-257.

Smith, B.D., Cranford, D., and Green, L. (2001). Hostility and caffeine: Cardiovascular effects during stress and recovery. *Personality and Individual Differences, 30*, 1125-1137.

Smith, T.W. (1994). Concepts and methods in the study of anger, hostility, and health. In A.W. Siegman and T.W. Smith (Eds.), *Anger, hostility and the heart* (pp. 23-42). Hillsdale, NJ: Lawrence Erlbaum.

Smith, T.W., Allred, K.D., Morrison, C.A., and Carlson, S.D. (1989). Cardiovascular reactivity and interpersonal influence: Active coping in a social context. *Journal of Personality and Social Psychology, 56*, 209-218.

Smith, T.W., Baldwin, M., and Christensen, A. (1990). Interpersonal influence as active coping: Effects of task difficulty on cardiovascular reactivity. *Psychophysiology, 27*, 429-437.

Smith, T.W., Gallo, L.C., and Ruiz, J.M. (2003). Toward a social psychophysiology of cardiovascular reactivity: Interpersonal concepts and methods in the study of stress and coronary disease.In J. Suls and K.A. Wallston (Eds.) *Social psychological foundations of health and illness* (pp. 335-366). Oxford: Blackwell.

Smith, T.W., Limon, J.P., Gallo, L.C., and Ngu, L.Q. (1996). Interpersonal control and cardiovascular reactivity: Goals, behavioral expression, and the moderating effect of sex. *Journal of Personality and Social Psychology, 70*, 1012-1024.

Smith, T.W., Ruiz, J.M., and Uchino, B.N. (2000). Vigilance, active coping, and cardiovascular reactivity during social interaction in young men. *Health Psychology, 19*, 382-392.

Steptoe, A., Willemsen, G., Kunz-Ebrecht, S.R., and Owen, N. (2003). Socioeconomic status and hemodynamic recovery from mental stress. *Psychophysiology, 40*, 184-191.

Suarez, E.C., Harlan, E., Peoples, M.C., and Williams, R.B. (1993). Cardiovascular and emotional responses in women: The role of hostility and harassment. *Health Psychology, 12*, 459-468.

Suarez, E.C., Kuhn, C.M., Schanberg, S.M., Williams, R.B., and Zimmerman, E.A. (1998). Neuroendocrine, cardiovascular, and emotional responses of hostile men: The role of interpersonal challenge. *Psychosomatic Medicine, 60*, 78-88.

Thomas, KM. S., Nelesen, R.A., and Dimsdale, J.E. (2004). Relationships between hostility, anger expression, and blood pressure dipping in an ethnically diverse sample. *Psychosomatic Medicine, 66*, 298-304.

Tomaka, J., Blascovich, J., Kelsey, R.M., and Leitten, C.L. (1993). Subjective, physiological, and behavioral effects of threat and challenge appraisal. *Journal of Personality and Social Psychology, 65*, 248-260.

Tomaka, J., and Palacios-Esquivel, R.L. (1997). Motivational systems and stress-related cardiovascular reactivity. *Motivation and Emotion, 21*, 275-296.

Tomaka, J., Palacios, R., Schneider, K.T., Colotla, M., Concha, J.B., and Herrald, M.M. (1999). Assertiveness predicts threat and challenge reactions to potential stress among women. *Journal of Personality and Social Psychology, 76*, 1008-1021.

Vella, E.J., and Friedman, B.H. (2009). Hostility and anger in: cardiovascular reactivity and recovery to mental arithmetic stress. *International Journal of Psychophysiology, 72*, 253-259.

Vitaliano, P.P., Russo, J., Paulsen, V.M., and Bailey, S.L. (1995). Cardiovascular recovery from laboratory stress: Biopsychosocial concomitants in older adults. *Journal of Psychosomatic Research, 39*, 361-377.

Wright, R.A. (1996). Brehm's theory of motivation as a model of effort and cardiovascular response. In: P.M. Gollwitzer, and J.A. Bargh (Eds.), *The psychology of action: Linking cognition and motivation and behavior.* New York: Guilford.

Wright, R.A., Dill, J.C., Geen, R.G., and Anderson, C.A. (1998). Social evaluation influence on cardiovascular response to a fixed behavioural challenge: Effects across a range of difficulty levels. *Annals of Behavioral Medicine, 20*, 277-285.

Wright, R.A. and Kirby, L.D. (2001). Effort determination of cardiovascular response: An integrative analysis with applications in social psychology. In M. Zanna (Ed.), *Advances in experimental social psychology* (vol.33, pp. 255-307). San Diego, CA: Academic Press.

Wright, R.A., and Kirby, L.D. (2003). Cardiovascular correlates of challenge and threat appraisals: A critical examination of the biopsychosocial analysis. *Personality and Social Psychology Review, 7*, 216-233.

Wright, R.A., and Lockard, S. (2006). Sex, outcome expectancy, and cardiovascular response to a masculine challenge. *Psychophysiology, 43*, 190-196.

Wright, R.A., Stewart, C.C., and Barnett, B.R. (2008). Mental fatigue influence on effort-related cardiovascular response: Extension across the regulatory (inhibitory)/non-regulatory performance dimension. *International Journal of Psychophysiology, 69*, 127-133.

In: Systolic Blood Pressure
Editor: Robert A. Arfi

ISBN: 978-1-61209-263-8
©2012 Nova Science Publishers, Inc.

Chapter II

From Poor Glucose Control to Stiff Arteries and Diabetic Complications

Daniel Gordin [1,2] *and Per-Henrik Groop* [*,1,2,3]

[1]Folkhälsan Institute of Genetics, Folkhälsan Research Center,
Biomedicum Helsinki, Finland
[2]Division of Nephrology, Department of Medicine,
Helsinki University Central Hospital, Finland
[3] The Baker IDI Heart and Diabetes Institute, Melbourne, Australia

Abstract

A strict control of the blood glucose level has been shown to be essential in order to prevent diabetic complications in patients with type 1 diabetes. However, the pathogenesis lying behind this complex cascade is far from clear. One pathway may lead via a toxic effect of glucose on the blood vessels resulting in a stiffening of the arteries and thus vascular complications.

To date diabetes affects more than 240 million people worldwide and the number is rapidly increasing. The majority of cases have type 2 diabetes, but also type 1 diabetes shows a remarkable increase. The incidence of type 1 diabetes, was recently shown to have doubled from 1980 to 2005 in Finnish children. The reason is still largely unknown.

The treatment of diabetes has markedly improved during recent years due to modern regimens. Despite better treatment it has not been able to eradicate the complications. Patients with type 1 diabetes are at increased risk of cardiovascular complications and diabetic nephropathy increases this risk markedly. As diabetic nephropathy influences one third of the patients, genetic predisposition seems evident. However, several studies have shown that diabetic kidney disease cannot exclusively be explained by genetic factors and a number of other players may be involved.

* Per-Henrik Groop, MD, DMSc, Folkhälsan Research Center, Biomedicum Helsinki, Haartmaninkatu 8, POB 63, FIN-00014 University of Helsinki, Finland, Phone: +358-9-19125459, Fax number: +359-9-19125452, E-mail: per-henrik.groop@helsinki.fi

Hyperglycemia causes extensive changes in the metabolic balance and has been shown to particularly influence the blood vessels. The track from a high blood glucose concentration to functional and structural arterial changes is long and various mechanisms seem to play their role. These include metabolic, hemodynamic and intracellular factors as well as growth factors and inflammatory components. Eventually, the function of the inner layer of the arteries, the endothelium, is disturbed.

Endothelial dysfunction is believed to be tightly linked to arterial stiffness, a surrogate marker for cardiovascular disease. An increase in the arterial stiffness causes a premature return of reflected waves in the late systolic phase, increasing central pulse pressure (PP) and thus systolic blood pressure (SBP). SBP increases the load on the left ventricle, increasing the oxygen demand of the myocardium. The increase in central PP and the decrease in diastolic BP (DBP) may directly cause subendocardial ischemia. The measurement of aortic stiffness, which integrates the alterations of the arterial wall, may also reflect parallel lesions present at the site of the coronary arteries.

Patients with type 1 diabetes have enhanced arterial stiffness even before clinically detectable diabetic complications compared to non-diabetic subjects. Arterial stiffness is further increased by micro- and macrovascular complications. Moreover, it has been shown in type 1 diabetes, that these patients suffer from premature arterial aging measured as increased PP, and the age – PP association was even steeper in the presence of diabetic nephropathy.

Epidemiological studies have shown arterial stiffness to play an independent role in the prediction of cardiovascular disease in selected patients groups. The predictive value is especially high for patients with type 2 diabetes, end stage renal disease, and coronary heart disease but it is also shown in hypertensive patients as well as in the general population. Whether an attenuation of the arterial stiffness also reduces cardiovascular disease has to be determined. Only a few pharmacological studies have provided data regarding this subject. Two drugs that inhibit the renin-angiotensin-system (RAS), perindopril and losartan, have been shown to decrease arterial stiffness and alongside this effect also provide a protective effect against cardiovascular events. No interventional study has yet elucidated the role of strict glucose control on arterial stiffness in patients with type 1 diabetes.

Tight metabolic and antihypertensive control are still the cornerstones in the prevention and treatment of diabetic complications. The specific role of tight glucose control cannot be emphasized enough. However, a need for a tool or surrogate marker to identify the patients at risk before clinically detectable complications is evident. One such marker may be arterial stiffness linking diabetes to increased cardiovascular risk. Future research will explore the mechanisms in more detail and hopefully provide the rationale for measures to retard the progression of arterial stiffness and thus diabetic complications.

1. Introduction

Diabetes and its complications have become a major burden for the patients and health-care systems worldwide. WHO has estimated that from year 2000 to 2030, the number of patients with diabeteswill increase by 114% while the world population increases by 37% [1]. Most of the patients with diabetes have type 2 but also type 1 diabetes shows a considerable increase. The highest incidence of type 1 diabetes in the world is found in Finland. It has increased from 31.4 per 100,000 per year in 1980 to 64.2 per 100,000 per year in 2005 in patients below 15 years [2].The reason for this trend is largely unknown but it is assumed that both genetic and environmental factors are involved. The concordance rate for monozygotic twins was shown to be 40%, while that for a first-degree relative was approximately 5% [3]. However, genetics by itself can hardly explain the rapid increase in the incidence. On the other hand, subjects carrying genetic susceptibility may be at increased risk and more vulnerable to environmental challenges. Consequently, early weight gain and childhood obesity have increased to a large extent during recent decades and may in part explain the finding [4, 5].

The diabetic complicationsare commonly divided into microvascular and macrovascular complications. The microvascular complications influence the smaller blood vessels; in the retina of the eyes (retinopathy), the kidney (nephropathy), and the nerves (neuropathy).The macrovascular complications affect the large vessels including those of the brain (cerebral), the heart (coronary), and the limbs.Although the treatment of diabetes has improved over recent years, it has not been able to eradicate the diabetes-related complications.We recently showed that excess mortality in patients with type 1 diabetes compared to non-diabetic subjects was confined to those with diabetic nephropathy [6]. Diabetic nephropathy influences about one third of the patients 15 to 20 years after onset of diabetes thus suggesting a genetic predisposition to the complications [7]. The search for susceptibility genes for diabetic nephropathy is ongoing and to date only a few genomic variants have conclusively been linked to diabetic nephropathy [8. 9]. These candidate genes associated with the angiotensin-converting enzyme, glomerular cells as well as the endothelium (also linked to arterial stiffness) [10]. However, most of the genomic variants that possibly increase the risk of diabetic nephropathy have still to be replicated. Large-scale genome wide association studies (GWAS) now ongoing might provide more insights in the near future. However, it is obvious that diabetic kidney disease cannot be explained exclusively by genetic factors and a number of non-genetic environmental players may be involved [11, 12]. These include metabolic changes, hypertension, diet, sedentary lifestyle, perinatal factors, age, and obesity [13].Nevertheless, the hyperglycemicmilieu is thought to play a crucial part in the pathogenesis in the complications of type 1 diabetes.

2. Hyperglycemia Leads to Complications

2.1. Biochemical and Molecular Pathogenesis

The glucose metabolism inpatients with type 1 diabetes is disturbed and contributes to the development of complications [14]. Several pathways have been shown to be involved on the route from hyperglycemia to arterial dysfunction [15]. Four of them have gained special interest. The aldose reductase pathway, the advanced glycation end-product (AGE) pathway, the hexosamine pathway, and the protein kinase-C (PKC) pathway cause both local and systemic changes in tissues [16]. Reactive glucose metabolites are generated as a consequence of the elevated glucose concentration at the blood and tissue level. This results in altered cell signaling and eventually cellular dysfunction and cell damage. Thus the events also associate with diabetic complications [17].

The aldose reductase pathway, also called the polyol pathway, involves the enzyme aldose reductase that in a normoglycemic environment reduces toxic agents and has a low affinity for glucose. However, in hyperglycemia it converts glucose into sorbitol meanwhile consuming the cofactor NADPH. This in turn results in a reduction of the essential antioxidant glutathione and the generation of harmful reactive oxygen species (ROS) [18, 19]. Attempts to inhibit the aldose reductase have shown promising results in animal models and for instance epalrestat was shown to decrease the decline in GFR in diabetic rats [20]. However, randomized clinical trials have been largely disappointing and no drugs are yet on the market.

The high blood glucose concentration also initiates the formation of AGEs that harm the environmentin several ways. They disturb gene transcription [21], cause cellular dysfunction, [22] and lead to the production of inflammatory agents and harmful growth factors [23, 24]. A few agents that inhibit AGEs have been studied in experimental models. Treating db/db mice with antagonists against glycated albumin reduced albuminuria and the decline in renal function compared to animals not given the treatment [25]. Another compound,aminoguanidine, inhibits the formation of AGEs and the development of diabetic nephropathy in long-term experimental diabetes in rats [26]. The effects of AGEs can also be inhibited by blocking its receptor, a phenomenon shown at least in mesangial cells [27]. Finally, AGE-cross-link breakers cleave covalent glucose-derived protein cross-links both in vitro and in vivo [28].

The hexosamine pathway is similarly activated by high intracellular glucose concentration. Thusfructose 6-phosphate is diverted from the glycolysis and converted into glucosamine 6-20phosphate by the enzyme GFAT (glutamine:fructose-6-phosphate amidotransferase) and finally toUDP N-acetyl glucosamine [29]. These biochemical changes are thought to disturb thefunction of cardiomyocytes [30] and modification of the endothelial cell proteinswas increased plaques in the carotid arteries of patients with type 2 diabetes [31].

Hyperglycemia also induces the synthesis of diacylglycerol that in turn activates the cofactor for protein kinase-C through the PKC pathway. PKC has a variety of effects on gene transcription, endothelial factors, inflammatory components as well as nitric oxide (NO), all harmful for the normal vascular function [32]. Inhibition of PKC-β prevents alterations in the diabetic eye and kidney in animal models[33]. However, in vivo studies blocking this pathway with PKC-β inhibitors (ruboxistaurin) have been unsuccessful in preventing the progression of diabetic retinopathy [34].

All these pathways seem to reflect hyperglycemia-induced overproduction of superoxide by the mitochondrial electron-transport chain. Excess superoxide partially inhibits the glycolytic enzyme GADPH, and hereby diverts upstream metabolites (glucose, fructose-6-phosphate, glyceraldehyde-3 phosphate) from the glycolysis. The inhibition of oxidative stress through these four pathways, may be a key to prevention of complications.

Notably, acute hyperglycemia increases oxidative stress in patients with type 1 diabetes [35]. Furthermore, superoxide production decreases in response to improved glycemic control in adult patients with type 1 diabetes [36]. Antioxidant treatmentis ableto prevent diabetic complications in animal models but not in large clinical trials[37]. A variety of antioxidants such as vitamin C, vitamin E, β-carotene, lipoic acids, have been used in animal models of diabetes, and in patients with diabetes [38]. These antioxidants have shown beneficial effects on cytokine expression, matrix synthesis, and cellular growth in animal models [39, 40] and Bursell et al. furthermore showed that vitamin E supplementation normalizes retinal blood flow and creatinine clearance in patients with type 1 diabetes [41]. However, large-scale studies such as the HOPE-study did not show beneficial effects of antioxidants in diabetic patients [42]. Therefore, a causal relationship between oxidative stress and vascular complications in patients with diabetes has still to be proven, although the association is rather likely.

2.2. Renin-Angiotensin System

The renin-angiotensin system (RAS) is a complex system of neuroendocrineinteractions that protects the heart, endothelium, brain, and kidney from sustained exposure to high blood pressure [43, 44]. The RAS has a central role in the control of blood pressure as it regulates fluid and electrolyte balance and modulates the growth of fibroblasts and myofibroblasts.In addition, it regulates the vascular response to injury and inflammation. Chronic activation of the RAS leads to hypertension and induces a cascade of proinflammatory, prothrombotic, and atherogenic effects associated with end-organ damage [45].

The juxtaglomerular cells in the kidney produce reninthat converts angiotensinogen into different variants of angiotensins (Ang) which in turn display a variety of functions.The angiotensin-converting enzyme (ACE) generates angiotensin I (Ang I) to angiotensin II (Ang II), the main mediator of the pro-fibrotic and vasoconstrictive effects of the RAS. In addition to this classical pathway it is now known that also other angiotensins are biologically active. Angiotensin converting enzyme 2 (ACE2) is a novel ACE homolog that binds to theMas receptor and converts Ang I and Ang II into the inactive Ang1-9 as well as into the vasodilative and antiproliferative Ang 1-7 [46].Ang-(1-7) can also be cleaved by ACE to another peptide Ang-(1-5), also biologically active [47]. These new data have resulted in an intensive research to findagents that target other components of the RAS than ACE and the Ang II.

ACE inhibitors and angiotensin II receptor blockers (ARBs) are the main drugs targeting the RAS and considered as the first-line treatment for hypertension in diabetic patients. Numerous studies support their therapeutic efficiency among them the LIFE study that demonstrated that the ARB losartan decreases cardiovascular morbidity and mortality in hypertensive patients with diabetes [48]. The ELITE trial was in turn the first large randomized study showing the effect of ARBs to improve the prognosis of patients with heart failure [49].

Furthermore, ACE inhibitors and ARBs may also prevent or delay the onset of type 2 diabetes, thus having beneficial effects beyond blood pressure control. The HOPE trial showed ramipril to reduce the risk of type 2 diabetes by 34% compared to placebo [50]. This may be due to improvement of insulin sensitivity, enhancement of insulin secretion, or direct effects on islet cell morphology. Other possible mechanisms may involve decreased sympathetic activity, adipocyte recruitment and differentiation, increased peroxisome proliferator-activated receptor-gamma activity, reduced glomerulosclerosis and tubulointerstitial fibrosis in the kidney, or reduction of vascular endothelial growthfactor [51].

Convincing data show beneficial effects of ACE inhibitors and ARBs in protecting the kidneys at all stages of diabetic nephropathy. The RENAAL study observed a significant improvement in the prognosis of patients with type 2 diabetes and diabetic nephropathy [52]. It reduced the risk for a composite endpoint (doubling of baseline serum creatinine, end-stage renal disease, or death) by 16% compared to the placebo group.These results are in line with those from the IDNT study where the risk for a composite endpoint was reduced by 20%

compared to placebo [53]. Similar results are available from patients with type 1 diabetes [54]. Notably the combination of an ACE inhibitor and ARB seemed to improve the renal outcome in type 2 diabetes, but not in type 1 diabetes [55, 56].

Interestingly, although renin was discovered already a long time ago by the Finnish scientists Robert Tigerstedt, not until now has renin been targeted by pharmacotherapy. Aliskiren, a direct renin inhibitor, combined with losartan have beneficial effects on diabetic nephropathy in type 2 diabetes that may go beyond blood-pressure-lowering effects [57]. Furthermore, both spironolactone andeplerenone, antagonise the effects of aldosterone at its receptor and have demonstrated clinical benefits in patients with hypertension, heart failure, and nephropathy.

Furthermore, both spironolactone andeplerenone, antagonize the effects of aldosterone at its receptor and have demonstrated clinical benefits in patients with hypertension, heart failure, and nephropathy.Recent experimental data proves that over-expression of ACE2 counterbalances the harmful effects of Ang II in the vasculature in diabetic animals [59], and that genetic deficiency or pharmacological inhibition of ACE2 causes increased prothrombotic, atherogenic and inflammatory activity [60, 61, 62]Despite the promising results in animal studies proposing that ACE2-enhancer drug, perhaps in combination with an ACE inhibitor, could be effective in reducing blood pressure it will take some time before the promise of ACE2 enhancement is clinically available.

2.3. Chronic Inflammation

The classical view considers atherosclerosis to be passive aggregation of cholesterol in the artery wall. This results in endothelial injury and platelet aggregation that in turn triggers the proliferation of smooth muscle cells in the intimal and medial layers. Eventually, the dysfunctional endothelium traps lipoproteins and forms an atherosclerotic plaque that is vulnerable to rupture [63]. However, the current view is slightly different. Immune cells and mediators are found in atherosclerotic lesions, supporting the view that there is also an inflammatory component involved in the disease process. A number of independent pathways have been recognized, that all show inflammation to be a key regulator of atherosclerosis and its complications [64]. Large scale studies have furthermore proven the predictive role of C-reactive protein in cardiovascular disease [65].

Chronic inflammation is thought to contribute to the development of diabetic vascular diseasesince CRP and IL-6 are increased in patients with diabetic nephropathy [66]. Furthermore, recent data from the FinnDiane Study show that CRP and mannose-binding lectin were associated with the progression of diabetic nephropathy [67].Soluble intercellular adhesion molecule 1 (ICAM-1) is in turn increased in patients with type 1 or type 2 diabetes [68, 29]and predicts cardiovascular disease in non-diabetic subjects [70]. Recent data from the DCCT study demonstrate that tight glycaemic control reduces ICAM-1concentrations [71]. Notably, in patients with type 1 diabetes elevated soluble receptor for advanced glycation end-product (sRAGE) concentrations are associated with cardiovascular disease and all-cause mortality [72].This finding was partially mediated by endothelial dysfunction and inflammation.

The American Diabetes Association recommends aspirin to be prescribed to all patients with type 1 diabetes>40 years or to those who have at least one cardiovascular disease risk factor [73]. It is however important to keep in mind the multifaceted effects of aspirin on the coagulation cascade and that the role of aspirin in primary prevention of diabetic complications remains unproven [74]Furthermore, the future will probably clarify the position of the statins as anti-inflammatory agents in the treatment of cardiovascular disease, but promising results are already available [75].

2.4. Growth Factors

Growth factors are known to be involved in the pathogenesis of diabetic vascular disease. As there are convincing data that linkthe vascular endothelial growth factor (VEGF), the growth hormone (GH), and the insulin like growth factors(IGF) to diabetic nephropathy the discussion will focus on these three, although other growth factors have also been studied [76].

VEGF stimulates endothelial cell proliferation and differentiation, increases vascular permeability, mediates endothelium-dependent vasodilatation, and plays a crucial role in angiogenesis [77]. It is associated with diabetic nephropathy both in experimental models and in human studies [78, 79]. In patients with type 1 diabetes, VEGF has been shown to correlate with the severity of diabetic nephropathy [80], although, contradictory data are also available [81]. Antibodies against VEGF have shown the most promising results so far in targeting this pathway [82].

Other important players seem to be growth hormone and insulin like growth factors. The GH/IGF system is active in most tissues, the extracellular space, and the circulation, where GH induces the formation of IGF-1 [83]. In the kidney, GH and IGF-1 play a role in renal hemodynamics and electrolyte, as well as water absorption [84].

Various agents that inhibit the GH/IGF system have been studied in the treatment of diabetic nephropathy. Somatostatin analogues suppress GH activity and the analogue (octreoide) was shown to prevent renal growth partly by inhibiting this pathway in diabetic mice [85]. GHR and IGF-1 antagonists have also been studied in experimental models, gaining promising results [86, 87]. Notably, aminoguanidine (AGE inhibitor) has positive effects on the diabetic kidney through the GH/IGF system thus linking different pieces of the complex puzzle together [88].

Pathogenesis of Arterial Stiffness

It is important to understand the mechanisms how hyperglycemia leads to the development of diabetic complications, in order to be able to develop new methods to treat the hyperglycemia-induced complications. Only a few of the mechanisms are described here but it is very likely that they all contribute to endothelial dysfunction and thus indirectly to the increase in arterial stiffness in patients with diabetes [89]. Arterial stiffness is strongly linked to cardiovascular disease and may therefore be considered an intermediate marker and link between hyperglycemia and vascular complications.

3.1. Pathophysiology

The central arterial pressure wave is composed of a forward traveling wave that is generated by the ejection of the heart and the later arriving wave that is reflected from the periphery. The forward wave caused by the left ventricle is dependent on the mechanical properties of the large central elastic arteries, but is not influenced by the wave reflection. The reflected wave is in turn, dependent on the elastic properties of the entire arterial tree (elastic, muscular arteries, and resistance arteries), the velocity of the wave and the distance to the major reflecting sites [90]. If arterial stiffness is increased, the reflected wave returns earlier from the periphery to the heart during systole. This phenomenon results in increased aortic pulse pressure, increased left ventricular afterload, increased LV massand oxygen demand, decreased stroke volume, and consequently potentiates the development of atherosclerosis [91].

The arterial tree can be separated into three anatomic regions,and since the heart is a pulsatile pump, each region has a distinct and separate function: (A) the large arteries(aorta, carotid, iliac) are elastic and possess a large buffering capacity. They conserve energy that is released by the heart during the systolic cardiac phase in order to maintain a steady blood flow during the entire cardiac cycle; (B) the intermediate-sized muscular arteries, especially those in the lower body (femoral, popliteal), modify the speed of the pressure wave by altering the smooth muscle tonein order to regulate the timing of the reflection wave; (C) the arterioles modify the mean arterial pressure, by regulatingtheir caliber, and thus peripheral resistance [92].

Changes in the central elastic arteries occur over a period of time, while changes in the muscular arteries and the arterioles often occur acutely [93]. The elastic fibers support the arterial wall at low pressure, whereas the collagen fibers are needed at higher pressure levels. A change in the stiffness of the muscular arteries is primarily due to acute changes in the smooth muscle tone as we have observed in our own studies [94]. Age and hypertensionhave little effect on the stiffness of muscular arteries, while drugs have little effect on the stiffness of elastic arteries [95].

3.2. Endothelial Dysfunction

The endothelium lines the inner wall of the arteries regardless of size. Arterial stiffness depends on the interplay between the endothelium and the smooth muscle cells of the arterial walls. The endothelium does not only serve as a barrier between the arterial wall and the blood, but it is also part of complex autocrine, paracrine and endocrine signaling. It regulates the composition of the subendothelial matrix, the permeability, the vascular tone, the coagulation cascade, and it activates the inflammatory response. It interacts with different crucial cell types such as smooth muscle cells, leucocytes, retinal pericytes, and renal mesangial cells [96]. The endothelium furthermore produces a number of substances that are involved its various functions. Such substances are e.g. nitric oxide (NO), VEGF, interleukins, tissue plasminogen activator,prostacyclin, endothelin, angiotensin converting enzyme (ACE) and von Willebrand factor. Many of them link hyperglycemia to arterial stiffness.

Endothelial dysfunction is characterized by loss of arterial NO-mediated endothelium-dependent vasodilatation. NO normally causes the smooth muscle to relax and decreased production of NO as well as decreased sensitivity to this substance is believed to play a role when the function of the endothelium becomes disturbed [97]. Notably, it is shown that patients with type 1 diabetes and microalbuminuria already display endothelial dysfunction. However, it seems that the phenomenon occurs even before microalbuminuria is present although the results are not consistent [98, 99, 100, 101, 102]. Acute hyperglycemia impairs endothelial function and increases arterial stiffness [103, 104]. Interestingly, a recent paper showed positive effects of renin inhibition on endothelial function and arterial stiffness in uncomplicated patients with type 1 diabetes [105].

Taken together, available data suggest that endothelial dysfunction is not only important in the pathogenesis of diabetic complications [106], but is also a central feature in the stiffening of the arteries [107, 108, 109].

3.3. Extracellular Proteins

The structural component of arterial stiffness depends largely on two extracellular proteins, elastin and collagen [110]. Enzymes called metalloproteases regulate the degradation of these two molecules. The amount of elastin in the arterial wall typically diminishes whereas the number of collagen fibers increases with age [111]. Collagen production is markedly stimulated by hypertension [112]. Furthermore, collagen is prone to nonenzymatic glycation due to its slow turnover and may therefore result in increased arterial stiffness in patients with diabetes [113]. Moreover, AGEs impair endothelial function by quenching nitric oxide (NO) and by increasing the generation of ROS [114]. By binding to specific receptors, AGEs initiate a variety of inflammatoryresponses that in turn may increase vascular stiffness via activation of metalloproteinases, a phenomenon that contributes to endothelial dysfunction and atherosclerosis [115].

3.4. Genetics of Arterial Stiffness

The heritability of arterial stiffness has been shown to range from 0.21 to 0.66 [116]. Genome-wide association studies (GWAS) have shown significant to suggestive linkages between chromosomal regions and pulse pressure, pulse wave velocity (PWV) as well as pulse wave analysis (PWA). In 2001 Atwood et al. found four regions to be associated with PP [117]. A few years later chromosome 8 was linked to PP but not to SBP suggesting that arterial stiffness may have a different genetic background than hypertension 118]. The results were supported by findings from the Framingham Study that showed that PWV and the reflected wave amplitude (PWA) were linked to chromosomes 2, 7, 13, and 15 [119, 120]. Interestingly, genetic loci for PP were also associated with coronary artery calcification [121]. It is likely that arterial stiffness is rather a cause than a consequence of cardiovascular risk. Thus, it is of interest to study whether these loci are associated with molecular determinants of arterial stiffness and other cardiovascular risk factors. The number of GWAS studies is yet low, while many studies have explored relationships between biologically relevant polymorphisms and arterial stiffness. Notably, a polymorphism of the angiotensin II type 1 receptor (AT1) genewas involved in the development of arterial stiffness in subjects with hypertension [122]. The effect of the angiotensin-converting enzyme (ACE) insertion/deletion (I/D) polymorphism on arterial stiffness is less clear [123]. Moreover, a number of studies have found relationships between matrix and metalloproteinase genes, endothelial cell related genes, as well as inflammatory genes, and the stiffness of the large arteries [124, 135, 126].

4. Risk Factors for Arterial Stiffness

The most important determinant of arterial stiffness is age. This is convincingly shown in large-scale studies [127, 128, 129]. As earlier pointed out, the large elastic arteries stiffen linearly with age, whereas the small muscular arteries do not [130].

An important risk factor for arterial stiffness is hypertension. Pulse wave velocity increases significantly less in well-controlled hypertensive patients than in patients with poor control [131]. Moreover, a longitudinal study showed that an important determinant of hypertension, low birth weight, is related to increased arterial compliance [132]. Dernellis et al. observed that aortic stiffness is a predictor of an increase in blood pressure in patients with normal blood pressure [133]. Not surprisingly, several epidemiological studies have shown that cigarette smoking has negative effects on large artery stiffness [134, 145]. Notably, acute smoking impairs regional arterial distensibility and increases PWV [136, 137]. Even passive smoking show similar effects [138]. Oncken et al. showed that smoking cessation decreases pulse pressure in postmenopausal women [139]. A recent paper shows that continuous smoking accelerates stiffening of large- and middle-sized arteries [140]. Physical activity protects against stiffness of the large arteries. This effect is at least in part mediated by the positive effects on cardiovascular risk factors [141]. However, it is of interest that arterial stiffness can be reduced by exercise [142, 143]. In contrast to aerobic training that reduces arterial stiffness, resistance training increases both arterial stiffness and pulse pressure [144]. The metabolic syndrome associates with pulse wave velocity as shown by Safar et al. [145]. Notably, similar findings were observed in young adults in the Bogalusa Heart Study [146]. Not surprisingly, hypercholesterolemic patients have stiffer arteries than subjects with normal cholesterol values [147]. Interestingly, acute systemic inflammation increases arterial stiffness in healthy subjects, and C-reactive protein is not unexpectedly associated with arterial stiffness [148, 149]. Finally, in kidney disease there is a stepwise increase in arterial stiffness with regard to the severity of the disease [150]. In type 2 diabetes, normal to elevated urinary albumin-to-creatinine ratio, creatinine clearance and carotid–femoral pulse wave velocity correlate inversely, independently of age. [151].

5. Diabetes and Arterial Stiffness

5.1. Type 1 Diabetes

Patients with type 1 diabetes have stiffer arteries than non-diabetic subjects [152, 153]. Similar findings have been observed in type 1 diabetic adolescents and children [154, 155], as well as adult patients without vascular complications [156].

Diabetic nephropathy further increases arterial stiffness in such patients [157, 158]. Recent data from the FinnDiane study show that arterial stiffness is increased in patients with diabetic retinopathy without any signs of nephropathy [159]. We have also shown that pulse pressure increases 15 to 20 years earlier in patients with type 1 diabetes compared to non-diabetic controls [160]. This observation was more pronounced in subjects with diabetic nephropathy but was also apparent in diabetic subjects with normal albumin excretion rate. The arterial stiffness correlates with the duration of diabetes and the exposure to hyperglycemia.

Thus, it is likely that the stiffening of the arteries is the result of chronic hyperglycemia and other chronic metabolic changes. In this respect it is of interest that a substudy of the FinnDiane study showed that the augmentation index as well as the brachial PWV increased in response to acute hyperglycemia in young patients with type 1 diabetes and no complications [161].

5.2. Type 2 Diabetes

Arterial stiffness is shown to be increased in patients with type 2 diabetes compared to non-diabetic subjects. The finding has been replicated many times using different methods [162, 163, 164, 165]. Notably, a decreased arterial elasticity is observed already in the pre-diabetic state, supporting the hypothesis that the risk for cardiovascular risk increases already before the actual debut of type 2 diabetes [166, 167, 168]. As for type 1 diabetes, complications further enhance arterial stiffness in type 2 diabetes [169, 170, 171]. Furthermore, an accelerated arterial aging has also been observed in patients with type 2 diabetes [172].

6. Estimates of Arterial Stiffness

6.1. Pulse Pressure

A crude surrogate marker for arterial stiffness is pulse pressure. It is defined as the difference between the systolic and diastolic blood pressure and is thus easily available even in larger population samples. Unfortunately, pulse pressure is rather an inaccurate measure in younger populations but the usability to predict cardiovascular disease increases with age. This was shown in the Framingham Heart Study and has been confirmed thereafter [173, 174, 175]. Furthermore, pulse pressure has been shown to predict cardiovascular and all-cause mortality in the general population.

A meta-analysis by Gasowsky et al. concludes that pulse pressure is a useful tool to predict fatal coronary events [176]. However, conflicting data has been provided by Dyer et al [177]. Franklin et al. compared different blood pressure indices in the Framingham study and reported that a combination of pulse pressure and mean arterial pressure is the strongest predictor of cardiovascular events [178].

6.2. Pulse Wave Velocity

Pulse wave velocity (PWV) is the speed at which the forward pressure wave is transmitted from the aorta through the vascular tree. In order to measure arterial stiffness in different-sized arteries, pressure waveforms are recorded sequentially between two points with known distance. The measurements are synchronized to the heart beats by a sequential ECG-recording in order to measure the speed of the pulse wave in a vessel. Different devices can be used for the purpose but an arterial tonometer is commonly used. The method is validated and reproducible [179].

PWV is an independent predictor of cardiovascular disease both in patients with hypertension or end-stage renal disease [180, 181]. PWV has also been shownto predict mortality in diabetic patients, in the elderly, and even in the general population [182, 183, 184]. Importantly, aortic PWV has recently been considered the "gold standard" of arterialstiffness [185].

6.3. Pulse Wave Analysis

Pulse wave analysis (PWA) can be measured non-invasively by applanation tonometer and other devices [186]. The recorded wave is measured from the radial artery and then transformed through a mathematical formula (transfer function) into aortic waveform. The validation of the transfer function is based upon a comparison with intra-arterial pressures in patients undergoing surgery [187]. The augmentation (AIx), is a measure of systemic arterial stiffness, and can be calculated as the difference between the second (causedby wave reflection) and the first systolic peak (caused by ventricular ejection) [188].

PWA is associated with coronary artery disease and the risk for cardiovascular disease in patients suffering from stable coronary artery disease [189, 190]. It is, moreover, a predictor of cardiovascular disease in patients with end-stage renal disease [191]. Age, height and gender are known confounding factors for PWA and have to be adjusted in the analyses. Moreover, PWA is a useful tool in short-term interventions as it is an estimate of systemic stiffness, strongly influenced by the interplay between smooth muscle cells and endothelium in the intermediate-sized arteries.

6.4. Other Methods

The compliance of large arteries can be measured by ultrasonography. The device registers the changes in the diameter of the vessel during the cardiac cycle. Compliance and distensibility can then be calculated using a formulaincluding blood pressure [192].

Similarly, distensibility of the aorta can be measured by magnetic resonance imaging. It is also possible to measure pulse wave velocity reliably with this technique [193].

The ambulatory arterial stiffness index (AASI) can be assessed by using a 24-hour ambulatory blood pressure device. AASI is calculated from the individual blood pressure readings as 1 minus the slope of diastolic on systolic pressure during 24-hour ambulatory monitoring [194].

Finally, the diastolic pulse contour analysis can be measured using a tonometer. The compliance of both large and small arteries can be examined by assessment of the diastolic portion of the pressure pulse contour utilizing a modified Windkessel model [195].

7. Treatments of Arterial Stiffness

7.1. Pharmacological Treatments

Laurent et al. have nicely reviewed a wide range of pharmacological and non-pharmacological treatmentsthat have an effect on arterial stiffness [196].Pharmacological treatments include antihypertensive drugs, lipid-lowering agents, and antidiabetic agents. Vasodilative drugs such as beta-blockers, calcium channel blockers, ACE-inhibitors, angiotensinreceptor blockers, and nitrates acutely decrease the augmentation index possibly through vasodilatation of the muscular arteries [197, 198, 199]. These agents have also effects on the elastic properties of the vessels.

Notably, trials using AGE breakers affecting the walls of the arteries have been promising. Aminoguanide decreased arterial stiffness and urine albumin excretion ratio in patients with diabetic nephropathy [200]. Kass et al. showed in a randomized, placebo-controlled study that alagebrium (ALT-711) improves arterial compliance in elderly people [201]. Similarly, the use of alagebrium is independently associated with aortic PWV in hypertensive patients [202]. It is of note that, alagebrium accumulates in the arterial wall rather than in the myocardium, suggesting the effects to be mediated by other than collagen-dependent pathways [203]. Nevertheless, the route for a pharmacological agent into clinical practice is long and despite these encouraging results the utility of AGE inhibition on diabetic complications remains to be established. Another peculiar question to answer is whether the agents break established crosslinks rather than prevent their formation.

Among the lipid-lowering agents it is the statins that are the most studied. Orr et al. observed destiffening of the arteries in response to atorvastatin in obese subjects [204]. Similar findings have been observed using fluvastatin [205]. Mäki-Petäjä et al. showed beneficial effects of ezetimibe and simvastatin on arterial stiffness, inflammation, and endothelial function in patients with rheumatoid arthritis [206]. However, also negative results are available and this issue needs to be further studied [207].

In patients with type 2 diabetes, the use of pioglitazone for three months reduced aortic PWV suggesting insulin-sensitizing agents to be beneficial for the vascular health [208] A similar study also showed with a follow-up time of 56 months, a beneficial effect of pioglitazone on arterial stiffness [209]. Interestingly, Ryan et al. observed a combined positive effect of fenofibrate and pioglitazone on endothelial function and arterial compliance in obese non-diabetic men [210]. Westerbacka et al. showed that supraphysiological doses of insulin decrease arterial stiffness measured as PWA [211]. Interestingly, this effect was reduced in insulin-resistant obese persons and patients with type 1 diabetes [212, 213].

Taken together, the data on the protective role of anti-diabetic agents on diabetic complications is still scarce although at least insulin seems to have a strong vasodilative effect on the vessels.

7.2. Non-Pharmacological Treatments

Non-pharmacological treatments include exercise, weight loss, low-salt diet, moderate alcoholconsumption, and hormone replacement therapy, as well as alternative treatment options such asgarlic powder, dark chocolate, and fish oil [214].Noteworthy, some of the effects seem to be mediated indirectly through other mechanisms. For example, the effect of unsaturated fatty acids in fish oil that decreases arterial stiffness in hypercholesterolemic patients is most likely mediated by lowering of trigycerides and LDL-cholesterol [215].

The role of antioxidants on diabetic complications was already earlier discussed. However, the direct effects of vitamin C and E on arterial compliance could be a consequence of a reduced peripheral resistance in type 2 diabetes and middle-aged subjects [216, 217]. On the contrary, a study by Escurza et al. showed that ascorbic acid did not improve arterial distensibility in young and older men [218] Similar results were reported by Kelly et al. where no effect of vitamin C on arterial stiffness, oxidative stress, or blood pressure was observed in healthy subjects [219].

The effects of weight loss on arterial stiffness have been speculated to be due to other beneficial effects on the metabolic system rather than directly on arterial stiffness [220]. However, a study by Barinas-Mitchell et al. showed that moderate weight loss reduces aortic pulse wave velocity in patients with type 2 diabetes independently of the effect on the blood pressure [221].

7.3. Interventional Studies

There are a few interventional studies targeting arterial stiffness as a primary endpoint. The CAFE study showed a difference in the augmentation index and central blood pressure in hypertensive patients with and without diabetestreated with beta-blockers compared with those taking calcium antagonists [32]. Beta-blockers did not reduce AIx and central BP, whereas calcium antagonists did. This may have been dueto the inability of beta-blockers to reduce the magnitude of the reflection wave [223]. This is inline with the results from the LIFE study showingthat ACE inhibitors reduce left ventricular hypertrophy andits consequences more effectively than beta-blockers [224]. Similar results are available from the REASON study where perindopril was more effective than atenolol [225]. Another ACE inhibitor, trandolapril, improved PWV but not the augmentation index in a trial with a follow-up of 52 months [226]. This was already earlier suggested by De Luca et al. in a small subset of patients (N=15) [227]. These results are not at contrast with the HOPE study, where ramipril showed beneficial effects on the left ventricular mass and function as well as cardiovascular events [228].These findings are also supported by experimental studies [229,230,231].

Angiotensinreceptor blockers have similar effects on arterial stiffness as ACE inhibitors. Agata et al. showed an improvement in PWV independently of blood pressure in a small set of hypertensive patients taking angiotensin II blockers [232]. The finding was later replicated in patients with type 2 diabetes [233]. A combination of valsartan and perindopril was more efficient than monotherapy of either agent in reducing arterial stiffness and left ventricular hypertrophy in hypertensive patients [234] Irbesartan improved arterial distensibility more effectively than lisinopril in fifteen hypertensive patients [235]. Interestingly, valsartan was more effective in reducing arterial stiffness than valsartan combined with a diuretic although the effect on blood pressure was equal [236]. Andreadis et al. showed that angiotensinII receptor blockers are more efficient than calcium channel blockers in lowering arterial stiffness although their effects on blood pressure are equal [237].

All in all, the number of large-scale randomized clinical trials on the effects of medication on arterial stiffness is still low. However, there seems to be an effect beyond lowering of blood pressure. ACE inhibitors and angiotensinreceptor blockers have so far been superior in improving arterial stiffness compared to other antihypertensive medications available. This goes in line with the predictive value of these drugs in the prevention of cardiovascular morbidity and mortality.

Conclusions

Tight metabolic and antihypertensive control is still the cornerstone in the prevention and treatment of diabetic complications. The specific role of tight glucose control cannot be emphasized enough. However, a need for a tool or surrogate marker to identify the patients at risk before clinically detectable complications is evident. One such marker may be arterial stiffness linking diabetes to increased cardiovascular risk. Future research will explore the mechanisms in more detail and hopefully provide the rationale for measures to retard the progression of arterial stiffness and thus diabetic complications.

Acknowledgments

The FinnDiane study was funded by the Folkhälsan Research Foundation, Wilhelm and Else Stockmann Foundation, Sigrid Juselius Foundation, European Commission, Medicinska Understödsföreningen Liv och Hälsa, Signe and Ane Gyllenberg Foundation, Waldemar von Frenckell Foundation, EVO governmental grants, and the National Institutes of Health. None of these groups had a role in data collection, analysis, or preparation of the manuscript.

Disclosure of Interests

No potential conflicts of interest relevant to this article were reported.

References

[1]   Wild S, Roglic G, Green A, Sicree R, King G. Global prevalence of diabetes. Estimates for the year 2000 and projections for 2030. *Diabetes Care*2004;27:1047–52.

[2]   Harjutsalo V, Sjöberg L, Tuomilehto J. Time trends in the incidence of type 1 diabetes in Finnish children: a cohort study. *Lancet* 2008;371:1777-82.

[3] Redondo MJ, Rewers M, Yu L, Garg S, Pilcher CC, Elliott RB, Eisenbarth GS. Genetic determination of islet cell autoimmunity in monozygotic twin, dizygotic twin, and non-twin siblings of patients with type 1 diabetes: prospective twin study. *Br Med J.* 1999;318:698-702.

[4] Speiser PW, Rudolf MC, Anhalt H, et al. Childhood obesity. *J Clin Endocrinol Metab*2005; 90: 1871–87.

[5] Kautiainen S, Rimpela A, Vikat A, Virtanen SM. Secular trends in overweight and obesity among Finnish adolescents in 1977–1999.*Int J Obes Relat Metab Disord*2002; 26: 544–52.

[6] Groop PH, Thomas MC, Moran JL, Wadèn J, Thorn LM, Mäkinen VP, Rosengård-Bärlund M, Saraheimo M, Hietala K, Heikkilä O, Forsblom C; FinnDiane Study Group. The presence and severity of chronic kidney disease predicts all-cause mortality in type 1 diabetes. *Diabetes* 2009;58:1651-8.

[7] Andersen AR, Christiansen JS, Andersen JK, Kreiner S, Deckert T. Diabetic nephropathy in Type 1 (insulin-dependent) diabetes: an epidemiological study. *Diabetologia* 1983;25:496-501.

[8] Trégouet DA, Groop PH, McGinn S, Forsblom C, Hadjadj S, Marre M, Parving HH, Tarnow L, Telgmann R, Godefroy T, Nicaud V, Rousseau R, Parkkonen M, Hoverfält A, Gut I, Heath S, Matsuda F, Cox R, Kazeem G, Farrall M, Gauguier D, Brand-Herrmann SM, Cambien F, Lathrop M, Vionnet N; EURAGEDIC Consortium. G/T substitution in intron 1 of the UNC13B gene is associated with increased risk of nephropathy in patients with type 1 diabetes. *Diabetes* 2008;57:2843-50.

[9] He B, Osterholm AM, Hoverfält A, Forsblom C, Hjörleifsdóttir EE, Nilsson AS, Parkkonen M, Pitkäniemi J, Hreidarsson A, Sarti C, McKnight AJ, Maxwell AP, Tuomilehto J, Groop PH, Tryggvason K. Association of genetic variants at 3q22 with nephropathy in patients with type 1 diabetes mellitus. *Am J Hum Genet* 2009;84:5-13.

[10] Hadjadj S, Tarnow L, Forsblom C, Kazeem G, Marre M, Groop PH, Parving HH, Cambien F, Tregouet DA, Gut IG, Théva A, Gauguier D, Farrall M, Cox R, Matsuda F, Lathrop M, Hager-Vionnet N; EURAGEDIC (European Rational Approach for Genetics of Diabetic Complications) Study Group. Association between angiotensin-converting enzyme gene polymorphisms and diabetic nephropathy: case-control, haplotype, and family-based study in three European populations. *J Am Soc Nephrol* 2007;18:1284-91.

[11] Mogensen CE, Christensen CK. Predicting diabetic nephropathy in insulin-dependent patients. *N Engl J Med* 1984;311:89-93.

[12] Chaturvedi N, Bandinelli S, Mangili R, Penno G, Rottiers RE, Fuller JH. Microalbuminuria in type 1 diabetes: rates, risk factors and glycemic threshold. *Kidney Int* 2001;60:219-27.

[13] Soedamah-Muthu SS, Chaturvedi N, Witte DR, Stevens LK, Porta M, Fuller JH; EURODIAB Prospective Complications Study Group. Relationship between risk factors and mortality in type 1 diabetic patients in Europe: the EURODIAB Prospective Complications Study (PCS). *Diabetes Care* 2008;31:1360-6.

[14] Klein R, Klein BE, Moss SE Relation of glycemic control to diabetic microvascular complications in diabetes mellitus. *Ann Intern Med* 1996;124:90-6

[15] Schrijvers BF, De Vriese AS, Flyvbjerg A. From hyperglycemia to diabetic kidney disease: the role of metabolic, hemodynamic, intracellular factors and growth factors/cytokines. *Endocr Rev* 2004;25:971-1010.

[16] Brownlee M. Biochemistry and molecular cell biology of diabetic complications. *Nature* 2001;414:813-20.

[17] Scott JA, King GL. Oxidative stress and antioxidant treatment in diabetes. *Ann N Y Acad Sci* 2004;1031: 204-213.

[18] Lee AY, Chung SS. Contributions of polyol pathway to oxidative stress in diabetic cataract. *FASEB J* 1999;13:23–30

[19] Engerman RL, Kern TS, Larson ME. Nerve conduction and aldose reductase inhibition during 5 years of diabetes or galactosaemia in dogs. *Diabetologia* 1994;37:141–144

[20] Itagaki I, Shimizu K, Kamanaka Y, Ebata K, Kikkawa R, Haneda M, Shigeta Y. The effect of an aldose reductase inhibitor (Epalrestat) on diabetic nephropathy in rats. *Diabetes Res Clin Pract* 1994;25:147–154

[21] Shinohara M, Thornalley PJ, Giardino I, Beisswenger P, Thorpe SR, Onorato J, Brownlee M. Overexpression of glyoxalase-I in bovine endothelial cells inhibits intracellular advanced glycation endproduct formation and prevents hyperglycemia-induced increases in macromolecular endocytosis. *J Clin Invest* 1998;101:1142–1147

[22] Charonis AS, Reger LA, Dege JE, Kouzi-Koliakos K, Furcht LT, Wohlhueter RM, Tsilibary EC. Laminin alterations after in vitro nonenzymatic glycosylation. *Diabetes* 1990;39:807– 814

[23] Abordo EA, Thornalley PJ. Synthesis and secretion of tumour necrosis factor-alpha by human monocytic THP-1 cells and chemotaxis induced by human serum albumin derivatives modified with methylglyoxal and glucose- derived advanced glycation endproducts. *Immunol Lett* 1997;58:139 –147

[24] Doi T, Vlassara H, Kirstein M, Yamada Y, Striker GE, Striker LJ. Receptorspecific increase in extracellular matrix production in mouse mesangial cells by advanced glycosylation end products is mediated via plateletderived growth factor. *Proc Natl Acad Sci U S A* 1992;89:2873–2877

[25] Cohen MP, Sharma K, Jin Y, Hud E, Wu VY, Tomaszewski J, Ziyadeh FN. Prevention of diabetic nephropathy in db/db mice with glycated albumin antagonists. A novel treatment strategy. *J Clin Invest* 1995;95:2338–2345

[26] Soulis-Liparota T, Cooper M, Papazoglou D, Clarke B, Jerums G. Retardation by aminoguanidine of development of albuminuria, mesangial expansion, and tissue fluorescence in streptozocininduced diabetic rat. *Diabetes* 1991;40:1328–1334

[27] Pugliese G, Pricci F, Romeo G, Pugliese F, Mene P, Giannini S, Cresci B, Galli G, Rotella CM, Vlassara H, Di Mario U. Upregulation of mesangial growth factor and extracellular matrix synthesis by advanced glycation end products via a receptor-mediated mechanism. *Diabetes* 1997;46:1881–1887

[28] Vasan S, Zhang X, Zhang X, Kapurniotu A, Bernhagen J, Teichberg S, Basgen J, Wagle D, Shih D, Terlecky I, Bucala R, Cerami A, Egan J, Ulrich P. An agent cleaving glucose-derived protein crosslinks in vitro and in vivo. *Nature* 1996;382:275–278

[29] Du XL, Edelstein D, Rossetti L, Fantus IG, Goldberg H, Ziyadeh F, Wu J, Brownlee M. Hyperglycemia-induced mitochondrial superoxide overproduction activates the hexosamine pathway and induces plasminogen activator inhibitor-1 expression by increasing Sp1 glycosylation. *Proc Natl Acad Sci U S A* 2000;97:12222–12226

[30] Clark RJ, McDonough PM, Swanson E, Trost SU, Suzuki M, Fukuda M, Dillmann WH. Diabetes and the accompanying hyperglycemia impairs cardiomyocyte calcium cycling through increased nuclear O-GlcNAcylation. *J Biol Chem* 2003;278:44230–44237

[31] Federici M, Menghini R, Mauriello A, Hribal ML, Ferrelli F, Lauro D, Sbraccia P, Spagnoli LG, Sesti G, Lauro R. Insulin-dependent activation of endothelial nitric oxide synthase is impaired by O-linked glycosylation modification of signaling proteins in human coronary endothelial cells. *Circulation* 2002;106:466–472

[32] Koya D, King GL. Protein kinase C activation and the development of diabetic complications. *Diabetes* 1998;47:859–866

[33] Koya D, Haneda M, Nakagawa H, Isshiki K, Sato H, Maeda S, Sugimoto T, Yasuda H, Kashiwagi A, Ways DK, King GL, Kikkawa R. Amelioration of accelerated diabetic mesangial expansion by treatment with a PKC beta inhibitor in diabetic db/db mice, a rodent model for type 2 diabetes. *FASEB J* 2000;14:439–447

[34] The PKC-DRS Study Group. The effect of ruboxistaurin on visual loss in patients with moderately severe to very severe nonproliferative diabetic retinopathy: initial results of the Protein Kinase C beta Inhibitor Diabetic Retinopathy Study (PKC-DRS) multicenter randomized clinical trial. *Diabetes* 2005;54:2188-97

[35] Gordin D, Forsblom C, Rönnback M, Parkkonen M, Wadén J, Hietala K, Groop PH. Acute hyperglycaemia induces an inflammatory response in young patients with type 1 diabetes. *Ann Med* 2008;40:627-33

[36] Ceriello A, Giugliano D, Quatraro A, Dello Russo P, Lefèvre PJ. Metabolic control may influence the increased superoxide generation in diabetic serum. *Diabet Med* 1991;8:540–542

[37] Scott JA, King GL. Oxidative stress and antioxidant treatment in diabetes. *Ann N Y Acad Sci* 2004;1031: 204-213.

[38] Kowluru RA,Kennedy A. Therapeutic potential of anti-oxidants and diabetic retinopathy. *Expert Opin Investig. Drugs* 2001;10:1665–1676.

[39] Montero A, Munger KA, Khan RZ, Valdivielso JM, Morrow JD, Guasch A, Ziyadeh FN, Badr KF F(2)-isoprostanes mediate high glucose-induced TGF-beta synthesis and glomerular proteinuria in experimental type I diabetes. *Kidney Int* 2000;58:1963-72.

[40] Koya D, Lee IK, Ishii H, Kanoh H, King GL. Prevention of glomerular dysfunction in diabetic rats by treatment with d-alpha-tocopherol. *J Am Soc Nephrol* 1997;8:426-35

[41] Bursell SE, Clermont AC, Aiello LP, Aiello LM, Schlossman DK, Feener EP, Laffel L, King GL. High-dose vitamin E supplementation normalizes retinal blood flow and creatinine clearance in patients with type 1 diabetes. *Diabetes Care* 1999;22:1245-51

[42] Lonn E, Yusuf S, Hoogwerf B, Pogue J, Yi Q, Zinman B, Bosch J, Dagenais G, Mann JF, Gerstein HC; HOPE Study; MICRO-HOPE Study. Effects of vitamin E on cardiovascular and microvascular outcomes in high-risk patients with diabetes: results of the HOPE study and MICRO-HOPE substudy. *Diabetes Care* 2002;25:1919-27

[43] Ferrario CM. Role of-angiotensin II in cardiovascular disease: Therapeutic implications of "more than a century of" research. *Renin Angiotensin Aldosterone Syst* 2006;7:3-14.

[44] Schrijvers BF, De Vriese AS, Flyvbjerg A. From hyperglycemia to diabetic kidney disease: the role of metabolic, hemodynamic, intracellular factors and growth factors/cytokines. *Endocr Rev* 2004;25:971-1010.

[45] Dielis AW, Smid M, Spronk HM, Hamulyak K, Kroon AA, ten Cate H, de Leeuw PW. The prothrombotic paradox of hypertension: Role of the renin-angiotensin and kallikrein-kinin systems. *Hypertension* 2005;46:1236-1242.

[46] Donoghue M, Hsieh F, Baronas E, Godbout K, Gosselin M, Stagliano N, Donovan M, Woolf B, Robison K, Jeyaseelan R, Breitbart RE, Acton S. A novel angiotensin-converting enzyme-related carboxypeptidase (ACE2) converts angiotensin I to angiotensin 1-9. *Circ Res* 2000;87:E1-9.

[47] Ferrario CM, Trask AJ, Jessup JA. Advances in biochemical and functional roles of angiotensin-converting enzyme 2 and angiotensin-(1-7) in regulation of cardiovascular function. *Am J Physiol Heart Circ Physiol* 2005;289:H2281-90.

[48] Dahlof B, Devereux RB, Kjeldsen SE Julius S, Beevers G, de Faire U, Fyhrquist F, Ibsen H, Kristiansson K, Lederballe-Pedersen O, Lindholm LH, Nieminen MS, Omvik P, Oparil S, Wedel H; LIFE Study Group. Cardiovascular morbidity and mortality in the Losartan Intervention For Endpoint reduction in hypertension study (LIFE): a randomised trial against atenolol. *Lancet* 2002;359:995-1003.

[49] Pitt B, Poole-Wilson PA, Segal R Martinez FA, Dickstein K, Camm AJ, Konstam MA, Riegger G, Klinger GH, Neaton J, Sharma D, Thiyagarajan B. Effect of losartan compared with captopril on mortality in patients with symptomatic heart failure: randomised trial--the Losartan Heart Failure Survival Study ELITE II. *Lancet* 2000;355:1582-7.

[50] Yusuf S, Sleight P, Pogue J, Bosch J, Davies R, Dagenais G; Heart Outcomes Prevention Evaluation Study Investigators. Effects of an angiotensin-converting-enzyme inhibitor, ramipril, on cardiovascular events in high-risk patients. *N Engl J Med* 2000;342:145–153.

[51] Scheen AJ. Renin-angiotensin system inhibition prevents type 2 diabetes mellitus. Part 2. Overview of physiological and biochemical mechanisms. *Diabetes Metab* 2004;30:498 –505.

[52] Brenner BM, Cooper ME, de Zeeuw D Keane WF, Mitch WE, Parving HH, Remuzzi G, Snapinn SM, Zhang Z, Shahinfar S; RENAAL Study Investigators. Effects of losartan on renal and cardiovascular outcomes in patients with type 2 diabetes and nephropathy. *N Engl J Med* 2001;345:861-9.

[53] Lewis EJ, Hunsicker LG, Clarke WRBerl T, Pohl MA, Lewis JB, Ritz E, Atkins RC, Rohde R, Raz I; Collaborative Study Group. Renoprotective effect of the Angiotensin-receptor antagonist irbesartan in patients with nephropathy due to type 2 diabetes. *N Engl J Med* 2001;345:851-60.

[54] Parving H-H, Hommel E, Jensen BR, Hansen HP 2001 Long-term beneficial effect of ACE inhibition on diabetic nephropathy in normotensive type 1 diabetic patients. *Kidney Int* 60:228–234

[55] Mogensen CE, Neldam S, Tikkanen I, Oren S, Viskoper R, Watts RW, CooperME. Randomised controlled trial of dual blockade of renin-angiotensin system in patients with hypertension, microalbuminuria, and non-insulin dependent diabetes: the candesartan and lisinopril microalbuminuria (CALM) study. *BMJ* 2000;321: 1440–1444

[56] Mann JF, Schmieder RE, McQueen M, Dyal L, Schumacher H, Pogue J, Wang X, Maggioni A, Budaj A, Chaithiraphan S, Dickstein K, Keltai M, Metsärinne K, Oto A, Parkhomenko A, Piegas LS, Svendsen TL, Teo KK, Yusuf S; ONTARGET

investigators. Renal outcomes with telmisartan, ramipril, or both, in people at high vascular risk (the ONTARGET study): a multicentre, randomised, double-blind, controlled trial. *Lancet* 2008;372:547-53.

[57] Parving HH, Persson F, Lewis JB, Lewis EJ, Hollenberg NK; AVOID Study Investigators. Aliskiren combined with losartan in type 2 diabetes and nephropathy. *N Engl J Med* 2008;358:2433-46.

[58] Parving HH, Persson F, Lewis JB, Lewis EJ, Hollenberg NK; AVOID Study Investigators. Aliskiren combined with losartan in type 2 diabetes and nephropathy. *N Engl J Med* 2008;358:2433-46.

[59] Zhong J, Basu R, Guo D, Chow FL, Byrns S, Schuster M, Loibner H, Wang XH, Penninger JM, Kassiri Z, Oudit GY.Angiotensin-Converting Enzyme 2 Suppresses Pathological Hypertrophy, Myocardial Fibrosis, and Cardiac Dysfunction. *Circulation* 2010 in press.

[60] Fraga-Silva RA, Sorg BS, Wankhede M, Dedeugd C, Jun JY, Baker MB, Li Y, Castellano RK, Katovich MJ, Raizada MK, Ferreira AJ. ACE2 activation promotes antithrombotic activity. *Mol Med* 2010;16:210-5.

[61] Thomas MC, Pickering RJ, Tsorotes D, Koitka A, Sheehy K, Bernardi S, Toffoli B, Nguyen-Huu TP, Head G, Fu Y, Chin-Dusting J, Cooper ME, Tikellis C. Genetic Ace2 Deficiency Accentuates Vascular Inflammation and Atherosclerosis in the ApoE Knockout Mouse. *Circ Res* 2010 in press

[62] Tikellis C, Bialkowski K, Pete J, Sheehy K, Su Q, Johnston C, Cooper ME, Thomas MC. ACE2 deficiency modifies renoprotection afforded by ACE inhibition in experimental diabetes. *Diabetes* 2008;57:1018-25.

[63] Ross R, Glomset JA. The pathogenesis of atherosclerosis. *N Engl J Med* 197612;295:369-77

[64] Libby P, Ridker PM, Hansson GK; Leducq Transatlantic Network on Atherothrombosis Inflammation in atherosclerosis: from pathophysiology to practice. *J Am Coll Cardiol* 2009;54:2129-38

[65] Ridker PM. C-reactive protein and the prediction of cardiovascular events among those at intermediate risk: moving an inflammatory hypothesis toward consensus. *J Am Coll Cardiol* 2007;49:2129-38

[66] Saraheimo M, Teppo AM, Forsblom C, Fagerudd J, Groop P-H. Diabetic nephropathy is associated with low-grade inflammation in Type 1 diabetic patients. *Diabetologia.* 2003;46:1402-7

[67] Hansen TK, Forsblom C, Saraheimo M, Thorn L, Wadén J, Høyem P, Østergaard J, Flyvbjerg A, Groop PH; FinnDiane Study Group. Association between mannose-binding lectin, high-sensitivity C-reactive protein and the progression of diabetic nephropathy in type 1 diabetes. *Diabetologia* 2010;53:1517-24

[68] Lechleitner M, Koch T, Herold M, Dzien A, Hoppichler F: Tumour necrosis factor alpha plasma level in patients with type 1 diabetes mellitus and its association with glycaemic control and cardiovascular risk factors. *J Intern Med* 2000;248:67–76

[69] Meigs JB, Hu FB, Rifai N, Manson JE. Biomarkers of endothelial dysfunction and risk of type 2 diabetes mellitus. *JAMA* 2004;291:1978–1986

[70] Ridker PM, Hennekens CH, Roitman-Johnson B, Stampfer MJ, Allen J. Plasma concentration of soluble intercellular adhesion molecule 1 and risks of future myocardial infarction in apparently healthy men. *Lancet* 1998;351:88–92

[71] Schaumberg DA, Glynn RJ, Jenkins AJ, Lyons TJ, Rifai M, Manson JE, Ridker PM, Nathan DM. *Effect of Intensive Glycemic Control on Levels of Markers of Inflammation in Type 1 Diabetes Mellitus in the Diabetes Control and Complications Trial.* 2005;111:2446-53

[72] Nin JW, Jorsal A, Ferreira I, Schalkwijk CG, Prins MH, Parving HH, Tarnow L, Rossing P, Stehouwer CD. Higher plasma soluble receptor for advanced glycation endproducts (sRAGE) levels are associated with incident cardiovascular disease and all-cause mortality in type 1 diabetes: a 12-yr follow-up study. *Diabetes* 2010 in press

[73] ADA. Standards of medical care in diabetes - 2008. *Diabetes Care* 2008;31:S12-54

[74] De Berardis G, Sacco M, Strippoli GF, Pellegrini F, Graziano G, Tognoni G, Nicolucci A. Aspirin for primary prevention of cardiovascular events in people with diabetes: meta-analysis of randomised controlled trials. *BMJ* 2009;6;339:b4531

[75] Ridker PM, Danielson E, Fonseca FA, Genest J, Gotto AM Jr, Kastelein JJ, Koenig W, Libby P, Lorenzatti AJ, MacFadyen JG, Nordestgaard BG, Shepherd J, Willerson JT, Glynn RJ; JUPITER Study Group Rosuvastatin to prevent vascular events in men and women with elevated C-reactive protein. *N Engl J Med* 2008;359:2195-207

[76] Cha DR, Kim NH, Yoon JW, Jo SK, Cho WY, Kim HK, Won NH. Role of vascular endothelial growth factor in diabetic nephropathy. *Kidney Int Suppl* 2000;77:S104–S112

[77] Neufeld G, Cohen T, Gengrinovitch S, Poltorak Z. Vascular endothelial growth factor (VEGF) and its receptors. *FASEB J* 1999;13:9–22

[78] Thomas S, Vanuystel J, Gruden G, Rodriguez V, Burt D, Gnudi L, Hartley B, Viberti G. Vascular endothelial growth factor receptors in human mesangium in vitro and in glomerular disease. *J Am Soc Nephrol* 2000;11:1236–1243

[79] Chiarelli F, Spagnoli A, Basciani F, Tumini S, Mezzetti A, Cipollone F, Cuccurullo F, Morgese G, Verrotti A, Vascularendothelial growth factor (VEGF) in children, adolescents and young adults with type 1 diabetes mellitus: relation to glycaemic control and microvascular complications. *Diabet Med* 2000;17:650–656

[80] Abdel Aziz MY, Ben Gharbia O, el-Sayed Mohamed K, Muchaneta-Kubara EC, El Nahas AM. VEGF and diabetic microvascular complications. *Nephrol Dial Transplant* 1997;12:1538

[81] Malamitsi-Puchner A, Sarandakou A, Tziotis J, Dafogianni C, Bartsocas CS. Serum levels of basic fibroblast growth factor and vascular endothelial growth factor in children and adolescents with type 1 diabetes mellitus. *Pediatr Res* 1998;44:873–875

[82] De Vriese AS, Tilton RG, Elger M, Stephan CC, Kriz W, Lameire NH. Antibodies against vascular endothelial growth factor improve early renal dysfunction in experimental diabetes. *J Am Soc Nephrol* 2001;12:993–1000

[83] Ballesteros M, Leung KC, Ross RJM, Iismaa TP, Ho KKY. Distribution and abundance of messenger ribonucleic acid for growth hormone receptor isoforms in human tissues. *J Clin Endocrinol* 2000;85:2865–2871

[84] Feld S, Hirschberg R. Growth hormone, the insulin-like growth factor system, and the kidney. *Endocr Rev* 1996;17:423–480

[85] Grønbæk H, Nielsen B, Schrijvers B, Vogel I, Rasch R, Flyvbjerg A. Inhibitory effects of octreotide on renal and glomerular growth in early experimental diabetes in mice. *J Endocrinol* 2002;172: 637–643

[86] Segev Y, Landau D, Rasch R, Flyvbjerg A, Phillip M. Growth hormone receptor antagonism prevents early renal changes in nonobese diabetic mice. *J Am Soc Nephrol* 1999;10:2374–2381

[87] Haylor J, Hickling H, El Eter E, Moir A, Oldroyd S, Hardisty C, El Nahas AM. JB3, an IGF-I receptor antagonist, inhibits early renal growth in diabetic and uninephrectomized rats. *J Am Soc Nephrol* 2000;11:2027–2035

[88] Bach LA, Dean R, Youssef S, Cooper ME. Aminoguanidine ameliorates changes in the IGF system in experimental diabetic nephropathy. *Nephrol Dial Transplant* 2000;15:347–354

[89] Duprez DA. Arterial stiffness and endothelial function: key players in vascular health. *Hypertension* 2010;55:612-3

[90] Nichols WW, O'Rourke MF: *McDonald's Blood Flow in Arteries. Theoretic, Experimental and Clinical Principles*. edn 4. London: Edward Arnold; 1998:23–40

[91] Marchais SJ, Guerin AP, Pannier BM, Levy BI, Safar ME, London GM. Wave reflections and cardiac hypertrophy in chronic uremia. Influence of body size. *Hypertension* 1993, 22:876–883

[92] Nichols WW, Edwards DG. Arterial elastance and wave reflection augmentation of systolic blood pressure: deleterious effects and implications for therapy. *J Cardiovasc Pharmacol Ther* 2001;6:5–21

[93] Boutouyrie P, Bussy C, Hayoz D, Hengstler J, Dartois N, Laloux B, Brunner H, Laurent S. Local pulse pressure and regression of arterial wall hypertrophy during long-term antihypertensive treatment. *Circulation* 2000, 101:2601–2606

[94] Gordin D, Rönnback M, Forsblom C, Heikkilä O, Saraheimo M, Groop PH. Acute hyperglycaemia rapidly increases arterial stiffness in young patients with type 1 diabetes. *Diabetologia* 2007;50:1808-14

[95] Bortolotto LA, Hanon O, Franconi G,Boutouyrie P, Legrain S, Girerd X. The aging process modifies the distensibility of elastic but not muscular arteries. *Hypertension* 1999, 34:889–892

[96] Cines DB, Pollak ES, Buck CA, Loscalzo J, Zimmerman GA, McEver RP, Pober JS, Wick TM, Konkle BA, Schwartz BS, Barnathan ES, McCrae KR, Hug BA, Schmidt AM, Stern DM. Endothelial cells in physiology and in the pathophysiology of vascular disorders. *Blood* 1998;91:3527-61

[97] De Caterina R. Endothelial dysfunctions: common denominators in vascular disease. *Curr Op Clin Nutr Met Care* 2000;3:453-467

[98] Mahmud FH, Van Uum S, Kanji N, Thiessen-Philbrook H, Clarson CL. Impaired endothelial function in adolescents with type 1 diabetes mellitus. *J Pediatr* 2008;152:557-62

[99] Schalkwijk CG, Poland DC, van Dijk W, Kok A, Emeis JJ, Dräger AM, Doni A, van Hinsbergh VW, Stehouwer CD. Plasma concentration of C-reactive protein is increased in type I diabetic patients without clinical macroangiopathy and correlates with markers of endothelial dysfunction: evidence for chronic inflammation. *Diabetologia* 1999;42:351-7

[100] Vervoort G, Lutterman JA, Smits P, Berden JH, Wetzels JF. Transcapillary escape rate of albumin is increased and related to haemodynamic changes in normo-albuminuric type 1 diabetic patients. *J Hypertens* 1999;17:1911–1916

[101] Huvers FC, De Leeuw PW, Houben AJ, De Haan CH, Hamulyak K, Schouten H, Wolffenbuttel BH, Schaper NC. Endothelium-dependent vasodilatation, plasma markers of endothelial function, and adrenergic vasoconstrictor responses in type 1 diabetes under near-normoglycemic conditions. *Diabetes* 1999;48:1300–1307

[102] O'Byrne S, Forte P, Roberts LJ 2nd, Morrow JD, Johnston A, Anggård E, Leslie RD, Benjamin N. Nitric oxide synthesis and isoprostane production in subjects with type 1 diabetes and normal urinary albumin excretion. *Diabetes* 2000;49:857–862

[103] Giugliano D, Marfella R, Coppola L, Verrazzo G, Acampora R, Giunta R, Nappo F, Lucarelli C, D'Onofrio F. Vascular effects of acute hyperglycemia in humans are reversed by L-arginine. Evidence for reduced availability of nitric oxide during hyperglycemia. *Circulation* 1997;95:1783–1790

[104] Gordin D, Rönnback M, Forsblom C, Heikkilä O, Saraheimo M, Groop PH. Acute hyperglycaemia rapidly increases arterial stiffness in young patients with type 1 diabetes. *Diabetologia* 2007;50:1808-14

[105] Cherney DZ, Lai V, Scholey JW, Miller JA, Zinman B, Reich HN. Effect of direct renin inhibition on renal hemodynamic function, arterial stiffness, and endothelial function in humans with uncomplicated type 1 diabetes: a pilot study. *Diabetes Care* 2010;33:361-5

[106] Schalkwijk CG, Stehouwer CD. Vascular complications in diabetes mellitus: the role of endothelial dysfunction. *Clin Sci* (Lond) 2005;109:143–159

[107] McEniery CM, Wallace S, Mackenzie IS, McDonnell B, Yasmin, Newby DE, Cockcroft JR, Wilkinson IB. Endothelial function is associated with pulse pressure, pulse wave velocity, and augmentation index in healthy humans. *Hypertension* 2006;48:602-8

[108] Kinlay S, Creager MA, Fukumoto M, Hikita H, Fang JC, Selwyn AP, Ganz P. Endothelium-derived nitric oxide regulates arterial elasticity in human arteries in vivo. *Hypertension* 2001;38:1049-1053

[109] Nigam A, Mitchell GF, Lambert J, Tardif JC. Relation between conduit vessel stiffness (assessed by tonometry) and endothelial function (assessed by flow-mediated dilatation) in patients with and without coronary heart disease. *Am J Cardiol* 2003;92:395-399

[110] Zieman SJ, Melanovsky V, Kass DA. Mechanisms, pathophysiology, and therapy of arterial stiffness. *Arterioscler Thromb Vasc Biol* 2005;25:932-943

[111] Greenwald SE. Ageing of the conduit arteries. *J Pathol* 2007;211:157e72

[112] Xu C, Zarins CK, Pannaraj PS, Bassiouny HS, Glagov S. Hypercholesterolemia superimposed by experimental hypertension induces differential distribution of collagen and elastin. *Arterioscler Thromb Vasc Biol* 2000;20:2566-2572

[113] Winlove CP, Parker KH, Avery NC, Bailey AJ. Interactions of elastin and aorta with sugars in vitro and their effects on biochemical and physical properties. *Diabetologia* 1996;39:1131-1139

[114] Rojas A, Romay S, Gonzalez D, Herrera B, Delgado R, Otero K. Regulation of endothelial nitric oxide synthase expression by albuminderived advanced glycosylation end products. *Circ Res* 2000;86:E50–E54

[115] Wendt T, Bucciarelli L, Qu W, Lu Y, Yan SF, Stern DM, Schmidt AM: Receptor for Advanced Glycation Endproducts (RAGE) and Vascular Inflammation: Insights into the Pathogenesis of Macrovascular Complications in Diabetes. *Curr Atheroscler Rep* 2002;4:228-237

[116] Lacolley P, Challande P, Osborne-Pellegrin M, Regnault V. Genetics and pathophysiology of arterial stiffness. *Cardiovasc Res* 2009;81:637-48

[117] Atwood LD, Samollow PB, Hixson JE, Stern MP, MacCluer JW. Genomewide linkage analysis of pulse pressure in Mexican Americans. *Hypertension* 2001;37:425–428

[118] Camp NJ, Hopkins PN, Hasstedt SJ, Coon H, Malhotra A, Cawthon RM, Hunt SC. Genome-wide multipoint parametric linkage analysis of pulse pressure in large, extended utah pedigrees. *Hypertension* 2003;42: 322–328

[119] DeStefano AL, Larson MG, Mitchell GF, Benjamin EJ, Vasan RS, Li J, Corey D, Levy D. Genome-wide scan for pulse pressure in the National Heart, Lung and Blood Institute's Framingham Heart Study. *Hypertension* 2004;44: 152–155

[120] Mitchell GF, DeStefano AL, Larson MG, Benjamin EJ, Chen MH, Vasan RS, Vita JA, Levy D. Heritability and a genome-wide linkage scan for arterial stiffness,wave reflection, and mean arterial pressure: the Framingham HeartStudy. *Circulation* 2005;112:194–199

[121] Turner ST, Peyser PA, Kardia SL, Bielak LF, Sheedy PF 3rd, Boerwinkle E, Bielak LF, Sheedy PF 3rd, Boerwinkle E, de Andrade M. Genomic loci with pleiotropic effects on coronary artery calcification. *Atherosclerosis* 2006;185:340–346

[122] Benetos A, Topouchian J, Ricard S, Gautier S, Bonnardeaux A, Asmar R, Poirier O, Soubrier F, Safar M, Cambien F. Influence of angiotensin II type 1 receptor polymorphism on aortic stiffness in never-treated hypertensive patients. *Hypertension* 1995;26:44–47

[123] Dima I, Vlachopoulos C, Alexopoulos N, Baou K, Vasiliadou C, Antoniades C, Aznaouridis K, Stefanadi E, Tousoulis D, Stefanadis C. Association of arterial stiffness with the angiotensinconverting enzyme gene polymorphism in healthy individuals. *Am J Hypertens* 2008;21:1354–1358

[124] Ye S. Influence of matrix metalloproteinase genotype on cardiovascular disease susceptibility and outcome. *Cardiovasc Res* 2006;69:636–645

[125] Lacolley P, Gautier S, Poirier O, Pannier B, Cambien F, Benetos A. Nitric oxide synthase gene polymorphisms, blood pressure and aortic stiffness in normotensive and hypertensive subjects. *J Hypertens* 1998;16:31–35

[126] Schnabel R, Larson MG, Dupuis J, Lunetta KL, Lipinska I, Meigs JB, Yin X, Rong J, Vita JA, Newton-Cheh C, Levy D, Keaney JF Jr, Vasan RS, Mitchell GF, Benjamin EJ. Relations of inflammatory biomarkers and common genetic variants with arterial stiffness and wave reflection. *Hypertension* 2008;51: 1651–1657

[127] Kelly RP, Hayward C, Avolio AP, O'Rourke MF. Non-invasive determination of agerelated changes in the human arterial pulse. *Circulation* 1989;80:1652-1659

[128] Vaitkevicius PV, Fleg JL, Engel JH, O'Connor FC, Wright JG, Lakatta LE, Yin FC, Lakatta EG. Effects of age and aerobic capacity on arterial stiffness in healthy adults. *Circulation* 1993;88:1456-1462, 1993

[129] Bortolotto LA, Blacher J, Kondo T, Takazawa K, Safar ME. Assessment of vascularm aging and atherosclerosis in hypertensive subjects: second derivative of photoplethysmogram versus pulse wave velocity. *Am J Hypertens* 2000;13:165-171

[130] van der Heijden-Spek JJ, Staessen JA, Fagard RH, Hoeks AP, Boudier HA, van Bortel LM. Effect of age on brachial artery wall properties differs from the aorta and is gender dependent: a population study. *Hypertension* 2000;35:637-642

[131] Benetos A, Adamopouolos C, Bureau J-M, Temmar M, Labat C, Bean K, Thomas F, Pannier B, Asmar R, Zureik M, Safar M, Guize L. Determinants of accelerated progression of arterial stiffness in normotensive subjects and in treated hypertensive subjects over a 6-year period. *Circulation* 2002;105:1202-1207

[132] J te Velde, Ferreira I, Twisk JW, Stehouwer CD, van Mechelen W, Kemper HC. Birthweight and arterial stiffness and blood pressure in adulthood--Results from the Amsterdam Growth and Health Longitudinal Study. *Int J Epidemiol* 2004;33:154-161

[133] Dernellis J, Panaretou M: Aortic stiffness is an independent predictor of progression to hypertension in nonhypertensive subjects. *Hypertension* 2005 ;45:426-431

[134] Failla M, Grappiolo A, Carugo S, Calchera I, Giannattasio C, Mancia G. Effects of cigarette smoking on carotid and radial artery distensibility. *J Hypertens* 1997;15:1659-1664

[135] Feely MA. Effect of smoking on arterial stiffening and pulse pressure amplification. *Hypertension* 2003;41:183-187

[136] Stefanadis C, Tsiamis E, Vlachopoulos C, Stratos C, Toutouzas K, Pitsavos C, Marakas S, Boudoulas H, Toutouzas P.Unfavorable effect of smoking on the elastic properties of the human aorta. *Circulation* 1997;95:31-8

[137] Rhee MY, Na SH, Kim YK, Lee MM, Kim HY. Acute effects of cigarette smoking on arterial stiffness and blood pressure in male smokers with hypertension. *Am J Hypertens* 2007;20:637-41

[138] Stefanadis C, Vlachopoulos C, Tsiamis E, Diamantopoulos L, Toutouzas K, Giatrakos N, Vaina S, Tsekoura D, Toutouzas P. Unfavorable effects of passive smoking on aortic function in men. *Ann Intern Med* 1998;128:426-434

[139] Oncken CA, White WB, Cooney JL, Van Kirk JR, Ahluwalia JS, Giacco S. Impact of smoking cessation on ambulatory blood pressure and heart rate in postmenopausal women. *Am J Hypertens* 2001;14:942-949

[140] Tomiyama H, Hashimoto H, Tanaka H, Matsumoto C, Odaira M, Yamada J, Yoshida M, Shiina K, Nagata M, Yamashina A.Continuous smoking and progression of arterial stiffening: a prospective study. *J Am Coll Cardiol* 2010;55:1979-87

[141] Paffenbarger RS Jr, Jung DL, Leung RW, Hyde RT. Physical activity and hypertension: an epidemiological view. *Ann Med* 1991;23:319-327

[142] Cameron JD, Dart AM. Exercise training increases total systemic arterial compliance in humans. *Am J Physiol* 1994;266:H693-H701

[143] Mustata S, Chan C, Lai V, Miller JA. Impact of an exercise program on arterial stiffness and insulin resistance in hemodialysis patients. *J Am Soc Nephrol* 2004;15:2713-2718

[144] Bertovic DA, Waddell TK, Gatzka CD, Cameron JD, Dart AM, Kingwell BA. Muscular strength training is associated with low arterial compliance and high pulse pressure. *Hypertension* 1999;33:1385-1391

[145] Safar ME, Thomas F, Blacher J, Nzietchueng R, Bureau J-M, Pannier B, Benetos A. Metabolic syndrome and age-Related progression of aortic stiffness. *J Am Coll Cardiol* 2006;47:72-75

[146] Li S, Chen W, Srinivasan SR, Berenson GS: Influence of metabolic syndrome on arterial stiffness and its age-related change in young adults: the Bogalusa Heart Study. *Atherosclerosis* 2005;180:349-354

[147] Wilkinson IB, Prasad K, Hall IR, Thomas A, MacCallum H, Webb DJ, Frenneaux MP, Cockcroft JR. Increased central pulse pressure and augmentation index in subjects with hypercholesterolemia. *J Am Coll Cardiol* 2002; 39:1005-1011

[148] Vlachopoulos C, Dima I, Aznaouridis K, Vasiliadou C, Ioakeimidis N, Aggeli C, Toutouza M, Stefanadis C. Acute systemic inflammation increases arterial stiffness and decreases wave reflections in healthy individuals. *Circulation* 2005;112:2193-2200

[149] Yasmin, McEniery CM, Wallace S, Mackenzie IS, Cockcroft JR, Wilkinson IB. Creactive protein is associated with arterial stiffness in apparently healthy individuals.*Arterioscler Thromb Vasc Biol* 2004;24:969-974

[150] Wang MC, Tsai WC, Chen JY, Huang JJ. Stepwise increase in arterial stiffness corresponding with the stages of chronic kidney disease. *Am J Kidney Dis* 2005;45:494-501

[151] Smith A, Karalliedde J, De Angelis L, Goldsmith D, Viberti G. Aortic pulse wave velocity and albuminuria in patients with type 2 diabetes. *J Am Soc Nephrol* 2005;16:1069–1075

[152] Brooks B, Molyneaux L, Yue DK. Augmentation of central arterial pressure in type 1 diabetes. *Diabetes Care* 1999;22:1722–1727

[153] Kool MJ, Lambert J, Stehouwer CD, Hoeks AP, Struijker Boudier HA, Van Bortel LM. Vessel wall properties of large arteries in uncomplicated IDDM. *Diabetes Care* 1995;18:618–624

[154] Urbina EM, Wadwa RP, Davis C, Snively BM, Dolan LM, Daniels SR, Hamman RF, Dabelea D. Prevalence of increased arterial stiffness in children with type 1 diabetes mellitus differs by measurement site and sex: the SEARCH for Diabetes in Youth Study. *J Pediatr* 2010;156:731-7

[155] Heilman K, Zilmer M, Zilmer K, Lintrop M, Kampus P, Kals J, Tillmann V. Arterial stiffness, carotid artery intima-media thickness and plasma myeloperoxidase level in children with type 1 diabetes. *DiabetesRes Clin Pract*. 2009;84:168-73

[156] Giannattasio C, Failla M, Piperno A, Grappiolo A, Gamba P, Paleari F, Mancia G. Early impairment of large artery structure and function in type I diabetes mellitus. *Diabetologia* 1999;42:987–994

[157] Lambert J, Smulders RA, Aarsen M, Donker AJ, Stehouwer CD. Carotid artery stiffness is increased in microalbuminuric IDDM patients. *Diabetes Care* 1998;21:99–103

[158] Tryfonopoulos D, Anastasiou E, Protogerou A, Papaioannou T, Lily K, Dagre A, Souvatzoglou E, Papamichael C, Alevizaki M, Lekakis J. Arterial stiffness in type 1 diabetes mellitus is aggravated by autoimmune thyroid disease. *J Endocrinol Invest* 2005;28:616–622

[159] Gordin D, Wadén J, Forsblom C, Thorn LM, Rosengård-Bärlund M, Heikkilä O, Saraheimo M, Tolonen N, Hietala K, Soro-Paavonen A, Salovaara L, Mäkinen VP, Peltola T, Bernardi L, Groop PH; for the FinnDiane Study Group. Arterial stiffness and vascular complications in patients with type 1 diabetes: The Finnish Diabetic Nephropathy (FinnDiane) Study. Ann Med 2010 in press

[160] Rönnback M, Fagerudd J, Forsblom C, Pettersson-Fernholm K, Reunanen A, Groop PH. Altered age-related blood pressure pattern in type 1 diabetes. *Circulation* 2004;110:1076–1082

[161] Gordin D, Rönnback M, Forsblom C, Heikkilä O, Saraheimo M, Groop PH. Acute hyperglycaemia rapidly increases arterial stiffness in young patients with type 1 diabetes. *Diabetologia* 2007;50:1808-14

[162] Taniwaki H, Kawagishi T, Emoto M, Shoji T, Kanda H, Maekawa K, Nishizawa Y, Morii H. Correlation between the intima-media thickness of the carotid artery and aortic pulse-wave velocity in patients with type 2 diabetes. Vessel wall properties in type 2 diabetes. *Diabetes Care* 1999;22:1851-7

[163] Brooks BA, Molyneaux LM, Yue DK. Augmentation of central arterial pressure in type 2 diabetes. *Diabet Med* 2001;18:374–380

[164] Ravikumar R, Deepa R, Shanthirani C, Mohan V. Comparison of carotid intima-media thickness, arterial stiffness, and brachial artery flow mediated dilatation in diabetic and nondiabetic subjects (The Chennai Urban Population Study [CUPS-9]). *Am J Cardiol* 2002;90:702–707

[165] Cameron JD, Bulpitt CJ, Pinto ES, Rajkumar C. The aging of elastic and muscular arteries: a comparison of diabetic and nondiabetic subjects. *Diabetes Care* 2003;26:2133–2138

[166] Henry RM, Kostense PJ, Spijkerman AM, Dekker JM, Nijpels G, Heine RJ, Kamp O, Westerhof N, Bouter LM, Stehouwer CD; Hoorn Study. Arterial stiffness increases with deteriorating glucose tolerance status: the *Hoorn Study Circulation* 2003;107:2089-95

[167] Ohnishi H, Saitoh S, Takagi S, Ohata J, Isobe T, Kikuchi Y, Takeuchi H, Shimamoto K. Pulse wave velocity as an indicator of atherosclerosis in impaired fasting glucose: the Tanno and Sobetsu study *Diabetes Care* 2003;26:437-40

[168] Schram MT, Henry RM, van Dijk RA, Kostense PJ, Dekker JM, Nijpels G, Heine RJ, Bouter LM, Westerhof N, Stehouwer CD. Increased central artery stiffness in impaired glucose metabolism and type 2 diabetes: the Hoorn Study. *Hypertension* 2004;43:176-81

[169] Hermans MM, Henry R, Dekker JM, Kooman JP, Kostense PJ, Nijpels G, Heine RJ, Stehouwer CD. Estimated glomerular filtration rate and urinary albumin excretion are independently associated with greater arterial stiffness: the Hoorn Study. *J Am Soc Nephrol* 2007;18:1942-52

[170] Cockcroft JR, Wilkinson IB, Evans M, McEwan P, Peters JR, Davies S, Scanlon MF, Currie CJ. Pulse pressure predicts cardiovascular risk in patients with type 2 diabetes mellitus. *Am J Hypertens* 2005;18:1463-7

[171] Schram MT, Kostense PJ, Van Dijk RA, Dekker JM, Nijpels G, Bouter LM, Heine RJ, Stehouwer CD. Diabetes, pulse pressure and cardiovascular mortality: the Hoorn Study. *J Hypertens* 2002;20:1743-51

[172] Knudsen ST, Poulsen PL, Hansen KW, Ebbehoj E, Bek T, Mogensen CE. Pulse pressure and diurnal blood pressure variation: association with micro- and macrovascular complications in type 2 diabetes. *Am J Hypertens* 2002;15:244–250

[173] Franklin SS, Khan SA, Wong ND, Larson MG, Levy D. Is pulse pressure useful in predicting coronary heart disease? The Framingham Heart Study. *Circulation* 1999;100:354- 360

[174] Mitchell GF, Moye LA, Braunwald E, Rouleau J-L, Bernstein V, Geltman EM, Flaker GC, Pfeffer MA. Sphygmomanometrically determined pulse pressure is a powerful

independent predictor of recurrent events after myocardial infarction in patients with impaired left ventricular function. *Circulation* 1997;96:4254-4260

[175] Benetos A, Safar M, Rudnichi A, Smulyan H, Richard J-L, Ducimetiere P, Guize L. Pulse pressure: a predictor of long-term cardiovascular mortality in a French male population. *Hypertension* 1997;30:1410-1415

[176] Gasowski J, Fagarda RH, Staessena JA, Grodzickib T, Pocockc S, Boutitied F, Gueyffier F, Boisseld JP for the INDANA Project Collaborators: Pulsatile blood pressure component as predictor of mortality in hypertension: a meta-analysis of clinical trial control groups *J Hypertens* 2002;20:145-151

[177] Dyer AR, Stamler J, Shekelle RB, Berkson DM, Paul O, Lepper MH, Lindberg HA: Pulse pressure-II. Factors associated with follow-up values in three Chicago epidemiologic studies. *J Chronic Dis* 1982;35:275-282

[178] Franklin SS, Lopez VA, Wong ND, Mitchell GF, Larson MG, Vasan RS, Levy D. Single versus combined blood pressure components and risk for cardiovascular disease: the Framingham Heart Study. *Circulation* 2009;119:243-50

[179] Wilkinson IB, Fuchs SA, Jansen IM, Spratt JC, Murray GD, Cockcroft JR, Webb DJ. Reproducibility of pulse wave velocity and augmentation index measured by pulse wave analysis. *J Hypertens* 1998;16:2079-84

[180] Laurent S, Boutouyrie P, Asmar R, Gautier I, Laloux B, Guize L, Ducimetiere P, Benetos A: Aortic stiffness is an independent predictor of all-cause and cardiovascular mortality in hypertensive patients. *Hypertension* 2001;37:1236- 1241

[181] Blacher J, Guerin AP, Pannier B, Marchais SJ, Safar ME, London GM: Impact of aortic stiffness on survival in endstage renal disease. *Circulation* 1999;99:2434-2439

[182] Cruickshank K, Riste L, Anderson SG, Wright JS, Dunn G, Gosling RG: Aortic pulse-wave velocity and its relationship to mortality in diabetes and glucose intolerance An integrated index of vascular function? *Circulation* 2002;106:2085-2090

[183] Sutton-Tyrrell K, Najjar SS, Boudreau RM, Venkitachalam L, Kupelian V, Simonsick EM, Havlik R, Lakatta EG,Spurgeon H, Kritchevsky S, Pahor M, Bauer D, Newman A: Health ABC Study. Elevated aortic pulse wave velocity, a marker of arterial stiffness, predicts cardiovascular events in well-functioning older adults. *Circulation* 2005; 111:3384-3390

[184] Meaume S, Benetos A, Henry OF, Rudnichi A, Safar ME: Aortic pulse wave velocity predicts cardiovascular mortality in subjects >70 years of age. *Arterioscler Thromb Vasc Biol* 2002;21:2046-2050

[185] Laurent S, Cockcroft J, Van Bortel L, Boutouyrie P, Giannattasio C, Hayoz D, Pannier B, Vlachopoulos C,Wilkinson I, Struijker-Boudier H. Expert consensus document on arterial stiffness: methodological issues and clinical applications. *Eur Heart J* 2006;27:2588 –2605

[186] Parati G, Bernardi L. How to assess arterial compliance in humans. *J Hypertens* 2006;24:1009-12.

[187] Chen CH, Ting CT, Nussbacher A, Nevo E, Kass DA, Pak P, Wang S, Chang M, Yin F. Validation of carotid artery tonometry as a means of estimating augmentation index of ascending aortic pressure. *Hypertension* 1996;27:168-175

[188] O'Rourke MF, Gallagher DE. Pulse wave analysis. *J Hypertens* 1996;14:147-157

[189] Weber T, Auer J, O'Rourke MF, Kvas E, Lassnig E, Berent R, Eber B. Arterial stiffness, wave reflections, and the risk of coronary artery disease. *Circulation* 2004;109:184-189

[190] Chirinos JA, Zambrano JP, Chakko S. Veerani A, Schob A, Willens HJ, Perez G, Mendez AJ: Aortic pressure augmentation predicts adverse cardiovascular events in patients with established coronary artery disease. *Hypertension* 2005;45:980-985

[191] London GM, Blacher J, Pannier B, Guerin AP, Marchais SJ, Safar ME: Arterial wave reflections and survival in endstage renal failure. *Hypertension* 2001;38:434-438

[192] Laurent S, Caviezel B, Beck L, Girerd X, Billaud E, Boutouyrie P, Hoeks A, Safar M. Carotid artery distensibility and distending pressure in hypertensive humans. *Hypertension* 1994;23:878-883

[193] Mohiaddin RH. Age-related changes of human aortic flow wave velocity measured non-invasively by magnetic resonance imaging. *J Appl Physiol* 1993;74:492-497

[194] Dolan E, Thijs L, Li Y, Atkins N, McCormack P, McClory S, O'Brien E, Staessen JA, Stanton AV. Ambulatory arterial stiffness index as a predictor of cardiovascular mortality in the Dublin Outcome Study. *Hypertension* 1006;47:365-370

[195] McVeigh GE, Bratteli CW, Morgan DJ, Alinder CM, Glasser SP, Finkelstein SM, Cohn JN: Age-related abnormalities in arterial compliance identified by pressure pulse contour analysis: aging and arterial compliance. *Hypertension* 1999;33:1392-1398

[196] Laurent S, Kingwell B, Bank A, Weber M, Struijker-Boudier H. Clinical applications of arterial stiffness: therapeutics and pharmacology. *Am J Hypertens* 2002;15:453-8

[197] Suzuki H, Nakamoto H, Okada H, Sugahara S, Kanno Y: A selective angiotensin receptor antagonist, valsartan, produced regression of left ventricular hypertrophy associated with a reduction of arterial stiffness. *Adv Perit Dial* 2003;19:59-66

[198] Pauca AL, Kon ND, O'Rourke MF: Benefit of glyceryl trinitrate on arterial stiffness is directly due to effects on peripheral arteries. *Heart* 2005;91:1428-1432

[199] Mitchell GF, Lacourciere Y, Arnold JMO, Dunlap ME, Conlin PR, Izzo JL Jr. Changes in aortic stiffness and augmentation index after acute converting enzyme or vasopeptidase inhibition. *Hypertension* 2005;46:1111-1117

[200] Bolton WK, Cattran DC, Williams ME, Adler SG, Appel GB, Cartwright K, Foiles PG, Freedman BI, Raskin P, Ratner RE, Spinowitz BS, Whittier FC, Wuerth JP: Randomized trial of an inhibitor of formation of advanced glycation end products in diabetic nephropathy. *Am J Nephrol* 2004;24:32-40

[201] Kass D, Shapiro E, Kawaguchi M, Capriotti A, Scuteri A, deGroof R, Lakatta E. Improved arterial compliance by a novel advanced glycation end-product crosslink breaker. *Circulation* 2001;104:1464-1470

[202] McNulty M, Mahmud A, Feely J. Advanced glycation end-products and arterial stiffness in hypertension. *Am J Hypertens* 2007;20:242-7

[203] Shapiro BP, Owan TE, Mohammed SF, Meyer DM, Mills LD, Schalkwijk CG, Redfield MM. Advanced glycation end products accumulate in vascular smooth muscle and modify vascular but not ventricular properties in elderly hypertensive canines. *Circulation* 2008;118:1002-10

[204] Orr JS, Dengo AL, Rivero JM, Davy KP Arterial destiffening with atorvastatin in overweight and obese middle-aged and older adults. *Hypertension* 2009;54:763-8

[205] Yokoyama H, Kawasaki M, Ito Y, Minatoguchi S, Fujiwara H. Effects of fluvastatin on the carotid arterial media as assessed by integrated backscatter ultrasound compared with pulse-wave velocity. *J Am Coll Cardiol* 2005;46:2031-7

[206] Mäki-Petäjä KM, Booth AD, Hall FC, Wallace SM, Brown J, McEniery CM, Wilkinson IB. Ezetimibe and simvastatin reduce inflammation, disease activity, and aortic stiffness and improve endothelial function in rheumatoid arthritis. *J Am Coll Cardiol* 2007;50:852-8

[207] Rizos EC, Agouridis AP, Elisaf MS. The Effect of Statin Therapy on Arterial Stiffness by Measuring Pulse Wave Velocity: A Systematic Review. *Curr Vasc Pharmacol* 2010 in press

[208] Satoh N, Ogawa Y, Usui T, Tagami T, Kono S, Uesugi H, Sugiyama H, Sugawara A, Yamada K, Shimatsu A, Kuzuya H, Nakao K. Antiatherogenic effect of pioglitazone intype 2 diabetic patients irrespective of the responsiveness to its antidiabetic effect. *Diabetes Care* 2003;26:2493–2499

[209] Harashima K, Hayashi J, Miwa T, Tsunoda T. Long-term pioglitazone therapy improves arterial stiffness in patients with type 2 diabetes mellitus. *Metabolism* 2009;58:739-45

[210] Ryan KE, McCance DR, Powell L, McMahon R, Trimble ER. Fenofibrate and pioglitazone improve endothelial function and reduce arterial stiffness in obese glucose tolerant men. *Atherosclerosis* 2007;194:e123-30

[211] Westerbacka J, Wilkinson I, Cockcroft J, Utriainen T, Vehkavaara S, Yki-Järvinen H. Diminished wave reflection in the aorta: a novel physiological action of insulin on large blood vessels. *Hypertension*. 1999;33: 1118–1122

[212] Westerbacka J, Uosukainen A, Mäkimattila S, Schlenzka A, Yki-Järvinen H Insulin-induced decrease in large artery stiffness is impaired in uncomplicated type 1 diabetes mellitus. *Hypertension* 2000;35:1043-8

[213] Westerbacka J, Vehkavaara S, Bergholm R, Wilkinson I, Cockcroft J, Yki-Järvinen H. Marked resistance of the ability of insulin to decrease arterial stiffness characterizes human obesity. *Diabetes* 1999;48:821-7

[214] Safar ME, O'Rourke MF. Arterial stiffness in hypertension In: *Handbook of Hypertension*, Vol. 23. Amsterdam: Elsevier; 2006

[215] McVeigh GE, Brennan GM, Cohn JN, Finkelstein SM, Hayes RJ, Johnston GD. Fish oil improves arterial compliance in non-insulindependent diabetes mellitus. *Arterioscler Thromb Vasc Biol* 1994;14:1425-1429

[216] Mullan BA, Young IS, Fee H, McCance DR. Ascorbic acid reduces blood pressure and arterial stiffness in type 2 diabetes. *Hypertension* 2002;40:804-809, 2002

[217] Mottram P, Shige H, Nestel P. Vitamin E improves arterial compliance in middle-aged men and women. *Atherosclerosis* 1999;145:399-404

[218] Eskurza I, Monahan KD, Robinson JA, Seals DR. Ascorbic acid does not affect large elastic artery compliance or central blood pressure in young and older men. *Am J Physiol Heart Circ Physiol* 2004;286:H1528-H1534

[219] Kelly RP, Poo Yeo K, Isaac HB, Lee CY, Huang SH, Teng L, Halliwell B, Wise SD. Lack of effect of acute oral ingestion of vitamin C on oxidative stress, arterial stiffness or blood pressure in healthy subjects. *Free Radic Res* 2008;42:514-22.

[220] Tanaka H, Safar ME. Influence of Lifestyle Modification on Arterial Stiffness and Wave Reflections. *Am J Hypertens* 2005;18:137-144

[221] Barinas-Mitchell E, Kuller LH, Sutton-Tyrrell K, Hegazi R, Harper P, Mancino J, Kelley DE. Effect of weight loss and nutritional intervention on arterial stiffness in type 2 diabetes. *Diabetes Care* 2006;29:2218-2222

[222] Williams B, Lacy PS, Thom SM, Cruickshank K, Stanton A, Collier D, Hughes AD, Thurston H, O'Rourke M; CAFE Investigators; Anglo-Scandinavian Cardiac Outcomes Trial Investigators; CAFE Steering Committee and Writing Committee. Differential impact of blood pressure-lowering drugs on central aortic pressure and clinical outcomes: principal results of the Conduit Artery Function Evaluation (CAFE) study. *Circulation* 2006;113:1213-25

[223] Oparil S, Izzo JL Jr. Pulsology rediscovered: commentary on the Conduit Artery Function Evaluation (CAFE) study. *Circulation* 2006;113:1213-25

[224] Dahlöf B, Devereux RB, Kjeldsen SE, for the LIFE Study Group. Cardiovascular morbidity and mortality in the Losartan Intervention For Endpoint reduction in hypertension study (LIFE): a randomized trial against atenolol. *Lancet* 2002;359: 995–1003

[225] Asmar RG, London GM, O'Rourke ME, Safar ME; REASON Project Coordinators and Investigators. Improvement in blood pressure, arterial stiffness and wave reflections with a very-low-dose perindopril/indapamide combination in hypertensive patient: a comparison with atenolol. *Hypertension* 2001;3:922-6

[226] Mitchell GF, Dunlap ME, Warnica W, Ducharme A, Arnold JM, Tardif JC, Solomon SD, Domanski MJ, Jablonski KA, Rice MM, Pfeffer MA; Prevention of Events With Angiotensin-Converting Enzyme Inhibition Investigators. Long-term trandolapril treatment is associated with reduced aortic stiffness: the prevention of events with angiotensinconverting enzyme inhibition hemodynamic substudy. *Hypertension* 2007;49:1271e7.

[227] De Luca N, Rosiello G, Lamenza F, Ricciardelli B, Marchegiano R, Volpe M, Marelli C, Trimarco B. Reversal of cardiac and large artery structural abnormalities induced by long-term antihypertensive treatment with trandolapril. *Am J Cardiol* 1992;70:52D–59D

[228] Lonn E, Shaikholeslami R, Yi Q, Bosch J, Sullivan B, Tanser P, Magi A, Yusuf S. Effects of ramipril on left ventricular mass and function in cardiovascular patients with controlled blood pressure and with preserved left ventricular ejection fraction: a substudy of the Heart Outcomes Prevention Evaluation (HOPE) *Trial. J Am Coll Cardiol* 2004;43:2200-2206

[229] Ahimastos AA, Natoli AK, Lawler A, Blombery PA, Kingwell BA. Ramipril reduces large-artery stiffness in peripheral arterial disease and promotes elastogenic remodeling in cell culture. *Hypertension* 2005;45:1194-1199

[230] Levy BI, Michel JB, Salzmann JL, Poitevin P, Devissaguet M, Scalbert E, Safar ME. Long-term effects of angiotensin-converting enzyme inhibition on the arterial wall of adult spontaneously hypertensive rats. *Am J Cardiol* 1993;71:8E–16E

[231] Ben Driss A, Himbert C, Poitevin P, Duriez M, Michel JB, Levy BI. Enalapril improves arterial elastic properties in rats with myocardial infarction. *J Cardiovasc Pharmacol* 1999;34:102–107

[232] Agata J, Nagahara D, Kinoshita S, Takagawa Y, Moniwa N, Yoshida D, Ura N, Shimamoto K. Angiotensin II receptor blocker prevents increased arterial stiffness in patients with essential hypertension. *Circ J* 2004;68:1194-8

[233] Karalliedde J, Smith A, DeAngelis L, Mirenda V, Kandra A, Botha J, Ferber P, Viberti G. Valsartan improves arterial stiffness in type 2 diabetes independently of blood pressure lowering. *Hypertension* 2008;51:1617-23

[234] Anan F, Takahashi N, Ooie T, Yufu K, Hara M, Nakagawa M, Yonemochi H, Saikawa T, Yoshimatsu H. Effects of valsartan and perindopril combination therapy on left ventricular hypertrophy and aortic arterial stiffness in patients with essential hypertension. *Eur J Clin Pharmacol* 2005;61:353-9

[235] Ali K, Rajkumar C, Fantin F, Schiff R, Bulpitt CJ. Irbesartan improves arterial compliance more than lisinopril. *Vasc Health Risk Manag* 2009;5:587-92

[236] Takami T. Evaluation of arterial stiffness in morning hypertension under high-dose valsartan compared to valsartan plus low-dose diuretic. *Hypertens Res* 2009;32:1086-90

[237] Andreadis EA, Sfakianakis ME, Tsourous GI, Georgiopoulos DX, Fragouli EG, Katsanou PM, Tavoularis EI, Skarlatou MG, Marakomichelakis GE, Ifanti GK, Diamantopoulos EJ. Differential impact of angiotensin receptor blockers and calcium channel blockers on arterial stiffness. *Int Angiol* 2010;29:266-72

In: Systolic Blood Pressure
Editor: Robert A. Arfi

ISBN: 978-1-61209-263-8
©2012 Nova Science Publishers, Inc.

Chapter III

Blood Pressure Changes in Patients with Migraines: Evidences, Controversial Views and Potential Mechanisms of Comorbidity

Sherifa Ahmed Hamed[*]

Department of Neurology and Psychiatry,
Assiut University Hospital, Assiut, Egypt

Abstract

Migraine and hypertension are common complaints and both have high prevalence worldwide.The comorbidity of migraine with hypertension is a common issue since 1913. Recent epidemiologic and population-based studies put some doubt regarding the association between migraine and hypertension, no association or even negative association was found by some authors. Authors who supported the positive association suggested that rennin-angiotensin system as a biological link between hypertension and CNS activities that are relevant for migraine pathogenesis. Authors who denied the association suggested a coincidental existence since any associationbetween two prevalent health conditions is likely to be detected in large series. Authors who supported the negative association suggested a central regulatory and homeostatic process resulting in reduction of sensitivity to pain(a phenomenon called hypertension-associated hypalgesia). Baroreflex stimulation, endogenous opioids, catecholamines and calcitonin peptide may influence blood pressure and pain sensitivity in patients with migraines and

---

[*] Corresponding Author: Dr. Sherifa Ahmed Hamed (M.D.), Consultant Neurologist, Associate Professor, Assiut University Hospital, Department of Neurology and Psychiatry, Floor # 4, Room # 4, Assiut, Egypt, P.O.Box 71516, Telephone:+2 088 237490, Fax: +2 088 2333327,+2 088 2332278, Email: hamed_sherifa@yahoo.com

lowers the number of migraine attacks in hypertensives. Despite the uncertainty still present in this field, a unifying view among most recent studies suggests that migraine is positively correlated with diastolic blood pressure but negatively correlated with systolic blood pressure and pulse pressure. Similar vascular risk profile and the abnormal properties of systemic as well as cranial arterial vessels exist in subjects with migraine and hypertension. On the other hand poor control of blood pressure may exacerbate the frequency and severity of migraine and other headaches. These evidences may suggest that both conditions may coexist as part of a systemic disease. Thus establishing the blood pressure should be a routine task in the assessment of all headache patients and the control of hypertension in migraine patients is an important factor for the success of migraine treatment and to lower cardio- and cerebro-vascular risks.

Introduction

Migraine is a common chronic presenting complaint encountered in Neurology and Internal Medicine clinics. A series of population-based studies based on the new operational International Headache Society (IHS) criteria, has found that migraine, although common, has a variable prevalence worldwide. In European and American studies the one-year period prevalence of migraine in adults is estimated at 10-15%, significantly more women are affected than men, in a ratio of 2-3:1 [1]; In Japan the reported prevalence is 8.4% [2]. In Africa, crude prevalence rate is estimated at 19 %, and specific rates of 26.8 % for women versus 9.4 % for men [3]. In Arab countries, the migraine prevalence was 2.6–5% in Saudi Arabia and 7.9% in Qatar, while the 1-year migraine prevalence was 10.1% in Oman [4]. In a study of Egyptian school children in Assiut, the prevalence of migraine is 16.6% (female to male ratio: 1.33) [5]. Overall, migraine prevalence varies by age, gender, race, and income. Before puberty, migraine prevalence is approximately 4%. As adolescence approaches, prevalence increases more rapidly in girls than in boys. Migraine is most common in the third decade of life and in lower socioeconomic groups. It increases until approximately age 40, and then declines. Migraine is more frequent in women than men [1,6]. Few studies of migraine incidence have been performed. A population-based study conducted by Rasmussen [6] showed that the annual incidence of migraine is 3.7 per 1,000 person years (women 5.8; men 1.6).

Hypertension and migraine are very prevalent disorders in general population and many old and recent studies suggested a relevant comorbidity between headache, migraine and arterial hypertension [7-11]. However, in some recent studies and textbooks, the relationship between migraine and hypertension is poorly characterized. Epidemiologic and population-based studies found no [12,13] or even negative [14] correlation between the two diseases.

In general, the relation between two disease states may be due to [15] 1) an artifact of diagnostic uncertainty when symptom profiles overlap or when diagnosis is not based on objective markers, 2) chance association or coincidental, 3) unidirectional causality, such as migraine resulting in blood pressure changes due to headache-specific treatment, 4) bidirectional causal association i.e. one disorder causes the other, 5) a shared environmental or genetic risk for the two disease states that increase the risk of both conditions, In such cases, understanding these shared risk factors may lead to greater understanding of the fundamental mechanisms of migraine, or 6) both conditions are manifestations of one systemic disease. However,the term comorbidity is used to refer to the greater than coincidental association of two conditions in the same individual [16].

The present article serves as an overview of the blood pressure changes encountered in patients with migraine. Studies in migraine literatures present in pubmed which highlighted migraine and blood pressure, migraine and hypertension, headache and blood pressure (publications till 2010) were checked. The reference lists of retrieved studies for additional reports of relevant studies were also checked. In this review, the evidences of comorbidity between migraine and high, low or normal blood pressure and the potential mechanisms of controversial views were discussed. It will be clear that despite the uncertainties regarding the presence of interictal blood pressure changes in patients with migraine, whether one condition leads to the other or both conditions are expression of similar systemic illness, both hypertension and migraine have to be carefully treated to avoid the development of cardio- and cerebrovascular complications.

Evidences of Blood Pressure Changes in Migraine

A) Evidences That Hypertension is Positively Associated with Migraine

Since several decades, the comorbidity of migraine with hypertension is a widely accepted issue despite the absence of confirmation by well-designed studies. In general, headache, particularly early-morning pulsating headache, is usually considered a symptom of hypertension and poor control of blood pressure may exacerbate the frequency and severity of migraine [17].

In 1913, Janeway [18] noted that migraine was common in subjects with arterial hypertensionand since then the relation between blood pressure and headache has been examined in many studies [8-11,19-26]. A higher prevalence of headache [27-30] and migraine [31,32] has been reported in hypertensive patients than among normo-tensive controls. On the other hand, a higher prevalence of hypertension has been reported in patients with headache [24,33-35]; or migraine [36-38]; than among headache free people.

Grebe et al. [39] retrospectively analyzed 64 files of headache outpatient clinic (Coimbra, Portugal), chosen randomly among patients suffering from migraine or tension headache. The authors found that the prevalence of hypertension was 35,9% among all patients (migrainous and non-migrainous headache), 28,5% among migraine patients and 44,8% among patients with tension headache. The prevalence of resistance to treatment was 39,8%, 34,3% and 41,3%, respectively. Of the patients resistant to treatment 60% were hypertensive and 62,5% of the hypertensive patients showed resistance to therapy. In the study of Prudenzano et al. [40], the authors found higher prevalence of hypertension in patients with tension headache. In 2005, Pietrini et al. [17] examined a total of 1486 consecutive outpatients with headache recruited from the department of Internal Medicine, Italy. In all headache groups, the prevalence of hypertension was higher than in general population. Hypertension was present in 28% of the patients, and was particularly common in medication-overuse headache (60.6%), chronic tension headache (55.3%), cluster headache (35%), episodic tension headache (31.4%), but less common in migraine without aura (23%) and migraine with aura (16.9%). In the preliminary case control study done by Hamed et al. [11] on 63 adult patients with migraine (n = 44) and tension headache (n = 19), the authors found higher systolic blood pressure in migraine without aura, transformed migraine compared to control subjects (p<0.045, p<0.002), while diastolic blood pressure was higher in patients with migraine with aura, transformed headache and tension headache (p<0.041, p<0.002, p<0.002) and in patients with tension headache than migraine with aura (p<0.024).

Information about the comorbidity of migraine and hypertension or hypertension frequency in migraine patients was also shown in large population based studies. In 2005, Scher et al. [41] studied 5,755 subjects from the Genetic Epidemiology of Migraine Study in the Netherlands and found higher blood pressure (systolic BP >140 mm Hg or diastolic BP >90 mm Hg) in individuals with migraine compared to those without migraine. In the population based study done by Gudmundsson et al. [42] evaluated 10,366 men and 11,171 women with migraine in a population-based study, the authors found that patients with migraine had higher diastolic blood pressure and lower systolic blood pressure and pulse pressure compared to controls. They also found that one standard deviation (1-SD) increase in diastolic blood pressure significantly increased the probability of migraine by 30% of women compared to 14% of men, while one standard deviation (1-SD) increase in systolic blood pressure and pulse pressure significantly decreased the probability of migraine by 19% and 13% of men and 25% and 14% of women, respectively.

The Possible Mechanisms of Comorbidity of Migraine with Hypertension

Shared biological mechanisms have been suggested as a link between migraine and hypertension. One such mechanism may be the rennin-angiotensin system, which is certainly involved in hypertension and has activities in the CNS that may be relevant for migraine pathogenesis [43-45].In support: **a)** attacks of migraine without aura and higher angiotensin converting enzyme activity are more frequent in subjects with angiotensin converting enzyme DD gene, and **b)** Clinical trials indicated that angiotensin-converting enzyme inhibitors as captobril and angiotensin II receptor blockers as Lisinopril are effective in the prophylactic treatment of migraine. In addition to their action on angiotensin-converting system, they alter sympathetic activity, inhibit free radical activity, increase prostacyclin synthesis and block the degradation of bradykinin, encephalin and substance P. All are implicated in the pathophysiology of migraine [44,45].

B) Evidences That Hypertension Is Not Associated with Headache

Most cross-sectional studies performed in unselected populations did not report significant association (negative or positive) between blood pressure and the prevalence of Headache. Chen et al. [46] found no association between migraine and hypertension in 508 young women with migraine and 3902 without migraine. In a cross sectional study of Wiehe et al. [12], the authors studied 1174 individuals older than 17 years, representative of inhabitants of Porto Alegre, RS, Brazil and complained of migraine or tension headache. The authors found that i) individuals with optimal or normal blood pressure complained of migraine more frequently than participants with high-normal blood pressure or hypertension, ii) episodic and chronic tension headache was not associated with hypertension in lifetime in the last year, and iii) individuals with migraine-like episodes of headache may have lower blood pressure than individuals without headache. In a cross-sectional study conducted in the hypertension clinic of a tertiary care University hospital in Brazil, Fuchs et al. [47], investigated 1763 subjects for the association between hypertension classified at moderate to severe stages and headache. The authors found that headache and hypertension was not associated. In addition, they found that pulse pressure and headache were inversely associated. In the large prospective study done by Hagen et al. [48], the authors estimated the relative risk of headache (migraine or non-migrainous headache) in relation to blood pressure at baseline in a total of 22 685 adults not likely to have headache, had their baseline blood pressure measured in 1984-6, and responded to a headache questionnaire at follow up 11 years later (1995-7). The authors found that subjects with a systolic blood pressure of 150 mm Hg or higher had 30% lower risk [risk ratio (RR) = 0.7, 95% CI 0.6-0.8] of having non-migrainous headache at follow up compared with those with systolic pressure lower than 140 mm Hg. For diastolic blood pressure, the risk of non-migrainous headache decreased with increasing values, and these findings were similar for both sexes, and were not influenced by use of antihypertensive medication. For migraine, there was no clear association with blood pressure. In the randomized sample of the Vobarno population done by Muiesan et al. [13] (Brescia, Italy), the authors evaluated the prevalence of headache in a general population sample (n = 301, 126 males, 175 females with age range 35-50 years) to determine its relationship to hypertension (diagnosed by office and/or 24 hours blood pressure). The authors found no differences in headache prevalence (58% vs 55%), migraine prevalence (32% vs 28%) and use of analgesic drugs in the presence of headache (82% vs 78%) between hypertensive (93.5% newly diagnosed, 6.5% treated) and normo-tensive subjects. The first population based study that uses International Headache Society (IHS) criteria for classification of headache found 11 % hypertension in 974 subjects [49]. However, the study did not report any difference on incidence of headache between hypertensives and non-hypertensives.

In addition to the above, there is a consensus agreement within the International Headache Society that chronic arterial hypertension of mild to moderate degree does not cause headache but this may not be the case in patients with hypertension classified at more severe stages. Severe hypertension in the setting of new acute headache may indicate a serious underlying cause and requires urgent investigation [50].

The Possible Factors or Reasons for the Denied Association between Migraine and Hypertension

The authors who found no association between migraine and arterial hypertension consider that the frequency rates of some common vascular risks (as hypertension) might be increased among patients with migraine which is also common (coincidental or chance association). Hypertension is also a common and consistent health problem in both developed and developing countries and its prevalence is currently rising steadily [51]. In general population, the prevalence of hypertension is 28.7% [52]. In economically developed countries, the prevalence of hypertension ranged between 20 and 50%. The prevalence of hypertension varies widely among different populations, with rates as low as 3.4% in rural Indian men and as high as 72.5% in Polish women [53]. The estimated prevalenceof hypertension in Egypt was 26.3%. Hypertension was slightlymore common in women than in men (26.9% versus 25.7%, respectively) [54]. Since both hypertension and migraine are frequent in population, any association between them is likely to be detected in large series. In fact individuals seeking medical care often show a high rate of association between two medical conditions which may be independent in the general population i.e., due to a Berkson's bias. In 10-20% of the population migraine and hypertension can be found together.

C) Evidences That Hypertension is Negatively Associated with Headache

Recent large-sample prospective and population-based studies showed a negative correlation between migraine and hypertension [12,48,55] with lower systolic pressure levels in migraine patients than in controls. Another indirect indication of this paradoxical link is suggested by the positive results of ACE inhibitors and sartans for migraine prophylaxis [56,57].

Hegan et al. [48] and Wiehe et al. [12] showed that migraine patients had lower values of blood pressure. Tzourio's et al. [55] found lower blood pressure and reduced carotid-intima media thickness (evidence of hypertension) in migraine patients. Recently, Tronvik and his colleagues [14], looked at the association between migraine and non-migrainous headache and various measures of blood pressure: systolic, diastolic, mean arterial pressure (average of diastolic and systolic), and pulse pressure (systolic minus diastolic). The authors used both cross-sectional and prospective data from two large epidemiologic studies covering 51,353 men and women over the age of 20 living in Trondheim, Norway. The reason for the study was to explore the link between blood pressure and headache frequency, and how blood pressure medication affects that relationship. The two large studies were called HUNT1 (Nord-Trøndelag Health Survey 1984-1986) and HUNT2 (Nord-Trøndelag Health Survey 1995-1997). The main topics of HUNT-1 included blood pressure, diabetes mellitus, and health related quality of life [58,59]. While HUNT-2 was more extensive than HUNT-1, and among several topics, HUNT-2 included 13 questions related to headache [58]. In HUNT study, Tronvik and his colleagues observed that: i) increasing systolic pressure was linked with decreasing prevalence of migraine and non-migrainous headache (people with higher systolic blood pressure were up to 40 per cent less likely to have headaches), ii) The most robust and consistent association was the link between increasing pulse pressure and decreasing prevalence of both migraine and non-migrainous headache, iii) This link was present for both men and women, in both studies, and iv) The finding was less clear in cases where people were also taking blood pressure medication.

The Possible Mechanisms of the Negative Association between Migraine and Hypertension

Researchers in Norway have shown that *high blood pressure* is linked to fewer *headaches*, possibly due to having stiffer artery walls which affects a homeostatic process that regulates blood pressure and decreases sensitivity to pain, i.e. a phenomenon called "hypertension-associated hypalgesia" (blood pressure linked reduction in pain sensitivity). In support: a) an inverse relationship between blood pressure levels and sensitivity to painful stimuli extends into the normo-tensive range [60], b) low pain sensitivity has been reported in hypertensive animals and humans and in groups deemed to be at an increased risk for the development of hypertension [61-63], and **c)** previous studies confirmed that increasing blood pressure was linked to decreasing amounts of chronic musculoskeletal pain in different parts of the body. In 2005, Hegan et al. [64] observed that individuals with a high blood pressure had a lower prevalence of chronic musculoskeletal complaints than individuals with a normal blood pressure. The authors also found that among 46 901 adults who participated in HUNT1 and HUNT 2 surveys, there was a strong linear trend of decreasing prevalence of chronic musculoskeletal complaints with increasing BP values (systolic and diastolic BP). The authors suggested that the phenomenon of hypertension-associated hypalgesia, may be one explanation for the negative association between migraine and musculoskeletal pains.

The mechanism for hypertension-associated hypalgesia is not clear. but data from humans and rats suggest an interaction between the cardiovascular and pain regulatory systems.

A role for baroreceptors in mediating the blood pressure-pain sensitivity relationship has received some experimental and clinical support. Stimulation of the baroreflex arch (a homeostatic process that helps to maintain blood pressure) in response to increased blood pressure is assumed to inhibit pain transmission at both spinal and supraspinal levels, possibly because of an interaction of the centers modulating nociception and cardiovascular reflexes in the brainstem [65]. The presence of the inverse association between blood pressure and pain sensitivity in the absence of clinical hypertension also support the view that some common central mechanism is underlying the antinociception and cardiovascular regulation rather than a specific effect of hypertension itself. Sanya et al. [66] assessed the baroreflex stimulations in 30 migraine patients in a headache-free phase. The authors applied oscillatory neck suction at 0.1 Hz (to assess the sympathetic modulation of the heart and blood vessels) and at 0.2 Hz (to assess the effect of parasympathetic stimulation on the heart) to assess the changes in power of the RR-interval and blood pressure fluctuations at the relevant stimulating frequency from the baseline values. The authors found that 0.1 Hz neck suction pressure were not significantly different between the patients and controls but the RR-interval oscillatory response to 0.2 Hz neck suction was significantly less in the migraine patients compared with the controls. This confirms that central autonomic changes are associated with the pathophysiology of migraine related blood pressure changes.

Although endogenous opioids are necessary for full expression of the relationship between resting blood pressure and pain sensitivity [60,61], however, the absence of the effect of opioid blockade on the blood pressure pain sensitivity relationship, leaves a doubtful role of endogenous opioid as explanation to the relationship between resting blood pressure and pain sensitivity in migraine [60]. Other neurotransmitters, like catecholamines, may also be involved [61]. It has been found that a polymorphism of catechol-O-methyltransferase (COMT) gene, of which its protein product is an important enzyme for the metabolism of catecholamines,may influence the response to pain [67] and may also be important also for blood pressure regulation [68]. In support, antihypertensive medications may have an influence on blood pressure-pain sensitivity relationship.

Hypotension and Headache: Is There a Relationship?

No studies reported hypotension in the inter-ictal period. However, hypotension is not excluded as comorbid with migraine. In fact, with hypotension, a painful headache is commonly experienced when one bend over and suddenly move upright his/her head. This is also called orthostatic and occurs with dramatic changes in cranial blood pressure. Once triggered, hypotensive headache presents itself just like migraine and most other headaches.

Ictal hypotension has been reported by some authors. Recently, Seçil et al. [69], recorded blood pressure at 3 times in 62 normo-tensive patients with migraine: (1) just before or very early, (2) during (when headache peaks), and (3) 1 hour after the attack. The authors detected diastolic hypotension in a considerable number of patients before or very early, during, and after migraine attack (5.1%). The authors hypothesized that pathophysiological mechanisms (as autonomic dysfunction) are involved in migraine, which are still largely unknown, could lead to a decrease in blood pressure. Autonomic dysfunction is also reported in many functional neuroimaging studies (fMRI and PET) with migraine [49]. It has been found that during migraine attacks, some substances are released especially calcitonin gene-related peptide (CGRP) (which is the main vasodilator) due to activation of contralateral locusceruleus, dorsal pontine area and dorsal raphe nucleus. This peptide could be the reason of diastolic and systolic hypotension during the entire attack [70].

The Current Opinion of the Comorbidity between Blood Pressure Changes and Migraine

Recent evidences suggest that during attacks of migraine and in the interictal period, migraine patients have changes in the properties of the systemic as well as cranial vasculature, including: generalized peripheral vasoconstriction [71], increased diameter and/or decreased distensibility of peripheral blood vessels [72], decreased brachial artery flow-mediated dilatation and increased nitrate-mediated response [73], increased brachial artery intima-media thickness [72], presence of microvascular retinal abnormalities [74] and reduced number and function of circulating endothelial progenitor cells (EPC) which are surrogate biologic markers of impaired vascular function and higher cardiovascular risk [75]. Nagai et al. [76] reported significant association between enhanced radial augmentation index and migraine. Augmentation index (AI) is a parameter of arterial stiffness that can be obtained from the central arterial waveform as the ratio of augmentation pressure by the reflection pressure wave to the pulse pressure. It has been reported that central AI is closely related to several risk factors for atherosclerosis and future cardiovascular events. AI can also be obtained from the radial arterial waveform. Since radial AI is closely associated with aortic AI, radial AI itself could provide information on vascular properties [77]. In the study of Hamed et al. [11], the authors found that brachial artery flow mediated dilatation was lower in patients with transformed headache and is inversely correlated with systolic and diastolic blood pressure and carotid artery intima-media thickness of all groups of headache patients (migrainous and non-migrainous).

Previous studies confirmed that hypertension is associated with modification of the physical properties of large arteries which are concerned the geometry, wall elasticity, and wall viscosity of cranial and peripheral vessels [78]. These properties are shared in patients with migraine and hypertension. Together with the evidences for the presence of vascular risk profile in some patients with migraine which include: high blood pressure [35], disturbed lipid profile [79], elevated body mass index (BMI) [80], insulinresistance [81], metabolic syndrome [82], hyperhomocysteinemia [83], ischemic cerebrovascular stroke [84] and coronary heart disease [85], all indicate the possibility of migraine being a local manifestation of a systemic vascular abnormality rather than a primary cerebral phenomenon.

Clinical Implications

1) Based on the above information and despite the fact that there is still uncertainty regarding the comorbidity of blood pressure changes with migraine, establishing the blood pressure should be a routine task in the assessment of all headache patients and the control of hypertension in migraine patients is an important factor for the success of migraine treatment and to lower cerebrovascular risk [86,87]. A unifying view among most recent studies suggests that migraine is positively correlated with diastolic blood pressure but negatively correlated with systolic blood pressure and pulse pressure [42,87,88]. Some evidence suggests that poor control of blood pressure may exacerbate the frequency and severity of migraine and other headaches [17].

2) Careful consideration of the therapeutic options is important for both migraine and hypertension. At present, acute treatment of migraine includes the use of non-steroidal anti-inflammatory drugs (NSAIDS) and triptans (5-HT agonists). However, some agents used to treat migraine can exacerbate hypertension and many of the drugs used to treat hypertension may cause headache. Triptans are vasoconstrictive and cannot be used in patients with cardiovascular diseases. A promising option is the use of antihypertensive drugs in migraine prophylactics. Recently, angiotensin converting enzyme inhibitors and blockers of angiotensin II provide beneficial results in migraine prophylaxis [44]. A very recent progress for migraine therapy includes the introduction of CGRP antagonist (MK-0974 or telcagepant) which shows high efficacy in treatment of migraine attacks with no adverse cardiovascular risk [89].

3) Addressing the vascular comorbidities with vascular risk profile with migraine in experimentally large sample sized studies could be a big step towards understanding vascular component of migraine attacks as well as systemic end points of attacks. It is important to point that the bidirectional association between migraine, hypertension and vascular risk factors may increase the risk of arterial endothelial damage resulting in cardio- and cerebrovascular complications [11].

References

[1]   Stewart, W.F., Lipton, R.B., Celentano, D.D., Reed, M.L. Prevalence of migraine headache in the United States. Relation to age, income, race, and other sociodemographic factors. *JAMA* 1992;267(1):64-69.

[2]   Sakai, F., Igarashi, H. Prevalence of migraine in Japan: a nationwide survey. *Cephalalgia*1997;17(1):15–22.

[3]   Marcellin, A.L., Yves, R.J., Prisca, A.O. Prevalence de la migraine a madagascar: resultats d'une enquete menee dans une population generale migraine prevalence in malagasy: results of a general population survey. *AJNS* 2005; 24 (1).

[4]   Benamer, H.T.S., Deleu, D.; Grosset, D. Epidemiology of headache in Arab countries. *The Journal of Headache and Pain.* 2010;11(1):1-3.

[5]   Ahmed, H.N., Farweez, H., Farghaly W.A., Kamel N.F., Bakhet, A. Prevalence of migraine among schoolchildren (primary and preparatory) in Assuit city, Egypt. *Eastern Mediterranean health journal* 1999;5:402–423.

[6]   Rasmussen, B.K. Epidemiology of headache in Europe. In: Olesen, J., ed. *Headacheclassification and Epidemiology*. New York: Raven Press; 1994, pp. 231-237.

[7]   Weiss, N.S. Relation of high blood pressure to headache, epistaxis, and selected other symptoms. *N Engl J Med* 1972;287(13):631–633.

[8]   Cooper, W.D., Glover, D.R., Hormbrey, J.M., Kimber, G.R. Headache and blood pressure: evidence of a close relationship. *J Hum Hypertens* 1989;3(1):41-44.

[9]   Couch, J.R., Hassanein, R.S. Headache as a risk factor in atherosclerosis-related diseases. *Headache* 1989;29(1):49–54.

[10] Mathew, N.T. Migraine and hypertension. *Cephalalgia* 1999;19 Suppl 25:17-19.

[11] Hamed, S.A., Hamed, E.A., Mahmoud, A.A., Mahmoud, N.M. Vascular risk factors, endothelial function and carotid thickness in patients with migraine: relationship to atherosclerosis. *J of stroke and cerebrovascular diseases* 2010;19(2):92-103.

[12] Wiehe, M., Fuchs, S.C., Moreira, L.B., Moraes, R.S., Fuchs, F.D. Migraine is more frequent in individuals with optimal and normal blood pressure: a population-based study. *Hypertens* 2002;20(7):1303-1306.

[13] Muiesan, M.L., Padovani, A., Salvetti, M., Monteduro, C., Poisa, P., Bonzi, B., Paini, A., Cottini, E., Agosti, C., Castellano, M., Rizzoni, D., Vignolo, A., Agabiti-Rosei, E. Headache: Prevalence and relationship with office or ambulatory blood pressure in a general population sample (the Vobarno Study). *Blood Press* 2006;15(1):14-19.

[14] Tronvik, E., Stovner, L.J., Hagen, K., Holmen, J., Zwart J-A. "High pulse pressure protects against headache: Prospective and cross-sectional data (HUNT study)." *Neurology* 2008;70(16):1329-1336.

[15] Hamed, S.A. The vascular risk associations with migraine: Relation to migraine susceptibility and progression. *Atherosclerosis* 2009;205(1):15-22.

[16] Feinstein, A.R. The pretherapeutic classification of comorbidity in chronic disease. *J Chron Dis* 1970; 23:455-468.

[17] Pietrini, U., De Luca, M., De Santis, G. Hypertension in headache patients? A clinical study. *Acta Neurol Scand* 2005;112:259-264.

[18] Janeway, T.C. A clinical study of hypertensive cardiovascular disease. *Arch Intern Med* 1913;12():755–798.

[19] Waters, W.E. Headache and blood pressure in the community. *BMJ* 1971;1(13):142–13.

[20] Weiss, N.S. Relation of high blood pressure to headache, epistaxis, and selected other symptoms. *N Engl J Med* 1972;287():631–633.

[21] Schéle, R., Ahlborg, B., Ekbom, K. Physical characteristics and allergic history in young men with migraine and other headaches. *Headache* 1978;18(2):80–86.

[22] Kottke, T.E., Tuomilehto, J., Puska, P., Salonen J.T. The relationship of symptoms and blood pressure in a population sample. *Int J Epidemiol* 1979;8(4):355–359.

[23] Abramson, J.H., Hopp, C., Epstein, L.M. Migraine and non-migrainous headaches: a community survey in Jerusalem. *J Epidemiol Community Health* 1980;34(3):188–193.

[24] Featherstone, H.J. Medical diagnosis and problems in individuals with recurrent idiopathic headaches. *Headache* 1985;25(4):136–140.

[25] Paulin, J.M., Waal-Manning, J., Simpson, F.O., Knight, R.G. The prevalence of headache in a small New Zealand town. *Headache* 1985;25(3):147–151.

[26] D'Alessandro, R.., Benassi, G., Lenzi, P.L., Gamberini, G., Sacquegna, T., De Carolis, P., Lugaresi, E. Epidemiology of headache in the republic of San Marino. *J Neurol Neurosurg Psychiatry* 1988;51(1):21–27.

[27] Gardner, J.W., Mountain, G.E., Hines, E.A. The relationship of migraine to hypertension and to hypertension headaches. *Am J Med Sci* 1940;200:50–53.

[28] Badran, RH., Weir, R.J., McGuiness, J.B. Hypertension and headache. *Scott Med J* 1970;15(2):48–51.

[29] Bulpitt, C.J., Dollery, C.T., Carne, S. Change in symptoms of hypertensive patients after referral to a hospital clinic. *Br Heart J* 1976;38(2):121–128.

[30] Jaillard, A.S., Mazetti, P., Kala, E. Prevalence of migraine and headache in a high-altitude town of Peru: a population-based study. *Headache* 1997;37(2):95–101.

[31] Markush, R.E., Herbert, R.K., Heyman, A., O'Fallon, W.M. Epidemiologic study of migraine symptoms in young women. *Neurology* 1975;25(5):430–435.

[32] Marcoux, S., Berube, S., Brisson, J., Fabia, J. History of migraine and risk of pregnancyinduced hypertension. *Epidemiology* 1992;3(1):53–56.

[33] Ziegler, D.K., Hassanein, R.S, Couch, J.R. Characteristics of life headache histories in a non-clinic population. *Neurology* 1977;27(3):265–269.

[34] Baldrati, A., Bini, L., D'Alessandro, R., Cortelli, P., de Capoa, D., De Carolis, P., Sacquegna, T. Analysis of outcome predictors of migraine towards chronicity. *Cephalgia* 1985; 5(S2):195-199.

[35] Cirillo, M., Stellanto, D., Lombardi, C., De Santo, N.G., Covelli, V. Headache and cardiovascular risk factors: positive association with hypertension. *Headache* 1999; 39(6): 409-416.

[36] Atkins J.B. Migraine as a sequel to infection by L icterohaemorrhagiae. *BMJ* 1955;1(4920):1011–1012.

[37] Merikangas, K.R., Fenton, B.T. Comorbity of migraine with somatic disorders in a large-scale epidemiological study in the United States. In: Olesen, J., eds. *Headache classification and epidemiology*. New York: Raven Press, 1994, pp. 301–314.

[38] Franceschi, M., Colombo, B., Rossi, P., Canal, N. Headache in a population-based elderly cohort. An ancillary study to the Italian longitudinal study of aging (ILSA). *Headache* 1997;37(2):79–82.

[39] Grebe, H.P., Nunes, da Silva, M.J., Diogo-Sousa, L. Role of arterial hypertension in comorbidity of chronic headaches. *Rev Neurol*2001;33(2):119-122.

[40] Prudenzano, M.P., Monetti, C., Merico, L., Cardinali, V., Genco, S., Lamberti, P., Livrea, P. The comorbidity of migraine and hypertension. A study in a tertiary care headache centre. *J Headache Pain* 2005;6(4):220-222.

[41] Scher, A.I., Terwindt, G.M., Picavet, H.S., Verschuren, W.M., Ferrari, M.D., Launer, L.J. Cardiovascular risk factors and migraine: the GEM population-based study. *Neurology*2005;64(4):614–620.

[42] Gudmundsson LS, Thorgeirsson G, Sigfusson N, Sigvaldason H, Johannsson M. Migraine patients have lower systolic but higher diastolic blood pressure compared with controls in a population-based study of 21,537 subjects. The Reykjavik Study. *Cephalalgia* 2006; 26(4):436-44.

[43] Paterna, S., Di Pasquale, P., D'Angelo, A., Seidita, G., Tuttolomondo, A., Cardinale, A., Maniscalchi, T., Follone, G., Giubilato, A., Tarantello, M., Licata, G. Angiotensin-converting enzyme gene deletion polymorphism determines an increase in frequency of

migraine attacks in patients suffering from migraine without aura. *Eur Neurol* 2000;43(3):133–136.

[44] Schrader, H., Stovner, L.J., Helde, G., Sand, T., Bovim, G. Prophylactic treatment of migraine with angiotensin converting enzyme inhibitor (lisinopril): randomised, placebo controlled, crossover study. *BMJ* 2001; 322(7277):19-22.

[45] Sliwka, U., Harscher, S., Diehl, R.R., van Schayck, R., Niesen, W.D., Weiller, C. Spontaneous oscillations in cerebral blood flow velocity give evidence of different autonomic dysfunctions in various types of headache. *Headache* 2001;41(2):157-163.

[46] Chen, T.C., Leviton, A., Edelstein, S., Ellenberg, J.H. Migraine and other diseases in women of reproductive age. The influence of smoking on observed associations. *Arch Neurol* 1987;44(10):1024–1028.

[47] Fuchs, F.D., Gus, M., Moreira, L.B., Moreira, W.D., Gonçalves, S.C., Nunes, G. Headache is not more frequent among patients with moderate to severe hypertension.*J Hum Hypertens* 2003;17(11):787-790.

[48] Hagen, K., Stovner, L.J., Vatten, L., Holmen, J., Zwart, J.A., Bovim, G. Blood pressure and risk of headache: a prospective study of 22 685 adults in Norway. *J Neurol Neurosurg Psychiat* 2002; 72(4):463-466.

[49] Breslau, N., Rasmussen, B.K. The impact of migraine: Epidemiology, risk factors, and co-morbidities. Neurology 2001;56 Suppl 1:S4-S12.

[50] Headache Classification Committee of the international Headache Society. Classification and diagnostic criteria for headache disorders, cranial neuralgias, and facial pain. *Cephalalgia* 1988;(suppl 7):1–96.

[51] World Health Report 2002: Reducing risks, promoting health life.Geneva, Switzerland: World Health Organization, 2002. *http://www.who.int/whr/2002/*

[52] Hajjar, I., Kotchen, T.A. Trends in prevalence, prevalence, awareness, treatment, and control of hypertension in the United States, 1988-2000.*JAMA* 2003;290(2):199-206.

[53] Kearney, P.M., Whelton, M., Reynolds, K. Whelton, P.K., He, J. Worldwide prevalenceof hypertension: a systematic review. *J Hypertens* 2004;22(1):11–19.

[54] Ibrahim, M.M., Rizk, H., Appel, LJ., El Aroussy, W., Helmy, S., Sharaf, Y., Ashour, Z., Kandil, H., Roccella, E., Whelton, PK., for the NHP Investigative Team. Hypertension Prevalence, Awareness, Treatment, and Control in Egypt. Results From the Egyptian National Hypertension Project (NHP). *Hypertension* 1995;26(6 Pt 1):886-890.

[55] Tzourio, C., Gagniere, B., El Amrani, M., Alpérovitch, A., Bousser, M.G. Relationship between migraine, blood pressure and carotid thickness. A population-based study in the elderly. *Cephalalgia* 2003;23(9):914–920.

[56] Charles, J.A., Jotkowitz, S., Byrd, L.H. Prevention of migraine with olmesartan in patients with hypertension/prehypertension. *Headache* 2006;46(3):503–507

[57] Tronvik, E., Stovner, L.J., Helde, G., Sand, T., Bovim, G. Prophylactic treatment of migraine with an angiotensin II receptor blocker. *JAMA* 2003;289(1):65–69.

[58] Hagen, K., Zwart, J.A., Vatten, L., Stovner, L.J., Bovim, G. Head-HUNT: validity and reliability of a headache questionnaire in a large population-based study in Norway. *Cephalalgia* 2000;20(4):244–251.

[59] Aamodt AH, Stovner LJ, Midthjell K, Hagen K, Zwart JA. Headache prevalence related to diabetes*Eur J Neurol*2007;14(7):738-744.

[60] Bruehl, S., Chung, O.Y., Ward, P., Johnson, B., McCubbin, J.A. The relationship between resting blood pressure and acute pain sensitivity in healthy normotensives and chronic back pain sufferers: the effect of opioid blockade. *Pain* 2002;100(1-2):191-201.

[61] Ghione, S. Hypertension-associated hypalgesia. Evidence in experimental animals and humans, pathophysiological mechanisms, and potential clinical consequences. *Hypertension* 1996;28(3):494–504.

[62] Schobel, H.P., Ringkamp, M., Behrmann, A., Forster, C., Schmieder, R.E., Handwerker, H.O. Hemodynamic and sympathetic nerve responses to painful stimuli in normotensive and borderline hypertensive subjects. *Pain*. 1996;66(2-3):117-124.

[63] al'Absi, M., Petersen, K.L., Wittmers, L.E. Blood pressure but not parental history for hypertension predicts pain perception in women. *Pain* 2000;88(1):61-68

[64] Hagen, K., Zwart, J.A., Holmen, J., Svebak, S., Bovim, G., Stovner, L.J., Nord-Trøndelag Health Study. Does hypertension protect against chronic musculoskeletal complaints? The Nord-Trøndelag Health Study. *Arch Intern Med* 2005 25;165(8):916-922.

[65] D'Antono, B., Ditto, B., Sita, A., Miller, S.B. Cardiopulmonary baroreflex stimulation and blood pressure–related hypoalgesia. *Biol Psychol* 2000;53(2-3):217-231.

[66] Sanya, E.O., Brown, C.M., von Wilmowsky, C., Neundörfer, B., Hilz, M.J. Impairment of parasympathetic baroreflex responses in migraine patients. *Acta Neurol Scand* 2005;111(2):102-107.

[67] Zubieta, J.K., Heitzeg, M.M., Smith, Y.R., Bueller, J.A., Xu, K., Xu, Y., Koeppe, R.A., Stohler, C.S., Goldman, D. COMT val158 met genotype affects μ-opioid neurotransmitter responses to a pain stressor. *Science* 2003;299(5610):1240-1243.

[68] Helkamaa, T., Männistö, P.T., Rauhala, P., Cheng, Z.J., Finckenberg, P., Huotari, M., Gogos, J.A., Karayiorgou, M., Mervaala, E.M. Resistance to salt-induced hypertension in catechol-O-methyltransferase-gene-disrupted mice. *J Hypertens* 2003;21(12):2365-2374.

[69] Seçil Y, Unde C, Beckmann YY, Bozkaya YT, Ozerkan F, Başoğlu M. Blood Pressure Changes in Migraine Patients before, during and after Migraine Attacks. *Pain Pract.* 2010 Feb 11. [Epub ahead of print]

[70] Juhasz, G., Zsombok, T., Modos, E.A., Olajos, S., Jakab, B., Nemeth, J., Szolcsanyi, J., Vitrai, J., Bagdy, G. NO-induced migraine attack:strong increase in plasma calcitonin gene-related peptide (CGRP) concentration and negative correlation with platelet serotonin release. *Pain* 2003;106(3):461-470.

[71] Iversen, H.K., Nielsen, T.H., Olesen, J., Tfelt-Hansen, P. Arterial responses during migraine headache. *Lancet*1990;336(8719):837–839.

[72] de Hoon, J.N., Willigers, J.M., Troost, J., Struijker-Boudier, H.A., van Bortel, L.M. Cranial and peripheral interictal vascular changes in migraine patients. *Cephalalgia*2003;23(2):96–104.

[73] Yetkin, E., Ozisik, H., Ozcan, C., Aksoy, Y., Turhan, H. Increased dilator response to nitrate and decreased flow-mediated dilatation in migraineurs.*Headache* 2007;47(1):104-110.

[74] Rose, K.M., Wong, T.Y., Carson., Couper, D.J., Klein, R., Sharrett, A.R. Migraine and retinal microvascular abnormalities: the Atherosclerosis Risk in Communities Study.*Neurology* 2007;68(20):1694-700.

[75] Lee, S.T., Chu, K., Jung, K.H., Kim, D.H., Kim, E.H., Choe, V.N., Kim, J.H., Im, W.S., Kang, L., Park., J.E., Park, H.J., Park, H.K., Song, E.C., Lee, S.K., Kim, M., Roh, J.K. Decreased number and function of endothelial progenitor cells in patients with migraine. *Neurology* 2008;70(17):1510-1517.

[76] Nagai, T., Tabara, Y., Igase, M., Nakura, J., Miki, T., Kohara, K. Migraine is associated with enhancedarterial stiffness. *Hypertens res* 2007;30():577–583.

[77] Nichols, W.W. Clinical measurement of arterial stiffness obtained from noninvasive pressure waveforms. *Am JHypertens* 2005;18(1 Pt 2):3S–10S.

[78] Armentano, R., Megnien, J.L., Simon, A., Bellenfant, F., Barra, J., Levenson, J. Effects of Hypertension on Viscoelasticity of Carotid and Femoral Arteries in Humans. *Hypertension*1995;26(1):48-54.

[79] Bic, Z., Blix, G.G., Hopp, H.P., Leslie, F.M., Schell, M.J. The influence of a low fat-diet on incidence and severity of migraine headaches. *J Women's Heath Gender-based Med* 1999;8():623-630.

[80] Bigal, M.E., Gironda, M., Tepper, S.J., Feleppa, M., Rapoport, A.M., Sheftell, F.D., Lipton, R.B. Headache prevention outcome and body mass index. *Cephalgia* 2006;26(4):445-450.

[81] Rainero, I., Limone, P., Ferrero, M., Valfrè, W., Pelissetto, C., Rubino, E., Gentile, S., Lo Giudice, R., Pinessi, L. Insulin sensitivity is impaired in patients with migraine. *Cephalgia* 2005;25(8):593-597.

[82] Watson, K.E., Peters Harmel, A.L., Matson, G. Atherosclerosis in type 2 diabetes mellitus: the role of insulin resistance. *J Cardiovasc Pharmacol Ther* 2003;8(4);253-260.

[83] Lea, R.A., Ovcaric, M., Sundholm, J., MacMillan, J., Griffiths, L.R. The methylenetetrahydrofolate reductase gene variant C677T influences susceptibility to migraine with aura. *BMD Medicine* 2004;2:3-10.

[84] Schwaag, S, Nabavi, DG, Frese, A, Husstedt, I.W., Evers, S. The association between migraine and juvenile stroke: A case-control study. *Headache.* 2003;43(2):90-93.

[85] Vanmolkot, F.H., Van Bortel, L.M., de Hoon, J.N. Altered arterial function in migraine of recent onset. *Neurology* 2007;68(19):1563-1570.

[86] Guasti, L, Zanotta, D, Diolisi, A, Garganico, D., Simoni, C., Gaudio, G., Grandi, A.M., Venco, A. Changes in pain perception during treatment with angiotensin converting enzyme-inhibitors and angiotensin II type 1 receptor blockade. *J Hypertens* 2002;20(3):485-491.

[87] Agostoni, E., Aliprandi, A. Migraine and hypertension.*Neurol Sci*2008;29 Suppl 1:S37-39.

[88] Rasmussen, B.K., Olesen, J. Symptomatic and non-symptomatic headaches in a general population. *Neurology* 1992;42(6):1225-1231.

[89] Farinelli, I., Missori, S., Martelletti, P. Proinflammatory mediators and migraine pathogenesis: moving towards CGRP as a target for a novel therapeutic class.*Expert Rev Neurother* 2008; 8(9):1347-1354.

In: Systolic Blood Pressure
Editor: Robert A. Arfi

ISBN: 978-1-61209-263-8
©2012 Nova Science Publishers, Inc.

Chapter IV

Impact of Blood Pressure on Coupled Ventricular and Vascular Stiffening, Related Cardiac Structural Remodeling and Eventually Functional Decay: Transition from Subclinical Systolic Dysfunction to Heart Failure

Chung-Lieh Hung[1,2], Yau-Huei Lai[1,2], Yih-Jer Wu[1,2,3] and Hung-I Yeh[1,2,3]

[1]Division of Cardiology, Department of Internal Medicine, Mackay Memorial Hospital, Taipei, Taiwan
[2]Department of Medicine, Mackay Medical College and Mackay Medicine Nursing and Management College, Taipei, Taiwan
[3]Mackay Medical College, Taipei, Taiwan

Abstract

In the recent years, heart failure (HF) with relatively preserved ejection fraction (EF) has gained much attention owing to largely unproved pathogenesis, high morbidity and the lack of efficient therapeutic approach. Hypertension, a leading cause and threat of HF and cardiovascular co-morbidities in developed society, is currently becoming more and more widely recognized. Increasing arterial load of long duration, when coupled with elevated ventricular wall stress and after-load, has been observed to be associated with ventricular-arterial stiffening and subsequent heart failure (HF) development.

Measure of ventricular contractility, such as end-systolic elastance, has been mentioned to be influenced by ventricular geometry. While myocardial contractility seemed to increase in asymptomatic hypertensive subjects in order to compensate for elevated arterial load, depressed contractility accompanied with increased passive myocardial stiffness was observed in the earlier stage HF patients. Indeed, it is well recognized that several systolic indices have actually declined in the earlier stage of HF though in this stage, conventional assessment of LV pumping in terms of ejection fraction (EF) may remain relatively unchanged.

Altered cardiac structure and function such as concentric remodeling before over hypertrophy has been widely assessed and recognized in earlier stage of HTN though the exact clinical significance is unclear so far. A more severe form, ventricular hypertrophy, denotes a useful clinical marker of target organ damage and remained as robust cardiovascular prognosticator. However, diastolic dysfunction when utilizing tissue Doppler imaging (TDI) in detecting early myocardial damage in earlier stage hypertension (HTN) has been well-documented. More recently, emerging imaging technology and modality such as deformation imaging have allowed detection of early ventricular systolic dysfunction clinically feasible. Evidence of systolic dysfunction, in terms of the decline of deformation has also been proved in the recent studies.

Even though, still there remained many issues unresolved regarding the interaction and mechanisms between ventricular remodeling and arterial adaptation in the transition from HTN to HF. A systemic approach and assessment to such link between ventricular remodeling, coupled ventricular-arterial stiffening and subclinical systolic dysfunction also remained to be established. More importantly, insights into the understanding of such transitional process may help identify subjects susceptible to HF development under increased arterial load and may warrant precise and earlier therapeutic intervention to prevent cascade of future unpleasant HF events.

General Introduction

The likelihood of survival in heart failure patients with reduced systolic function has improved in the recent decades partially may be due to the shifts in population demographics, changes in the risk factors, and the evolution of therapeutic strategies [1, 2]. Among them, heart failure with preserved ejection fraction (HFpEF) has gained much attention owing to largely unproved pathogenesis, high morbidity and the lack of efficient therapeutic approach. HFpEF actually comprises nearly one-half of all HF patients and has been shown to be associated with grave prognosis [3]. Diastolic dysfunction, characterized by abnormalities of ventricular filling, including decreased diastolic distensibility and impaired relaxation, is thought to represent an important pathophysiological intermediate between hypertension and heart failure, especially in HFpEF.

Hypertension, a leading cause and threat of cardiovascular co-morbidities in developed societies, is currently becoming more and more widely recognized. It is among one of the most commonly encountered disease entities in daily clinical practice. Both chronic hypertension and aging has been well known for their dominant impact and risk for the development of heart failure with a normal ejection fraction [4]. Patients with hypertension have increased risk of developing structural changes in the myocardium, leading to target organ damage [5], myocardial fibrosis and heart failure [6].Although myocardial infarction (MI) still carries the greatest relative risk for HF among all risk factors (hypertension, diabetes, MI, valvular diseases), the far greater prevalence of hypertension translates to a greater population-attributable risk [7]. Fifty years ago, before the widespread availability of effective antihypertensive drug treatment, overt heart failure remained one of the most common complications of hypertension accounting for 40% of associated deaths.In the Framingham Heart Study, during more than 20 years of follow-up, hypertension has been observed to produce a twofold hazard for heart failure incidencein men and a threefold hazard in women[8].

Etiology

The main factors responsible for the development of LV hypertrophy (LVH) are chronic pressure and volume overload [9]. To compensate for pressure overload, activated biological process including various hormones, growth factors (eg: catecholamines, angiotensin II, endothelin) and cytokinesalso contribute protein genesis by promoting vascular and cardiomyocytes growth leading to structural modifications and remodeling [9]. On the one hand, LV wall thickness increases in order to normalize wall tensionin cases of chronic pressure overload based on Laplace law [10]. In concentric hypertrophy, the myofibrils increase in diameter, whereas they increase in length in eccentric hypertrophy. Concentric hypertrophy occurs most commonly in hypertension and is more likely associated with normal or reduced LV end-diastolic volume (LVEDV). On the other hand, LVEDV often increases with eccentric hypertrophy [11]. A mixed geometric phenotype and a possible dynamic transition among various patterns may result from combined chronic pressure and volume overload which make the exact diagnosis of early stage of cardiac functional disturbanceless accurate and objective quantificationdifficult [12].

When early stage diastolic dysfunction occurs without overt systolic dysfunction with simultaneous geometric alterations, it usually occurs in elderly patients with ventricular collagen deposition, fibrosis, and ischemia. [13] This coupling of ventricular and vascular stiffening processes not only results in ventricular geometric alterations [14], more importantly, may also lead to load-dependent impairment of systolic as well as diastolic ventricular function [15, 16].

In untreated hypertension, progression from LVH to HF is usually associated with ischemia, ventricular stiffness, myocytes apoptosis or fibrosis, and eventually systolic dysfunction [17]. It has thus been suggested that HFpEF may be the result of coupled ventricular and vascular functional changes, which progresses with hypertension duration or aging [14].However, in those patients effectively treated with antihypertensive medications, concentric hypertrophy may be manifested by preserved systolic function with diastolic impairment [18].

Pathogenesis

Two major mechanisms have been proposed for the association of hypertension and HF so far. First, hypertension is a risk factor for MI, which is associated with LV systolic dysfunction. Second, hypertension promotes LVH, which is associated with diastolic dysfunction [19] (Figure 1).

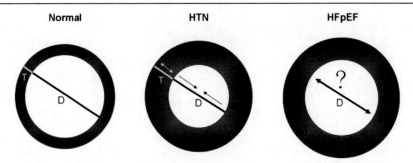

Figure 1. Assumptions on ventricular geometric alterations at end-diastolic phase and the transition from normal subjects, hypertensive patients to heart failure with preserved ejection fraction (HFpEF). Progressive increased ventricular wall thickness (T) or relative wall thickness (RWT=2T/D) with minor reduced lumen diameter (D) at early stage hypertension (HTN) patients may result in geometric pattern of "Concentric Remodeling". During the process of HTN to HFpEF, global ventricular mass may increase but the exact mechanisms involved still remains inconclusive.

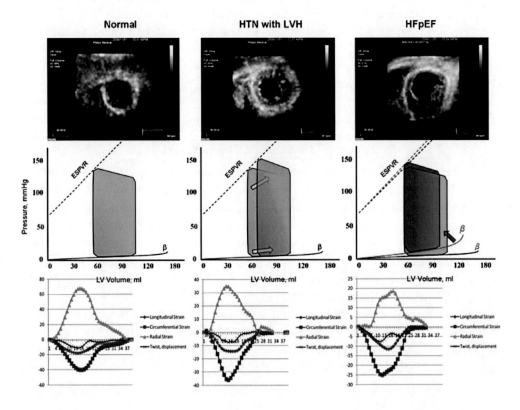

Figure 2. The representative LV wall geometries and structures were demonstrated from normal, hypertensive subject (HTN) to heart failure patients with preserved ejection fraction (HFpEF) from left to right. Note the increased LV wall thickness and increased wall-LV-diameter ratio presented as three-dimensional (3D) illustrations in the HTN and HFpEF subjects. The shift of end-systolic pressure-volume relations (ESPVR) and the load-independent diastolic function derived from the end-diastolic-systolic PV relationship with exponential fitting to obtain the chamber stiffness constant (LV stiffness constant, β) were displayed in these three different clinical scenarios, respectively. In addition, corresponding deformation imaging (longitudinal, circumferential and radial strain) from three different cardiac motions and ventricular twistby speckle-tracking techniques were shown. While radial strain and longitudinal function started to deteriorate in the HTN subjects, short-axis function including circumferential strain and twist remained relatively unchanged. In the HFpEF subjects, all parameters seemed to become worse except for cardiac twist behavior.

As the left ventricle progressively hypertrophies in response to increased afterload, its systolic pumping reserve may become diminishedpredisposing to subsequent heart failure development with underlying preserved ejection fraction [8, 20, 21, 22,23]. In early stages, the hypertrophied left ventricle becomes stiffer and thicker with diastolic filling impairment develops due to ventricular fibrosis. To compensate for persistently elevated LV end-diastolic pressure, the left atrium enlarges and thickens in order to maintain adequate diastolic filling. In the later stage, systolic dysfunction and overt heart failure becomes apparent.At the same time, valvular insufficiency ensues due to unfavorable cardiac sphericity which then further exacerbate the deteriorated heart pumping [24].

Diastolic function can be defined by the relation between LV filling rates and pressures. Noninvasive methods, such as echocardiography, mainly divide diastolic filling in two filling phases [25]. Early diastolic filling is predominantly influenced by active myocardial relaxation whereas the late diastolic filling is affected by ventricular stiffness, relative wall thickness, or LA-to-LV pressure gradient [26].

When LVH manifests with pathologically prolonged LV relaxation with underlying increased stiffness, the left ventricle can no longer accommodate the rise in intra-ventricular volume. As a result, LV filling pressure rises in order to maintain efficient filling and subsequent emptying. Eventually, impaired LV filling lowers cardiac output and promotes arterial underfilling, thereby increasing preload [27].

It is now well recognized that several systolic indices have actually declined in the earlier stage of HF, even though conventional assessment of LV pumping in terms of ejection fraction (EF) may remain relatively unchanged [28].While myocardial contractility by measuring mid-wall mechanics seemed to increase in asymptomatic hypertensive subjects in order to compensate for elevated arterial load, depressed contractility accompanied with increased passive myocardial stiffness was observed in the earlier stage HF patients. It is not known whether impaired LV relaxation invariably leads to elevated pulmonary capillary wedge pressure during exercise [29].On the other hand, elevation of LV filling pressures seems to be a more direct cause of decreased exercise tolerance. It is important to gain a better understanding of why some patients with delayed LV relaxation develop higher LV filling pressures than others.

Exerciseintolerance in HFpEF patients might be associated with higher LVEDP at a similar end-diastolic volume, suggesting the underlying failure ofthe Frank-Starling mechanism [30].Diastolic dysfunction may or may not be present in HFpEF. One recent study assessed end-diastolic pressure-volume relations (EDPVR) from data measured before and after right heart/pericardial unloading[6]. At rest, the EDPVR curve was shifted upward and somewhat left-ward with a higher stiffness coefficient during the early filling. This may be related to higher left atrial pressures thatdetermine the pressure at the moment of mitral valve opening [31].Frankly speaking, these EDPVR changes suggest a more prominent role of loading in the development of heart failure representing. Instead, concepts of end-systolic stiffness may reflect ventricular contractility under various after-load status at a given end-systolic volume [32, 33] which piloted the concept of ventricular-arterial interaction. True myocardial contractility expressed as the maximal velocity from an unloaded, isolated myofiber in a vivo beating heart was first introduced by Suga and Sagawa et al [34]. Known as pressure-volume relationship (ESPVR or Ees), this estimate of end-systolic stiffness and cardiac contractility is invasive, highly accurate by measuring parameters at the end of systolic phase using a conductance catheterbut maybe somewhat technically demanding [35,

24] (Figure 2). Smaller end-systolic volume and higher end-systolic pressure may denote typical markers of higher contractility while those with counter-directional values may represent compromised contractility. In patients suffering from HFpEF, a steeper end-systolic pressure-volume relationship has been shown [8, 36]. Formula or equations simulating this measure by non-invasive modalities have been developed [37] and may be applicable in recent large population-based studies.

Pathophysiology of Systolic-Ventricular and Arterial Stiffening

Combined systolic-ventricular and arterial stiffening caninfluence cardiovascular function in several ways. The coupled physiologic interaction between ventricle and peripheral artery system makes the chronic adaptation of ventricular function to prolonged, elevated after-load induced by hypertension mandatory. Increased sensitivity of changes in blood pressure to circulating volume is common in HFpEF patients and may triggerrapid-onset pulmonary edema [38]. Although ascribed to low LVdiastolic compliance, similar blood pressure sensitivity is notobserved in systolic-depression with elevated EDP. Rather,combined ventricular-arterial stiffening more directlypredicts enhanced pressure-load dependence[39], which redistributes the blood flowinto more compliant pulmonaryveins.

Another consequence of ventricular-arterial stiffening is the increase in myocardial oxygen consumption[40], which may limit cardiac reserve in those with concomitant coronary artery disease.Finally, increased ventricular-arterial stiffening and theconsequent rise in systolic pressure during stress can worsendiastolic function.Cardiac relaxation is delayed by elevated systolic pressureand can translate into increased LVEDP and limited ventricular filling,which exacerbate hypertensive stress responses[16].

Elevated peripheral arterial resistancehas been considered an adaptive response to impaired ventricular contractility and end-organ perfusion [41]. It is commonly found in advanced heart failure. Decreased arterial compliance is one of the earliest detectable structural changes in the vessel wall. Stiffening in medium-sized and large elastic arteries is associated with multiple cardiovascular risk factors-including hypertension, dyslipidemia, obesity, smoking, diabetes, and aging [42]. Recent investigations have sought to confirm the presence of arterial stiffening during the early stages of myocardial dysfunction to identify its potential role in the development of HFpEF [43].

One recent study showed a constant association between carotid arterial stiffness and impaired regional LV function in a cohort of asymptomaticindividuals without previously diagnosed cardiovascular disease [44]. Impaired aortic elastic properties, even in the pre-hypertension stage, was associated with reduced vascular wall strain reflecting lower aortic distensibility and potentially increased stiffness [45]. By using the distensibility coefficient, a direct measure of carotid vascular compliance, the authors further confirmed the presence of arterial stiffness in the setting of sub-clinical myocardial dysfunction. The prognostic significance of such asymptomatic alterations in myocardial contractility has yet to be determined.

Because arterial stiffness correlateswell with the severity of atherosclerosis, impaired arterial complianceis associated with ventricular dysfunction through atherosclerosis and related ischemic events. Sub-clinical atherosclerosis is also associated with regional myocardial dysfunction [46]. Conduit vessel resistance, particularly in the setting of coronary stenosis, may increase myocardial vulnerability to falls in coronary perfusion, resulting in sub-endocardial ischemia[47].Furthermore, the association between arterial stiffening and myocardial dysfunction can be regional in nature, and heterogeneously located plaques may influence the distribution of ventricular dysfunction.

There are several mechanisms that also may contribute to the relationship between arterial stiffening and myocardial dysfunction. Hyperactivity of the renin-angiotensin-aldosterone system (RAAS) may produce both vascular and ventricular damage and adverse remodeling [48].Drops in diastolic blood pressure due to arterial stiffness may compromise coronary bloodflow, even in the absence of significant coronary stenotic lesions [49]. Impaired myocardial oxygenation, especially at the level of small coronary vessels, may lead to myocardial fibrosis and deposition of vascular collagen [50].

A reasonable explanation for the relationship between decreased arterial compliance and LV dysfunction involves persistent hypertension, chronic pulsatileloading, and subsequent ventricular hypertrophy predisposing to impaired myocardial function. In the Fernandes study[23],carotid arterial compliance was negatively associated with regional myocardial function even after antihypertensive therapy. Therefore, it appears that arterial stiffness *per se*, rather than its sequelae, are directly associated with alterations in regional myocardial function. This finding coincides with recent work demonstrating that arterial-ventricular stiffening can progress even in the absence of cardiac hypertrophy[51]. The coupling effects of vascular and ventricular stiffening increase the response of systolic pressure to changes in filling volume.[18].In addition to baroreflex and autonomic dysfunction, combined stiffening could furtherexaggerated pressure drop with diuretics and postural shifts in the elderly [18,51].

Measure of Myocardial Stiffness, Remodeling and Subclinical Systolic Dysfunction

Measure of ventricular contractility, such as end-systolic elasticity, has been mentioned to be influenced by ventricular geometry. Evidences supporting diastolic dysfunction or chamber stiffness in hypertensive subjects with HFpEF by echocardiography are based on conventional, noninvasive analysis Doppler findings such as relaxationdelay, increased velocity of E-wave deceleration, and reversed E/A ratio [53, 54]. Recent studies on invasive analysis have also shown a high prevalence of LVEDP elevation and relaxation delay [55], thoughstudies of the association between HF and more direct measures of vascularstiffness have been less consistent. E/A reverse is often seen in asymptomatic elderly or hypertensive people, which do not meet the defined criteria for heart failure. In addition, such estimates are prone to load changes and have biphasic stage based on early and late mitral inflow ratio and can be misleading in some occasions. Therefore, some investigators have hypothesized that impaired relaxation is a precursor to overt heart failure, meaning that symptoms of heart failure can be revealed during stress tests in these patients[56].

Surrogate of estimating myocardial damage, conventionally measured by longitudinal myocardial velocity as tissue velocity or tissue Doppler imaging, has long been used for objective assessment of diastolic dysfunction [57, 58, 59]. Impaired ventricular filling due to worse compliance by combination usage of conventional Doppler and tissue Doppler imaging has been validated with invasive catheterization data [60]. Diastolic dysfunction detected by tissue Doppler imaging as a useful clinical tool in the early evaluation of earlier stage myocardial dysfunction as a progression from hypertension, diastolic dysfunction to diastolic heart failure accompanied with ventricular geometric remodeling or functional disturbances has been well known. Such easy measure in the detection of myocardial longitudinal motion as a reliable evaluation of myocardial contraction and relaxation velocity in hypertensives may be sensitive to "subtle" myocardial damage and has been shown to reflect improvement of myocardial dysfunction after treatment before ventricular geometric changes [61, 62, 63]. Atrial pumping, assessed by peak late-diastolic mitralannular velocity utilizing pulsed-wave tissue Doppler imaging has also been introduced, which was reported to be capable of identifying hypertensive patients with a history of atrial fibrillation [64].

Recently developed, emerging myocardial imaging technique such as deformationimaging including strain (S) or strain rate (SR) has been used to quantify the intrinsic cardiac contractility and relaxation [65, 66]. Before the introduction of such deformation imaging, tissue velocity has been used for this purpose as mentioned above. Theoretically, strain rate (SR) imaging examines the velocity gradient between 2 adjacent points of pre-defined distance along the ultrasound beam separated by a fixed distance which then generate data in units of inverse seconds. The integration of SR with time would lead to strain formation, expressed as percentage, representing the normal myocardial deformation in the region of interest.These advanced techniques can actually analyze cardiac motion and deformation irrespective of echo beam direction which may thus provide a very good chance in the detailed understanding of cardiac mechanics from all portions not limited to ventricle [67, 68, 69].

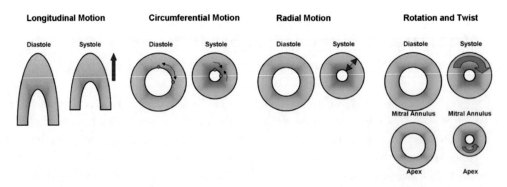

Figure 3. Various cardiac motion and deformation patterns displayed from left to right. Longitudinal motion denotes upward contraction from mitral annulus plane result in shortening of longitudinal axis.
Circumferential motion denotes shortening of cardiac curvature due to decreased LV diameter during cardiac systole while radial motion denotes systolic myocardial thickening from short-axis planes. Contra-lateral cardiac rotation from different short-axis planes (mitral annulus versus apex) results in cardiac twist behavior during systolic process.

Though still remained controversial in some ways, most researchers do believe that these novel imaging techniques own several advantages in the aspect of clinical practice and are able to provide more accurate, dimensionless information which may render objective myocardial quantification possible without related confounding biological anthropometrics

[55, 70]. In addition, a more reasonable approach of cardiac contractile function by using these techniques (SR) may be due to their less load-independent features in some studies which may represent true myocardial contractility rather than effect of tethering [71, 72]. Also, these techniques also provide a measure which tends to be less tethered or influenced by cardiac motion or translational movement as assessed by tissue velocity modality [73, 74, 75].

By utilizing these advanced techniques, one can assess the objective quantification of myocardial performance of regional or global function at simultaneous cardiac cycle by off-line analysis. Due to the myocardial structure and spatial distribution, as least three different cardiac motions and thus derived strain and strain rates (longitudinal, circumferential and radial) can be quantified and assessed by such imaging modalities(Figure 3).

According to Torrent-Guasp's muscle band theory [76], the whole cardiac was wrapped into a continuous muscle band resulting in a characteristic helical architecture. The descending limb rising from mitral annulus to ventricular apex whirling back as ascending segment back to mitral annulus forms left-handed sub-epicardium and right-handed sub-endocardium separated by mid-wall circumferential fiber sheets [77] (Figure 4). Simultaneous contra-lateral (clockwise and counter-clockwise) and circular rotation of the ventricular basal (mitral annulus plane) and apical part from myocardial short-axis planes during systole may thus generate twist behavior – an important cardiac mechanics involved while contraction and unwrapping (Figure 3). Correlation between ventricular twist behavior and invasive hemodynamic data has been made, and has been shown to provide even better estimate than ejection fraction [78].

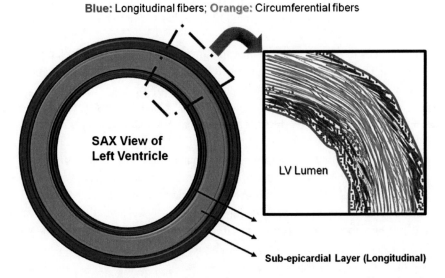

Figure 4. The heart is a complex biologic pump in part because of the complex orientation and architecture of transmural myofibers arrangement in the ventricular wall. The myofiber helix angle changes continuously from the more longitudinally distributed subendocardium to the obliquely distributed subepicardium, forming a right- to a left-handed oblique helix with a more circumferentially oriented midwall myofiber in between. Mathematical models have shown that this counterdirectional helical arrangement of muscle fibers in the heart is energetically efficient with synergistic use of inversely oriented skeletal muscle pairs which may help maintain stability and minimizes energy expenditure. The role and clinical significance of such myofiber sheets arrangement are not yet understood very well.

This unique anatomy and spatial configuration of LVactually reflects complicated cardiac mechanics and may help explain the highly efficient cardiac performance facilitating abrupt lumen emptying and susequent early diastolic suction in a very short period.As mentioned above, the obliqually arranged longitudinal fiber lining the right-handed, sub-endocardial layer susceptible to early myocardial damage may be the main target of longitudinal functional measure.

Deteriorated left atrial function, assessed by similar techniques, has also been reported to be a sensitive marker of early stage diastolic dysfunction [79]. Several recent exploratory studies utilizing such techniques have successfully identified subjects with HFpEF with global reduction in the value as compared to those with hypertension or normal controls [80]. Moreover, this parameter not only acts as a clinically feasible tool in the detection of deteriorated heart function in hypertensive subjects, but also may act as a useful guide inheart failure improvement responsive to therapy beyond blood pressure control. Frankly speaking, longitudinal function has been observed to be influenced earlier than short-axis function or twist in the heart failure subjects with relatively preserved ejection fraction [81] (Figure 2). One possible reason for this observation may come from that oblique endocardial fibers are more susceptible to myocardial ischemia or interstitial fibrosis from micro-injuries in subjects with potentially higher cardiovascular risks including hypertension or coronary artery disease [82, 83, 84]. Indeed, minor LV geometric changes were observed to accompany with reduced global longitudinal strain by Kuznetsova et al [85].

Factors influencing various myocardial strain or strain rate based on different direction may be different when different software or modality introduced. To what extent of such assessment from various directions remained inconclusive, however, a common consensus could be inconclusive.

Newer advances in magnetic resonance imaging techniques using displacement encoding with stimulated echo (DENSE), a validated MRI-based, phase-shift displacement technique in combination with phase contrast velocity mapping [86] or tagging techniques have also rendered objective quantification of regional and global stress/strain relationship and deformationwhich is currently ready for daily clinical practice and examined in large clinical studies [87, 88]. The basic utilization of tagging skills have allowed precise cardiac motion tracking which is capable of generating strain and strain rate data using identical pulse sequences with additional application of spatial modulation of magnetization (SPAMM). Recent multi-ethnic study by using magnetic resonance imaging (MRI) showed that in early stage atherosclerosis, concentric ventricular geometries were actually related to worsening myocardial systolic function in terms of circumferential S/SR, and subjects with reduced S/SR were observed to be associated with higher clinical events including heart failure hospitalization and mortality [89, 90, 91].

Such concentric ventricular phenotype changes, typically reflecting an earlier stage or minor form cardiac remodeling before hypertrophy, actually represents the cardiac adaptation process to elevated after-load. One important lesson form this study, however, could be the issue regarding heart failure with normal ejection fraction may come from those with geometric alterations. This finding, when combined with other associated studies, implied that potential diastolic or sub-clinical systolic dysfunction may come from those with ventricular phenotypic abnormalities in terms of concentric remodeling before overt ventricular hypertrophy. This longitudinal study, so far the largest prospective study with the most patient population enrolled, provide with the direct clue between diastolic heart failure and objective measures that could be steadily assessed by current imaging techniques.

Intriguingly, this assessment can be utilizedin a number of clinical scenarios associated with ealry stage disorders. Sironi et al ever reported that metabolic derangement linked to increased visceral fat deposition was associated with minor systolic dysfunction by measuring circumferential deformation [92]. Di Bello et al. also demonstrated that pre-HTN was associated with reduced global systolic function in terms of longitudinal myocardial strain imaging [93]. On the one hand, subjectswith cardiomyopathy or minor stable angina may demonstrate trivial myocardial dysfunction by utilizing such deformation imaging. On the other hand, systemic diseases such as HTN or diabetes were also shown to have deteriorated myocardial performance.

One major limitation in these studies, however, could be due to the lack of longitudinal data translating such imaging information into clinical outcomes in different populations from large scale studies. One possibility may be due to the relative time-consuming process of image analysis that can hardly put into daily practice.

HF Regression through Antihypertensive Therapy

Though advances in the current medical therapies and efforts have been made, the improvement of clinical outcomes of HFpEF remains limited, partially because of limited understanding of the underlying cardiac mechanisms and that earlier steps should be taken to prevent disease progression before a "point of no return" [94].

An increasing number of echo-based studies have identified associations between LVH regression and a lowered cardiac event rate, suggesting that LVH regression should be a treatment goal in hypertension [95,96].The recognition that arterial-ventricular systolic stiffness contribute to the hyperactivity of systolic pressures to ventricular volume changes may also have important therapeutic significance [18].

Though no available treatment can directly improve LV diastolic filling through its primary drug action and mechanisms involved, many clinical trials have documented the regression of LVH in response to antihypertensive therapy [97,98].It remains controversial whether there are differential drug effects and clinical outcomes. Regarding individual drug choices, available trial data favor ARB, ACEI, and long-acting calcium-channel-blocker (CCB) in that order[99, 100].In patients with small LV chamber size, high EF, and poor relaxation, slowing the heart rate with beta-blockers or CCBs may be beneficial [101]. Diuretics and sodium restriction may exacerbate this condition due to volume depletion.Combining negative inotropic agents to reduce systolic stiffness with vasodilators to lower vascular stiffness would be expected to substantially diminish these sensitivities of blood pressure and cardiac work to volume change. Thus, in elderly patients in whom volume management is problematic, or arterial pressures display marked liability with salt loading, diuretics, fluid intake or exertional stress, the combination vasodilator/negative inotropic therapy might prove beneficial[19].Because restrictive filling is often associated with myocardial fibrosis, aldosterone antagonists may have a role in reducing fibrosis through their hormonal effects [102].

Several co-morbidities, including diabetes, has been mentioned to participate or, aggravated such alterations with subsequent heart failure development [103]. Some diabetic patients may still have macrovascular (myocardial infarction, stroke) or microvascular (retinopathy, nephropathy, neuropathy) disease progression even under tight sugar control [104]. The potential role of sub-clinical LV structural and functional improvement after such hypertension and blood sugar control has not yet been demonstrated so far. There is little information regarding the difference of such potential functional improvement in hypertensive patients with or without diabetes after pharmacological therapy. However, vascular endothelial dysfunction and remodeling under such circumstances may lead to vascular stiffness and worsen cardiovascular risk [105]. Up to 50% of patients with a history of hypertension have evidence of diastolic dysfunction[106], which represents an attractive target for heart failure prevention. A link between the persistent pressure overloading of the interaction of heart and vascular load in combination with diabetes or not, and also by intrinsic changes in the heart itself, and common co-morbidities such as diabetes, hypertension, renal disease, and neurohumoral stress that impact both systems. Importantly, such combined stiffening not only alters the heart-arterial interactions at rest, but particularly under stress by exertional demands, salt loading, and abrupt changes in heart function. In this broad sense, combined ventricular-arterial stiffening has a large impact on cardiovascular reserve, blood pressure liability and diastolic dysfunction, coronary and peripheral flow regulation, endothelial function, mechanical signaling, and other factors.

References

[1] Roger VL, Weston SA, Redfield MM, et al. Trends in heart failure incidence and survival in a community-based population. *JAMA* 2004;292:344-50.

[2] Redfield MM. Heart failure - an epidemic of uncertain proportions. *N Engl J Med* 2002;347:1442-4.

[3] Davis BR, Kostis JB, Simpson LM, et al. Heart failure with preserved and reduced left ventricular ejection fraction in the Antihypertensive and Lipid-Lowering Treatment to Prevent Heart Attack Trial. *Circulation* 2008;118:2259–2267.

[4] Owan TE, Redfield MM. Epidemiology of Diastolic Heart Failure. *Prog Cardiovasc Dis*. 2005;47:320-332.

[5] Willenheimer R, Dahlöf B, Rydberg E, Erhardt L: AT$_1$-receptor blockers in hypertension and heart failure: clinical experience and future directions. *Eur Heart J* 1999 , 20:997-1008.

[6] Querejeta R, López B, González A, et al. Increased collagen type I synthesis in patients with heart failure of hypertensive origin. Relation to myocardial fibrosis*Circulation* 2004;110:1263-1268.

[7] He J. Ogden LG, Bazzano LA et al. Risk factors for congestive heart failure in US men and women: NHANES I epidemiologic follow-up study. *Arch Intern Med*. 2001;161:996-1002.

[8] Levy D, Larson MG, Vasan RS, et al. The progression from hypertension to congestive heart failure. *JAMA* 1996;275:1557-1562.

[9]   De Simone G, Pasanisi F, Contaldo F. Link of nonhemodynamic factors to hemodynamic determinants of left ventricular hypertrophy. *Hypertension* 2001;38:13-18.

[10]   Mayet J, Hughes A. Cardiac and vascular pathophysiology in hypertension. *Heart*. 2003 Sep;89(9):1104-9.

[11]   Verma A, Medris A, Hicham S, et al. Prognostic implications of left ventricular mass and geometry following myocardial infarction. *J Am Coll Cardiol Img*. 2008; 1:582-591.

[12]   Berenji K, Drazner MH, Rothermel BA, Hill JA. Does load-induced ventricular hypertrophy progress to systolic heart failure? *Am J Physiol Heart Circ Physiol*. 2005 Jul;289(1):H8-H16.

[13]   Frohlich ED. Fibrosis and ischemia: the real risks in hypertensive heart disease. *Am J Hypertension* 2001;14:194S-199S

[14]   Roman MJ, Ganau A, Saba PS, Pini R, Pickering TG, Devereux RB. Impact of arterial stiffening on left ventricular structure. *Hypertension*. 2000 Oct;36(4):489-94.

[15]   Mottram PM, Haluska B, Leano R, Cowley D, Stowasser M, Marwick TH. Effect of aldosterone antagonism on myocardial dysfunction in hypertensive patients with diastolic heart failure. *Circulation*. 2004 Aug 3;110(5):558-65.

[16]   Kawaguchi M, Hay I, Fetics B, et al. Combined Ventricular Systolic and Arterial Stiffening in Patients With Heart Failure and Preserved Ejection Fraction: Implications for Systolic and Diastolic Reserve Limitations. *Circulation* 2003;107:714-720

[17]   Fortuno MA, Ravassa S, Fortuno A, et al. Cardiomyocyte apoptotic cell dath in arterial hypertension: mechanisms and potential management. *Hypertension* 2001;38:1406-1412.

[18]   Devereux RB, Wachtell K, Gerdts E, et al. Prognostic significance of left ventricular mass change during treatment of hypertension. *JAMA* 2004;292:2350-2356.

[19]   Vasan RS, Levy D. The role of hypertension and the pathogenesis of heart failure. A clinical mechanistic overview. *Arch Intern Med*. 1996;156:1789-1796.

[20]   Redfield MM, Jacobsen SJ, Borlaug BA, Rodeheffer RJ, Kass DA. Age- and gender-related ventricular-vascular stiffening: a community-based study. *Circulation*. 2005 Oct 11;112(15):2254-62.

[21]   Borlaug BA, Lam CS, Roger VL, Rodeheffer RJ, Redfield MM. . Contractility and Ventricular Systolic Stiffening in Hypertensive Heart Disease: Insights into the Pathogenesis of Heart Failure with Preserved Ejection Fraction. *J Am Coll Cardiol*. 2009 Jul 28;54(5):419-21.

[22]   Westermann D, Kasner M, Steendijk P, Spillmann F, Riad A, Weitmann K, Hoffmann W, Poller W, Pauschinger M, Schultheiss HP, Tschöpe C. Role of left ventricular stiffness in heart failure with normal ejection fraction.*Circulation*. 2008 Apr 22;117(16):2051-60.

[23]   Lam CS, Roger VL, Rodeheffer RJ, Bursi F, Borlaug BA, Ommen SR, Kass DA, Redfield MM. Cardiac structure and ventricular-vascular function in persons with heart failure and preserved ejection fraction from Olmsted County, Minnesota.*Circulation*. 2007 Apr 17;115(15):1982-90.

[24]   Yiu SF, Enriquez-Sarano M, Tribouilloy C, Seward JB, Tajik AJ. Determinants of the degree of functional mitral regurgitation in patients with systolic left ventricular dysfunction: A quantitative clinical study. *Circulation*. 2000 Sep 19;102(12):1400-6.

[25] Benjamin EJ, Levy D, Anderson KM, Wolf PA, Plehn JF, Evans JC, et al. Determinants of Doppler indexes of left ventricular diastolic function in normal subjects (the Framingham Heart Study). *Am J Cardiol*. 1992;70:508–15.

[26] Izzo JL Jr, Sica DA, Black HR. *Hypertension Primer: the essentials of high blood pressure*. Fourth edition. Chapter C150.

[27] Izzo JL Jr, Sica DA, Black HR. *Hypertension Primer: the essentials of high blood pressure*. Fourth edition. Chapter A60.

[28] Redfield MM, Jacobsen SJ, Burnett JC Jr, et al. Burden of systolic and diastolic ventricular dysfunction in the community: appreciating the scope of the heart failure epidemic. *JAMA* 2003;289:194-202.

[29] Skaluba SJ, Litwin SE. Mechanisms of exercise intolerance: Insights from tissue Doppler imaging. *Circulation* 2004;109:972-977.

[30] Kitzman DW, Higgenbotham MB, Cobb FR, et al. Exercise intolerance in patients with heart failure and preserved left ventricular systolic function: failure of the Frank-Starling mechanism. *J Am Coll Cardiol*. 1991;17:1065–1072.

[31] Leite-Moreira AF, Correia-Pinto J, Gillebert TC. Afterload induced changes in myocardial relaxation: a mechanism for diastolic dysfunction. *Cardiovasc Res*. 1999;43:344–353.

[32] Suga H, Sagawa K: Instantaneous pressure/volume relationships and their ratio in the excised, supported canine left ventricle. *Circulation Research* 1974, 35:117-126.

[33] Grossman W, Braunwald E, Mann T, McLaurin LP, Green LH: Contractile state of the left ventricle in man as evaluated from end-systolic pressure-volume relations. *Circulation* 1977, 56:845-852.

[34] Suga H, Sagawa K, Shoukas AA: Load independence of the instantaneous pressure/volume ratio of the canine left ventricle and effects of epinephrine and heart rate on the ratio. *Circulation Research* 1973, 32:314-322.

[35] Kass DA, Midei M, Graves W, Brinker JA, Maughan WL: Use of a conductance (volume) catheter and transient inferior vena cava occlusion for rapid determination of pressure-volume relationship in man. *Cathet Cardiovasc Diagn* 1988, 15:192-202.

[36] Baicu CF, Zile MR, Aurigemma GP, Gaasch WH. Left ventricular systolic performance, function, and contractility in patients with diastolic heart failure. *Circulation* 2005;111:2306 –12.

[37] Chen CH, Fetics B, Nevo E, et al. Noninvasive single-beat determination of left ventricular end-systolic elastance in humans. *J Am Coll Cardiol*. 2001;38:2028–2034.

[38] Gandhi SK, Powers JC, Nomeir AM, et al. The pathogenesis of acute pulmonary edema associated with hypertension. *N Engl J Med*. 2001;344:17–22.

[39] Chen CH, Nakayama M, Nevo E, et al. Coupled systolic-ventricular and vascular stiffening with age: implications for pressure regulation and cardiac reserve in the elderly. *J Am Coll Cardiol*. 1998;32:1221–1227.

[40] Kelly RP, Tunin R, Kass DA. Effect of reduced aortic compliance on cardiac efficiency and contractile function of in situ canine left ventricle. *Circ Res*. 1992;71:490–502.

[41] Gaasch WH, Zile MR. Left ventricular diastolic dysfunction and diastolic heart failure. *Annu Rev Med*. 2004;55:373–394.

[42] Sharrett AR, Ding J, Criqui MH, et al. Smoking, diabetes, and blood cholesterol differ in their associations with subclinical atherosclerosis: the Multiethnic Study of Atherosclerosis (MESA). *Atherosclerosis*. 2006;186:441–447.

[43] Haider AW, Larson MG, Franklin SS, Levy D. Systolic blood pressure, diastolic blood pressure, and pulse pressure as predictors of risk for congestive heart failure in the Framingham Heart Study. *Ann Intern Med*. 2003;138:10 –16.

[44] Fernandes VR, Polak JF, Cheng S, et al. Arterial stiffness is associated with regional ventricular systolic and diastolic dysfunction: the Multi-Ethnic Study of Atherosclerosis. *Arterioscler Thromb Vasc Biol*. 2008;28;194-201.

[45] Celik T, Iyisoy A, Kursaklioglu H, Turhan H, Cagdas Yuksel U, Kilic S, Kutsi Kabul H, Genc C. Impaired aortic elastic properties in young patients with prehypertension. *Blood Press Monit*. 2006 Oct;11(5):251-5.

[46] Fernandes VR, Polak JF, Edvardsen T, et al. Subclinical atherosclerosis and incipient regional myocardial dysfunction in asymptomatic individuals: the Multi-Ethnic Study of Atherosclerosis (MESA). *J Am Coll Cardiol*. 2006;47:2420 –2428.

[47] Kass DA, Saeki A, Tunin RS, Recchia FA. Adverse influence of systemic vascular stiffening on cardiac dysfunction and adaptation to acute coronary occlusion. *Circulation* 1996;93:1533–1541.

[48] Mahmud A, Feely J. Arterial stiffness and the renin-angiotensin-aldosterone system. *J Renin Angiotensin Aldosterone Syst*. 2004;5:102–108.

[49] Benetos A, Rudnichi A, Safar M, Guize L. Pulse pressure and cardiovascular mortality in normotensive and hypertensive subjects. *Hypertension* 1998;32:560 –564.

[50] Strauer BE. Development of cardiac failure by coronary small vessel disease in hypertensive heart disease? *J Hypertens Suppl*. 1991;9:S11–S20.

[51] Kass DA. Age-related changes in venticular-arterial coupling: pathophysiologic implications. *Heart Fail Rev*. 2002;7:51– 62.

[52] White M, Roden R, Minobe W, et al. Age-related changes in betaadrenergic neuroeffector systems in the human heart. *Circulation* 1994;90:1225–38.

[53] Díez J, Querejeta R, López B, González A, Larman M, Martínez Ubago JL. Losartan-dependent regression of myocardial fibrosis is associated with reduction of left ventricular chamber stiffness in hypertensive patients. *Circulation*. 2002 May 28;105(21):2512-7.

[54] Hatle L. How to diagnose diastolic heart failure a consensus statement. *Eur Heart J*. 2007;28(20):2421–3.

[55] Zile MR, Gaasch WH, Carroll JD, et al. Heart failure with a normal ejection fraction: is measurement of diastolic function necessary to make the diagnosis of diastolic heart failure? *Circulation* 2001;104:779–782.

[56] Caruana L, Petrie MC, Davie AP, et al. Do patients with suspected heart failure and preserved left ventricular systolic function suffer from "diastolic heart failure" or from misdiagnosis? A prospective descriptive study. *BMJ* 2000;321:215–218.

[57] MacIver D, Townsend M. A novel mechanism of heart failure with normal ejection fraction. *Heart* 2008;94:446.

[58] Yu CM, Lin H, Yan H, et al. Progression of systolic abnormalities in patients with "isolated" diastolic heart failure and diastolic dysfunction. *Circulation* 2002 Mar 12;105(10):1195-201.

[59] Vinereanu D, Nicolaides E, Tweddel A, Fraser A. "Pure" diastolic dysfunction is associated with long-axis systolic dysfunction. Implications for the diagnosis and classification of heart failure. Eur J Heart Fail 2005;7:820–8.

[60] Ommen SR, Nishimura RA, Appleton CP, Miller FA, Oh JK, Redfield MM, et al. Clinical utility of Doppler echocardiography and tissue Doppler imaging in the estimation of left ventricular filling pressures: A comparative simultaneous Dopplercatheterization study. *Circulation*. 2000;102(15):1788–94.

[61] Derumeaux G, Ovize M, Loufoua J, et al. Doppler tissue imaging quantitates regional wall motion during myocardial ischemia and reperfusion. Circulation 1998;97:1970– 7.

[62] Solomon S, Janardhanan R, Verma A, Bourgoun M, Daley W, Purkayastha, D, et al. Effect of angiotensin receptor blockade and antihypertensive drugs on diastolic function in patients with hypertension and diastolic dysfunction: a randomised trial. *Lancet* 2007;369:2079-87.

[63] Vinereanu D, Florescu N, Sculthorpe N, Tweddel AC, Stephens MR, Fraser AG. Differentiation between pathologic and physiologic left ventricular hypertrophy by tissue Doppler assessment of long-axis function in patients with hypertrophic cardiomyopathy or systemic hypertension and in athletes. *Am J Cardiol* 2001;88:53– 8.

[64] Toh N, Kanzaki H, Nakatani S, Ohara T, Kim J, Kusano KF, Hashimura K, Ohe T, Ito H, Kitakaze M. Left atrial volume combined with atrial pump function identifies hypertensive patients with a history of paroxysmal atrial fibrillation. *Hypertension*. 2010 May;55(5):1150-6.

[65] D'hooge J, Heimdal A, Jamal F, Kukulski T, Bijnens B, Rademakers F, Hatle L, Suetens P, Sutherland GR. Regional strain and strain rate measurements by cardiac ultrasound: principles, implementation and limitations. *Eur J Echocardiogr*. 2000 Sep;1(3):154-70.

[66] Edvardsen T, Gerber BL, Garot J, Bluemke DA, Lima JA, Smiseth OA. Quantitative assessment of intrinsic regional myocardial deformation by Doppler strain rate echocardiography in humans: validation against three-dimensional tagged magnetic resonance imaging. *Circulation* 2002;106:50–6.

[67] Langeland S, D'hooge J, Wouters PF, et al. Experimental validation of a new ultrasound method for the simultaneous assessment of radial and longitudinal myocardial deformation independent of insonation angle. *Circulation* 2005;112:2157-62.

[68] Leitman M, Lysyansky P, Sidenko S, et al. Two-dimensional strain-a novel software for real-time quantitative echocardiographic assessment of myocardial function. *J Am Soc Echocardiogr* 2004;17:1021-9.

[69] Amundsen BH, Helle-Valle T, Edvardsen T, et al. Noninvasive myocardial strain measurement by speckle tracking echocardiography: validation against sonomicrometry and tagged magnetic resonance imaging. *J Am Coll Cardiol* 2006; 47:789-93.

[70] Aurigemma GP, Zile MR, Gaasch WH. Contractile Behavior of the Left Ventricle in Diastolic Heart Failure: With Emphasis on Regional Systolic Function. *Circulation* 2006;113;296-304.

[71] Weidemann F, Jamal F, Sutherland GR, Claus P, Kowalski M, Hatle L, De Scheerder I, Bijnens B, Rademakers FE. Myocardial function defined by strain rate and strain during alterations in inotropic states and heart rate. *Am J Physiol Heart Circ Physiol* 283: H792–H799, 2002.

[72] Edvardsen T, Gerber BL, Garot J, Bluemke DA, Lima JA, Smiseth OA. Quantitative assessment of intrinsic regional myocardial deformation by Doppler strain rate

echocardiography in humans: validation against three-dimensional tagged magnetic resonance imaging. *Circulation* 2002;106:50–6.

[73] Paulus WJ, Tschope C, Sanderson JE, Rusconi C, Flachskampf FA, Rademakers FE et al. How to diagnose diastolic heart failure: a consensus statement on the diagnosis of heart failure with normal left ventricular ejection fraction by the Heart Failure and Echocardiography Associations of the European Society of Cardiology. *Eur Heart J* 2007;28:2539–50.

[74] Nagueh SF, Appleton CP, Gillebert TC, Marino PN, Oh JK, Smiseth OA et al. Recommendations for the evaluation of left ventricular diastolic function by echocardiography. *Eur J Echocardiogr* 2009;10:165–93.

[75] Abraham TP, Dimaano VL, Liang HY. Role of tissue Doppler and strain echocardiography in current clinical practice. *Circulation* 2007;116:2597–609.

[76] Torrent-Guasp F, Buckberg GD, Clemente C, Cox JL, Coghlan HC, Gharib M. The structure and function of the helical heart and its buttress wrapping. I. The normalmacroscopic structure of the heart. *Semin Thorac Cardiovasc Surg* 2001;13(4):301-319.

[77] Sosnovik DE, Baldwin SL, Lewis SH, Holland MR, Miller JG. Transmural variation of myocardial attenuation measured with a clinical imager. *Ultrasound Med Biol* 2001;27:1643–50.

[78] [1] Kim WJ, Lee BH, Kim YJ, et al. Apical rotation assessed by speckle-tracking echocardiography as an index of global left ventricular contractility. Circ Cardiovasc Imaging 2009;2:123-31.

[79] Otani K, Takeuchi M, Kaku K, Haruki N, Yoshitani H, Tamura M, Abe H, Okazaki M, Ota T, Lang RM, Otsuji Y. Impact of Diastolic Dysfunction Grade on Left Atrial Mechanics Assessed by Two-Dimensional Speckle Tracking Echocardiography. *J Am Soc Echocardiogr.* 2010 Jul 26.

[80] Maeder MT, Kaye DM. Heart failure with normal left ventricular ejection fraction. *J Am Coll Cardiol* 2009;53:905–18.

[81] Wang J, Khoury DS, Yue Y, et al. Preserved left ventricular twist and circumferential deformation, but depressed longitudinal and radial deformation in patients with diastolic heart failure. *Eur Heart J.* 2008 April;29(10):1283-1289.

[82] Mundhenke M, Schwartzkopff B, Strauer BE. Structural analysis of arteriolar and myocardial remodelling in the subendocardial region of patients with hypertensive heart disease and hypertrophic cardiomyopathy. Virchows Arch 1997;431:265– 73.

[83] Vinereanu D, Nicolaides E, Tweddel AC, et al. "Pure" diastolic dysfunction is associated with long-axis systolic dysfunction. Implications for the diagnosis and classification of heart failure. *Eur J Heart Fail* 2005;7:820–8.

[84] Shan K, Bick RJ, Poindexter BJ, et al. Relation of tissue Doppler derived myocardial velocities to myocardial structure and beta-adrenergic receptor density in humans. *J Am Coll Cardiol* 2000;36:891– 6.

[85] Kuznetsova T, Herbots L, Richart T, D'hooge J, Thijs L, Fagard RH, et al. Leftventricularstrainandstrainrateinageneralpopulation. *European Heart Journal* 2008 29(16):2014-2023.

[86] Wen H, Bennett E, Epstein N, Plehn J. Magnetic resonance imaging assessment of myocardial elastic modulus and viscosity using displacement imaging and phase-contrast velocity mapping. *Magn Reson Med.* 2005 Sep;54(3):538-48.

[87] Kim D, Gilson WD, Kramer CM, Epstein FH. Myocardial tissue tracking with two-dimensional cine displacement-encoded MR imaging: development and initial evaluation. *Radiology*. 2004 Mar;230(3):862-71.

[88] Petitjean C, Rougon N, Cluzel P. Assessment of myocardial function: a review of quantification methods and results using tagged MRI. *J Cardiovasc Magn Reson*. 2005;7(2):501-16.

[89] Rosen BD, Edvardsen T, Lai S, Castillo E, Pan L, Jerosch-Herold M, Sinha S, Kronmal R, Arnett D, Crouse JR 3rd, Heckbert SR, Bluemke DA, Lima JA. Left ventricular concentric remodeling is associated with decreased global and regional systolic function: the Multi-Ethnic Study of Atherosclerosis.*Circulation*. 2005 Aug 16;112(7):984-91.

[90] Bluemke DA, Kronmal RA, Lima JA, Liu K, Olson J, Burke GL, Folsom AR. The relationship of left ventricular mass and geometry to incident cardiovascular events: the MESA (Multi-Ethnic Study of Atherosclerosis) study. *J Am Coll Cardiol*. 2008 Dec 16;52(25):2148-55.

[91] Fernandes VR, Polak JF, Cheng S, Rosen BD, Carvalho B, Nasir K, McClelland R, Hundley G, Pearson G, O'Leary DH, Bluemke DA, Lima JA. Arterial stiffness is associated with regional ventricular systolic and diastolic dysfunction: the Multi-Ethnic Study of Atherosclerosis.*Arterioscler Thromb Vasc Biol*. 2008 Jan;28(1):194-201.

[92] Sironi AM, Pingitore A, Ghione S, De Marchi D, Scattini B, Positano V, Muscelli E, Ciociaro D, Lombardi M, Ferrannini E, Gastaldelli A. Early hypertension is associated with reduced regional cardiac function, insulin resistance, epicardial, and visceral fat. *Hypertension*. 2008 Feb;51(2):282-8.

[93] Di Bello V, Talini E, Dell'Omo G, Giannini C, Delle Donne MG, Canale ML, Nardi C, Palagi C, Dini FL, Penno G, Del Prato S, Marzilli M, Pedrinelli R. Early left ventricular mechanics abnormalities in prehypertension: a two-dimensional strain echocardiography study. *Am J Hypertens*. 2010 Apr;23(4):405-12.

[94] Zhang Q, Fung JW, Yip GW, et al. Improvement of left ventricular myocardial short-axis, but not long-axis function or torsion after cardiac resynchronization therapy: an assessment by two-dimensional speckle tracking. *Heart* 2008;94:1464-71.

[95] Wachtell K, Bella JN, Rokkedal J, et al. Change in diastolic left ventricular function after one year of antihypertensive treatment: the LIFE trial. *Circulation* 2002;105:1071-1076.

[96] Frey N, Katus HA, Olson EN, et al. Hypertrophy of the heart a new therapeutic target? *Circulation* 2004;109:1580-1589.

[97] Okin PM, Devereux RB, Jern S, et al. Regression of electrocardiographic left ventricular hypertrophy during antihypertensive treatment and the prediction of major cardiovascular events: the LIFE study. *JAMA* 2004;292:2343-2349.

[98] Matthew J, Sleight P, Lonn E, et al. Reduction of cardiovascular risk by regression of electrocardiographic markers of left ventricular hypertrophy by the angiotensin-converting enzyme inhibitor ramipril. *Circulation* 2001;104:1615-1621.

[99] Devereux RB, Dahlof B, Gerdts E, et al. Regression of hypertensive left ventricular hypertrophy by losartan compared with atenolol. *Circulation* 2004;110:1456-1462.

[100] Heart Failure Society of America. Executive summary: HFSA 2006 Comprehensive heart failure practice guideline.*J Card Fail*. 2006;12(1):10-38.

[101] Kass DA, Wolff MR, Ting CT, et al. Diastolic compliance of hypertrophied ventricle is not acutely altered by pharmacologic agents influencing active processes. *Ann Intern Med.* 1993;119:466-73.

[102] Lea WB, Kwak ES, Luther JM, et al. Aldosterone antagonism or synthase inhibition reduces end-organ damage induced by treatment with angiotensin and high salt. *Kidney Int.* 2009;75:936-44.

[103] van Heerebeek L, Hamdani N, Handoko ML, Falcao-Pires I, Musters RJ, Kupreishvili K, Ijsselmuiden AJ, Schalkwijk CG, Bronzwaer JG, Diamant M, BorbÉly A, Velden J, Stienen GJ, Laarman GJ, Niessen HW, Paulus WJ: Diastolic stiffness of the failing diabetic heart: importance of fibrosis, advanced glycation end products, and myocyte resting tension. *Circulation* 2008, 117:43-51.

[104] Patel A, Chalmers J, Chaturvedi V, et al. Diabetes and vascular disease: a new international trial. *Asian Cardiovasc Thorac Ann.* 2003;11:180-184.

[105] ijan S, Hayward RA. Treatment of hypertension in type 2 diabetes mellitus: blood pressure goals, choice of agents, and setting priorities in diabetes care. *Ann Intern Med.* 2003;138:593-602.

[106] Shah SJ, Gheorghiade M. Heart failure with preserved ejection fraction: treat now by treating comorbidities. *JAMA* 2008;300:431-433.

In: Systolic Blood Pressure   ISBN: 978-1-61209-263-8
Editor: Robert A. Arfi   ©2012 Nova Science Publishers, Inc.

Chapter V

Antihypertensive Drugs Association: An Update

M. Destro, F. Cagnoni and A. D'Ospina

Centro Diagnosi e Cura Ipertensione Arteriosa –
Ospedale Unificato Broni Stradella- Stradella (PV) - Italy

Introduction

It is well established that chronic, poorly controlled hypertension is an independent risk factor for cardiovascular morbidity and mortality, stroke and renal failure and in consequence controlling high blood pressure can reduce complications such as heart attack, heart failure, stroke, kidney failure and premature death. Confirming this statement, a prospective analysis of the 36-year follow-up data from the Framingham Heart Study demonstrated that hypertension (Systo-Diastolic blood pressure $\geq$ 140/90 mm Hg) is an important risk factor contributing to all major atherosclerotic CVD outcomes, including CHD, stroke, peripheral artery disease, and heart failure (1). Although a common and treatable risk factor for cardiovascular morbidity and mortality, hypertension is still highly prevalent, affecting approximately 1 billion individuals worldwide. Though awareness and treatment of hypertension has increased over the years, substantial improvements in blood pressure control rates are still lacking, despite availability of multiple antihypertensive agents with various pharmacological mechanisms of action and relatively few side effects. As a matter of facts because of the high prevalence of hypertension in the general population, approximately 35% of atherosclerotic CVD events may be attributable to hypertension.

In addition to being a powerful risk factor for cardiovascular disease, hypertension in elderly patients increases the risk of decline in cognitive function (2).

Due to the complex nature of hypertension, it is not surprising that single antihypertensive agents normalize blood pressure for less than a majority of hypertensive patients, and to lower the risk of complications from uncontrolled high blood pressure it is vital to treat patients early and aggressively.

Given the just mentioned poor blood pressure control rates observed worldwide, it is important to carefully examine the numerous factors that influence blood pressure control. One important factor is the efficacy of the antihypertensive agent prescribed: it is important to choose an effective agent in order to maximize the chances of achieving goal blood pressure.

Patient adherence is another critically important factor influencing blood pressure control. No matter how well an antihypertensive agent works in a short-term clinical trial, it will not be effective in the clinical setting if patients do not continue to take it over the long term. One of the most important factor that may impact control is convenience of dosing.

The tolerability profile of an agent can have a major impact on patient adherence.

Hypertension is generally asymptomatic for most patients; thus, a poorly tolerated drug with troublesome side effects may cause patients to feel worse while taking the drug than they did prior to the initiation of therapy; this fact will likely lead them to discontinue treatment, which, in turn, will lead to poor blood pressure control.

An antihypertensive agent should, therefore, be effective and also have an excellent safety and tolerability profile and a simple, convenient dosing schedule. As we said, the lack of overt symptomatology in hypertension (until it progresses) makes side effects even more intolerable to patients; if the adverse events observed with many antihypertensive drugs occur too frequently or are too severe, patients often skip or completely discontinue their blood pressure medication altogether.

If blood pressure medications are not taken as directed, drug efficacy is severely compromised, and a compromise in efficacy leads to uncontrolled blood pressure and, eventually, elevations above target range.

There are many mechanisms involved in hypertension and it's now absolutely clear that one class of drug alone does not target all mechanisms at the same time; monotherapy is often insufficient to bring blood pressure down to a safe range.

Actually several evidences coming from wide Clinical Studies confirm that the majority of hypertensive patients require two or more agents to reach blood pressure goal, and for those patients with stage 2 hypertension (or blood pressure > 20/10 mmHg above goal), it is recommended that treatment is initiated with a combination of two drugs from different classes; consequently most of the treatment guidelines for hypertension recommend that patients with baseline blood pressure ≥160/100 mmHg should be given a combination of two molecules from different drug classes as initial therapy.

The renin-angiotensin-aldosterone system plays a crucial role in blood pressure regulation and hypertension-related complications. Angiotensin-converting enzyme inhibitors were the first to be used to block the RAAS and now have many compelling indications in the treatment of hypertension and its cardiovascular and renal complications. Angiotensin II receptor blockers, introduced 20 years later, have been shown to be equally as effective as antihypertensive (2-4)treatment also in particular categories of patients (3, 5-7) and are also associated with a lower number of side effects. Furthermore, in clinical trials ARBs and ACEIs were associated with comparable benefits for their most typical indications.

In addition, due to the development of direct renin inhibitors, blockade of the renin–angiotensin–aldosterone system at the level of theinteraction of renin with a substrate has become a clinical reality; the potential of renin inhibition must be viewed in the context of the remarkable efficacy of both angiotensin converting enzyme inhibition and angiotensin receptor blockers.There is an approximately linear relationship between relative risk of cardiovascular events and level of blood pressure, at least at levels between about 115/75 and

180/105 mmHg (8-10).Randomized clinical trials have demonstrated a 20% to 30% *relative* reduction in overall cardiovascular risk with antihypertensive treatment across this wide range of blood pressure levels (11-17). More importantly, the absolute cardiovascularrisk reduction is directly related to the pre-treatment blood pressure levels.

Although specific clinical trial evidence only confirms the value of systolic blood pressure reduction to 140 mmHg, the totality of available evidence supports the benefit of blood pressure reduction to even lower levels in individuals at high risk(12-13, 18-19).On the other hand, the benefits of lowering systolic blood pressure below that level in patients with mildly elevated blood pressure but at low absolute risk, are small. Multiple trials have addressed the question of whether more aggressive treatment of blood pressure improves outcomes. For instance, in the Hypertension Optimal Treatment (HOT) trial (20), the targeted blood pressure separations were not sufficient to determine whether "the lower" was "the better"; on the other hand in the United Kingdom Prospective Diabetes Study (UKPDS) (19) a tighter control of blood pressure resulted in better cardiovascular disease outcome in individuals with diabetes. Although the available data are consistent with the notion that lower blood pressure levels, within the usual range seen in clinical settings, are beneficial, few clinical data currently support treatment to a level <140/90 mmHg in the overall population(10).

The ESH/ESC 2007 Guidelines underlined that regardless of the drug employed, monotherapy allows to achieve blood pressure target in only a limited number of hypertensive patients and that the use of more than one agent is necessary to achieve target blood pressure in the majority of patients. A vast array of effective and well tolerated combinations is available; the ESH/ESC 2007 Guidelines also suggested that a combination of two drugs at low doses should be preferred as first step treatment when initial blood pressure is in the grade 2 or 3 range or if total cardiovascular risk is high or very high. Moreover, these Guidelines consider that in several patients blood pressure control is not achieved by two drugs, so introducing the concept that a combination of three or more drugs is sometimes required.

Two-Drugs Combination
Antihypertensive Treatment

The practice of combining agents that counteract different mechanisms is the most likely explanation for the fact that most available two-drugs combinations have an agent that addresses renin secretion and/or angiotensin II action (e.g.: beta blockers, angiotensin converting enzyme inhibitors [ACE's], angiotensin II receptor blockers [ARBs] or direct direct renin inhibitors) combined with another one that that is more effective in rennin-independent hypertension (e.g.: diuretics, dihydropiridine or non dihydropiridine calcium channel blockers [CCBs]).

For example, considering a combination of an ARB with a CCB, a well conducted Randomized Clinical Study (21) showed that the combination of olmesartan (ARB) and amlodipine (CCB) resulted in significantly greater blood pressure lowering in patients not achieving adequate blood pressure control with olmesartan monotherapy, thus allowing a significantly greater proportion of patients to achieve blood pressure goal. In fact blood pressure goal rates were significantly higher with olmesartan/amlodipine 20 mg/5 mg and olmesartan/amlodipine 20 mg/10 mg (44.5% and 45.8%,) vs. olmesartan/placebo (28.5%).

Another study has assessed the effect of irbesartan (ARB) and irbesartan/hydrochlorotiazide (HCTZ) on blood pressure in 14,200 patients with uncontrolled hypertension with or without the Metabolic Syndrome (22-23). Both irbesartan and irbesartan/HCTZ produced significant reductions in systolic blood pressure and diastolic blood pressure over the 9-month study period (irbesartan monotherapy, 26.8/13.3 mmHg,; irbesartan/HCTZ, 27.9/14.2 mmHg,), and blood pressure normalization was achieved by 66% of patients receiving monotherapy and 79% of those receiving irbesartan/HCTZ.

Considering a particular group of hypertensive patients, in the ATHOS Study (24) has been made a comparison of the associations telmisartan (ARB) / HCTZ vs amlodipine/HCTZ in older patients with predominantly systolic hypertension: systolic blood pressure was significantly reduced with telmisartan/ HCTZ compared with amlodipine /HCTZ in the 24 h, morning and daytime examined periods.

Still using HCTZ but in combination with another ARB, other another Randomized Clinical Study (25-26) investigated the efficacy and tolerability of valsartan or hydrochlorothiazide (HCTZ) monotherapy and higher-dose combinations (val 320/HCTZ 12.5 mg or val 320/HCTZ 25 mg) in patients with essential hypertension. Both combinations resulted in a significantly greater proportion of responders at study than monotherapy. In addition, a dose-response was observed with increasing dose of HCTZ with respect to mean sitting systolic blood pressure. Both dosages were well tolerated and the combination of valsartan and HCTZ at high dosage (320/12.5 mg and 320/25 mg) increased antihypertensive efficacy in patients with mild-to-moderate hypertension inadequately controlled with valsartan 320 mg monotherapy, without compromising tolerability. In addition, the valsartan/HCTZ combinations were associated with an attenuation of the potassium increase usually seen when using RAAS inhibitors.

In one of our Study (27) we compared efficacy and safety of amlodipine/valsartan with amlodipine monotherapy in patients with stage 2 hypertension. Amlodipine/valsartan 10/160 mg was found to be more effective than amlodipine 10 mg in stage 2 hypertension. The results were statistically significant and showed that dual mechanism CCB/ARB therapy with amlodipine/valsartan was associated with significant improvements, compared mean reduction from baseline in mean sitting systolic blood pressure, providing additional support for the rationale of combining drugs with complementary mechanisms of action, such as amlodipine/valsartan, for the treatment of patients withstage 2 hypertension.

Again considering combination treatmentvs. monotherapy, we repute very interesting a prespecified secondary analysis of the COACH study (28) based on baseline hypertension severity and prior antihypertensive medication use and a post-hoc efficacy analysis of the subset of patients with baseline mean seated systolic blood pressure ≥ 180 mmHg; the efficacy and safety of placebo, amlodipine (5 or 10 mg/day), olmesartan medoxomil (10, 20, or 40 mg/day), and all possible combinations of the drugs were evaluated for 8 weeks. In each subgroup, ≥ 1 dosage combination of amlodipine + olmesartan significantly reduced mean seated diastolic and systolic blood pressure compared with constituent monotherapies. Combinations produced the greatest mean blood pressure reductions in patients with baseline mean seated systolic blood pressure ≥180 mm Hg and, finally, more patients with stage 1 than stage 2 hypertension achieved blood pressure goal.

More recently two Studies investigated the efficacy, safety and tolerability of the direct renin inhibitor aliskiren in association with HCTZ in patients non-responsive to HCTZ monotherapy (29-30). In both Studies Aliskiren/HCTZ treatment showed similar tolerability to HCTZ alone and a numerically lower incidence of potassium changes, while providing clinically significant blood pressure reductions and improved blood pressure control rates in patients who are non-responsive to HCTZ monotherapy.

Other Authors (31) investigated the blood pressure lowering effects of the oral direct renin inhibitor aliskiren, alone or in combination with the angiotensin receptor blocker valsartan; at first aliskiren monotherapy provided anti-hypertensive efficacy and placebo-like tolerability in patients with hypertension, meanwhile secondary analysis showed that aliskiren and valsartan in combination may provide additive blood pressure-lowering effects with maintained tolerability.

Finally, several Clinical Studies have suggested suboptimal persistence and adherence to thiazide diuretic monotherapy making them somewhere and somehow still recommended as initial treatment for hypertension; on this issue an interesting analysis compared patient persistence and adherence with hydrochlorothiazide monotherapy to fixed-dose combinations containing HCTZ (32); the study cohort consisted of 48,212 patients; 72.5% used HCTZ, 13.2% ACEI/HCTZ, 9.3% ARB/HCTZ, and 5.0% BB/HCTZ; mean age was 53.7 years and 66.5% were female. Results reported that a significantly lower proportion of patients using HCTZ (29.9%) remained persistent with therapyat 12 months compared with ARB/HCTZ, ACEI/HCTZ and BB/HCTZ; similarly, PDC was lower for HCTZ patients (32.5%) as compared to ARB/HCTZ (53.7%), ACEI/HCTZ (50.9%), and BB/HCTZ (51.3%). MPR was also significantly lower for HCTZ patients as compared to those using fixed-dose combination therapies. All these data seemed to confirm that initiating HCTZ fixed-dose combination therapy with an ACEI, ARB, or BB was associated with greater persistence and adherence in comparison with HCTZ monotherapy.

Three-Drugs Combination Antihypertensive Treatment

About 23-54% of patients require ≥3 drugs to control their blood pressure (BP). This data has been confirmed by Clinical trials including ALLHAT, ACCOMPLISH, INVEST, and LIFE, which have reported that 23% to 54% patients require three or more antihypertensive agents for BP control and target-level maintenance (<140/90 or <130/80 mmHg depending on cardiovascular risk) (33-36).

Combination therapy with complementary mechanisms of action increases the probability of treatment success. Numerous single-pill combinations with two drugs are available but BP largely remains uncontrolled, more so in the elderly, black, diabetic, obese, and severely hypertensive patients (19,37-38). Because the different double combinations of RAAS blockers, amlodipine and HCTZ have shown to give good result in lowering blood pressure, but considering that about 23-54% of patients require ≥3 drugs to control their blood pressure, a Study (39) was performed to evaluate the efficacy and safety of a triple combinations of the three above mentioned molecules: results showed that triple therapy was significantly superior to all of the dual therapies in reducing mean sitting systolic blood pressure and mean sitting diastolic blood pressure from baseline to end point. The addition of HCTZ in this design followed the general clinical practice of adding another agent only if the patients are unable to achieve a target BP level. Significantly more patients on triple therapy achieved overall blood pressure control (<140/90 mm Hg) and systolic and diastolic control compared with each dual therapy; Aml/Val/HCTZ was well tolerated and the benefits of triple therapy over dual therapy were observed regardless of age, sex, race, ethnicity, or baseline mean sitting systolic blood pressure.

Substantially the same results were obtained in a *post hoc* analysis (40) of the EX-EFFeCTS Study (27) by which the efficacy and safety of amlodipine/valsartan/ hydrochlorothiazide and Aml/HCTZ combinations in the subgroup of patients receiving add-on HCTZ were evaluated; also in this case it has been demonstrated that therapies combining drugs with complimentary mechanisms of actionlike a CCB, an ARB and a thiazide diuretic have been shown to achieve better blood pressure control and attenuate adverse events like peripheral edema and hyperkalemia (38,41-42).

Finally, we can argue that initiation of antihypertensive treatment with combination therapy is recommended in patients with BP ≥20/10 mmHg above goal (44-45). On average, 3.2 drugs might be needed to achieve BP control (46). Studies using a design similar to clinical practice that involves a sequential treatment algorithm of dual therapy followed by triple therapy, have reported 80-90% of stage 2 hypertensive patients achieving BP goals by the end of treatment (47).

Special Features and Comorbility: Hypertension, Diabetes and Nephropathy

It has been observed that as many as 60% of patients with diabetes also have hypertension(48); blood pressure control rates are poor among diabetic persons, and blood pressure targets are not reached in approximately two thirds of these patients (49). Given the severe cardiovascular and renal complications associated with both diabetes and hypertension, the lack of blood pressure control is a major concern (50). According to the ESH/ESC 2007 guidelines in these patients goal should be <130/80 mmHg and the antihypertensive treatment may be started already when blood pressure is in the high-normal range.

In patients with type 2 Diabetes Mellitus and albuminuria, overactivation of the RAAS occurs and angiotensin II mediates a number of effects from increased collagen synthesis to proliferation of smooth muscle cells, arterial wall fibrosis, accumulation and activation of inflammatory cells, and increased vascular permeability, which result in premature vascular and renal complications (51).

Increased (intra)renal activity of the renin-angiotensin system may cause a persistent increase in renovascular resistance and intraglomerular pressure especially in patients with diabetes, thus contributing to the development of diabetic renal damage.

The ideal treatment strategy in hypertensive patients with diabetes remains to be defined. An exploratory analysis (52) was undertaken comparing results in the diabetic and non-diabetic cohorts from 3 randomized multicenter trials (Val-MARC, VALOR and VELOCITY) (53-55) that evaluated different blood pressure-lowering treatment strategies with ARB monotherapy and/ or ARB plus hydrochlorothiazide combination therapy. Across all 3 studies, combination treatment was, as expected, consistently more effective compared with monotherapy in both diabetic and non-diabetic patients.

To evaluate the effect of dual blockage of the renin-angiotensin system by adding maximal recommended dose of ARB with maximal recommended dose of ACE inhibitors in type 2 diabetic patients with diabetic nephropathy a Clinical Study (56) was performed. Tthe examined population included type 2 diabetic patients with UPCr > 0.5 gm/gm and hypertension who received maximal recommended dose of ACE inhibitors (enalapril 40 mg/day) over three months; at the end of this period the subjects were randomized to two groups: ARB group received adding maximal recommended dose of ARB (telmisartan 80 mg/day) and control group received previous ACE inhibitors only for 24 weeks. The results showed that adding maximal recommended dose of ARB with maximal recommended dose of ACE inhibitors in type 2 diabetic patients can reduce proteinuria more than ACE inhibitors alone; no serious adverse events were reported during both treatments.

Special Features and Comorbility: Hypertension and Left Ventricular Hypertrophy (LVH)

In patients with hypertension and LVH, both an angiotensin converting enzyme inhibitor and an angiotensin type 1 receptor antagonist regress LVH; however, it remains controversial whether dual blockade of the renin-angiotensin system will regress LVH using a combination of ACE inhibitor and AT1 antagonist in these particular group of patients.

To help in solving the last question a Clinical Study has been performed: the results showed that both ACE inhibitors and AT1 antagonists benefit the regression of LVH in diabetic patients who start dialysis therapy(57); moreover, combination therapy with ACE inhibitors and AT1 antagonists would provide more beneficial effects on LVH in these patients than monotherapy. To explore new strategies and the effect of aliskiren, the first orally active direct renin inhibitor, the angiotensin-receptor blocker losartan, and their combination on the reduction of LV mass in hypertensive patients, a Study was recently completed and published (58); the Authors randomized 465 patients with hypertension, increased ventricular wall thickness, and body mass index>25 kg/m^2 to receive aliskiren 300 mg, losartan 100 mg, or their combination daily for nine months.Aliskiren resulted as effective as losartan in promoting LV mass regression; reduction in LV mass with the combination of aliskiren plus losartan was not significantly different from that with losartan monotherapy, independent of blood pressure lowering. These findings seem to suggest that aliskiren is as effective as an angiotensin receptor blocker in attenuating the measure of myocardial end-organ damage in hypertensive patients with LV hypertrophy.

Special Features and Comorbility: Hypertension Diabetes and Cardiometabolic Syndrome (CMS)

Cardiometabolic Syndrome is quite frequently associated with hypertension and diabetes and hypertensive patients with the cardiometabolic syndrome are at increased risk for type 2 diabetes and cardiovascular disease.

Some Authors examined the effects of valsartan and hydrochlorothiazide combined and alone on insulin sensitivity (using homeostasis model assessment-insulin resistance), and inflammatory/metabolic biomarkers in pre-diabetic hypertensive subjects with CMS (59). Eligible patients entered 16-week therapy with valsartan 320 mg/daily, HCTZ 25 mg/daily, or valsartan/HCTZ 320/25 mg/daily. At the end point, there were no statistically significant differences in HOMA-IR among the 3 groups; HCTZ significantly increased HbA1c and triglyceride concentrations and lowered serum potassium levels *vs.* valsartan and also increased plasma aldosterone and C-reactive protein levels. Blood pressure reduction and blood pressure control rates were highest with valsartan/HCTZ meanwhile there were no differences between combination valsartan/HCTZ or monotherapies on a measure of insulin sensitivity; however, the negative metabolic effects of HCTZ were absent with valsartan/HCTZ, indicating an ameliorating effect of the ARB on these measures.

Particular Features and Comorbility: Hypertension and "Non Diabetic Nephropathy"

To slow and/or prevent the progression of kidney diseases independent from diabetes different strategies involve the use of ARBs alone or in combination. Although dual blockade of the renin-angiotensin-aldosterone system with the combination of an angiotensin-converting enzyme inhibitor and angiotensin II receptor blocker is generally well-established as a treatment for nephropathy, this treatment is not fully effective in some patients.

Based on the evidence implicating aldosterone in renal disease progression a 1-year randomized, open-label, multicenter, prospective controlled study Study was conducted to examine the efficacy of blockade with three different mechanisms by adding an aldosterone blocker in patients who do not respond adequately to the dual blockade. Results reported that triple blockade of the RAAS was effective for the treatment of proteinuria in patients with non-diabetic nephropathy whose increased urinary protein had not responded sufficiently to a dual blockade (60).

Some other Authors performed a Study with the aim to evaluate the renoprotection and blood pressure lowering effect of low-dose hydrochlorothiazide added to intensive renin-angiotensin inhibition in non-diabetic hypertensive patients with chronic kidney disease (61). The results demonstrated that a low dose of hydrochlorothiazide had a renoprotective effect due to its blood pressure-lowering effect; the Authors accordingly propose that a low dose of hydrochlorothiazide should be administered to those patients in whom the blood pressure is not well controlled by intensive renin-angiotensin system inhibition therapy using the maximum recommended doses of angiotensin II Type I receptor blockers and angiotensin I-converting enzyme inhibitors.

Particular Features and Comorbility: Hypertension and Cardiopathy

Several studies have demonstrated that a prolonged over-activation of neurohormonal mechanisms contributes to drive structural and functional abnormalities of the cardiovascular system and leads to poor prognosis especially in patients with congestive heart failure. In particular, activation of the renin-angiotensin-aldosterone system leads to increased levels of angiotensin II and plasma aldosterone, and promote development of arterial vasoconstriction and remodelling, sodium retention, oxidative process, and cardiac fibrosis. Angiotensin II receptor blockers may modulate this excessive over-activity and improve survival in those patients.

In the CHARM-Added Study addition of ARB to ACE inhibitors reduces the risk of CV death and CHF hospitalisation in patients with CHF; CHARM-Added was a prospective analysis in patients who were receiving an optimum dose of ACE inhibitors at baseline. Patients were chosen at random to receive either candesartan or placebo in addition to their ACE treatment. Over the 41-month follow-up period, candesartan reduced the risk of the primary endpoint (CV death or CHF hospitalisation) by 15% compared with ACE inhibitor alone treatment (62).

The VALIANT Study (63)was a double-blind, active-controlled, trial, which compared the effect of the angiotensin-receptor blocker valsartan, the ACE inhibitor captopril, and the combination of the two on mortality in patients with acute myocardial infarction complicated by heart failure, left-ventricular dysfunction, or both; the results showed that valsartan is as effective as captopril in patients who are at high risk for cardiovascular events after myocardial infarction, but combining valsartan with captopril increased the rate of adverse events without improving survival.

The JIKEY Hearth Study (64) demonstrated that in Japanese patients with hypertension, coronary heart disease and/or heart failure, valsartan given on top of conventional therapy improves the combined endpoint of morbidity and mortality vs. non-ARB therapy, with the same level of blood pressure lowering efficacy after an average of 3.1 years follow-up. Similar results on the same asian population were obtained in the Kyoto Study (65).

Still looking at the comorbility of hypertension and cardiopathy, butfrom a relative new point of view, quite recent evidences indicate that increased arterial stiffness, involving accelerated vascular aging of the aorta, is a powerful and independent risk factor for early mortality and provides prognostic informations above and beyond traditional CVD risk factors such as blood pressure itself, age, gender, diabetes, smoking, and cholesterol (66-67). As arterial stiffness is the principal determinant of pulse pressure, any increase would result in unfavourable hemodynamics which affect ventricular afterload and impair coronary perfusion.Starting from these acquisitions, another Study (68) examined whether the combination of an ARB with HCTZ would improve arterial stiffness to a greater extent than an equivalent antihypertensive medication, the calcium channel blocker amlodipine, in type 2 Diabetes Mellitus patients with systolic hypertension and albuminuria. Treatment with Valsartan/HCTZ reduced Ao-PWV by 0.9 m/s more than amlodipine in patients with type 2 Diabetes Mellitus, systolic hypertension, and albuminuria despite similar attained brachial and central aortic PP in both groups at the end of the study.

Conclusions: Current and Future Developments

According to a recent review of published literature, approximately a quarter of the adult population worldwide (26.4%) was hypertensive in 2000 and this is expected to increase to 29.2% by 2025 (69). Appropriate management of hypertension is therefore an Important priority worldwide, especially given the impact that effective blood pressure control can have on morbidity and mortality. Despite the availability of many antihypertensive drugs, at least 50% of patients do not achieve blood pressure targets and thus remain at increased cardiovascular risk.

Many evidences could confirm that the majority of patients will require two or more antihypertensives drugs to achieve blood pressure goal and significant reduction of CV risk. Currently available fixed-dose agents include several combinations with complementary pharmacodynamic activity, and practically with most of them it has been shown that administering two drugs in a single-dose formulation substantially improves patient compliance as compared with separate agent administration.

Among antihypertensive agents, inhibitors of the renin-angiotensin system (angiotensin-II receptor blockers, direct renin inhibitors and angiotensin converting enzyme inhibitors) and long-acting dihydropyridine calcium channel blockers have been shown to provide safe, effective and well-tolerated blood pressure control. These agents have also been proven as effective as, and in some cases superior to, other classes of agents in reducing cardiovascular morbidity and mortality. As the majority of high-risk patients require at least two and possibly even three medications to achieve the target blood pressure, combination therapy with these two classes of drugs is a rational approach to therapy(70-72).

Also administering fixed-dose combinations of three agents with complementary modes of action, such as an ARB plus a CCBs and a thiazide diuretic, has been found to produce clinical benefits not associated with merely increasing the dose of a single agent. These benefits include greater bloodpressure reductions, more rapid blood pressure control, and improved compliance without an increase in overall tolerability concerns, which may be particularly valuable in patients with moderate to severe hypertension or additional CV risk factors.

Furthermore other Studies have shown that in some cases RAAS blocker plus a dihydropyridine CCB is superior to older diuretic-based combinations for preventing cardiovascular events.

Limiting their analysis to trials concluded before June 2008, a group of Authors (73)performed a very interesting systematic review of published clinical trials evaluating dual intervention with ACE inhibitors and ARBs, and compared these with trials of DRI/ACE inhibitor or DRI/ARB combinations. Their conclusions seem fine, and particularly that ACE inhibitor/ARB combinations show equivocal effects on clinical outcomes and DRI/ACE inhibitor and DRI/ARB combinations reduced markers of organ damage indeed, but still longer-term trials are required to establish whether more complete renin-angiotensin-aldosterone system control with aliskiren-based therapy translates into improved outcome clinical benefits.

In conclusion, data coming from a wide number of Studies suggest that, for clinical decision making, should be better if physicians rely on how the agents perform when administered together in add-on studies and how each component performs as monotherapy in reducing blood pressure, achieving blood pressure goals and reducing outcomes, as well as considering patient factors such as response to and tolerance of such agents as monotherapy and cost. Finally, the availability of effective and well tolerated fixed-dose combination of antihypertensive agents should encourage primary-care physicians to be more willing to use such therapies in a timely manner when blood pressure goals are not being achieved with monotherapy.

References

[1] Kannel, W.B., Fifty years of Framingham Study contributions to understanding hypertension. *J Hum Hypertens*, 2000. 14(2): p. 83-90.

[2] Dahlof, B., et al., Cardiovascular morbidity and mortality in the Losartan Intervention For Endpoint reduction in hypertension study (LIFE): a randomised trial against atenolol. *Lancet*, 2002. 359(9311): p. 995-1003.

[3] Goodfriend, T., M. Elliott, and K. Catt, Angiotensin receptors and their antagonists. *N Engl J Med*, 1996. 334: p. 1649-1654

[4] Lewis, E.J., et al., Renoprotective effect of the angiotensin-receptor antagonist irbesartan in patients with nephropathy due to type 2 diabetes. *N Engl J Med*, 2001. 345(12): p. 851-60.

[5] Lithell, H., et al., The Study on Cognition and Prognosis in the Elderly (SCOPE): principal results of a randomized double-blind intervention trial. *J Hypertens*, 2003. 21(5): p. 875-86.

[6] Brenner, B.M., et al., Effects of losartan on renal and cardiovascular outcomes in patients with type 2 diabetes and nephropathy. *N Engl J Med*, 2001. 345(12): p. 861-9.

[7] Cohn, J., G. Tognoni, and V.H.F.T. Investigators., A randomized trial of the angiotensin-receptor blocker valsartan in chronic heart failure. *N Engl J Med*, 2001.

[8] Lewington, S., et al., Age-specific relevance of usual blood pressure to vascular mortality: a meta-analysis of individual data for one million adults in 61 prospective studies. *Lancet*, 2002. 360(9349): p. 1903-13.

[9] Law, M.R. and N.J. Wald, Risk factor thresholds: their existence under scrutiny. *BMJ*, 2002. 324(7353): p. 1570-6.

[10] van den Hoogen, P.C., et al., The relation between blood pressure and mortality due to coronary heart disease among men in different parts of the world. Seven Countries Study Research Group. *N Engl J Med*, 2000. 342(1): p. 1-8.

[11] Neal, B., S. MacMahon, and N. Chapman, Effects of ACE inhibitors, calcium antagonists, and other blood-pressure-lowering drugs: results of prospectively designed overviews of randomised trials. Blood Pressure Lowering Treatment Trialists' Collaboration. *Lancet*, 2000. 356(9246): p. 1955-64.

[12] Yusuf, S., et al., Effects of an angiotensin-converting-enzyme inhibitor, ramipril, on cardiovascular events in high-risk patients. The Heart Outcomes Prevention Evaluation Study Investigators. *N Engl J Med*, 2000. 342(3): p. 145-53.

[13] Randomised trial of a perindopril-based blood-pressure-lowering regimen among 6,105 individuals with previous stroke or transient ischaemic attack. *Lancet*, 2001. 358(9287): p. 1033-41.

[14] Neaton, J.D. and D. Wentworth, Serum cholesterol, blood pressure, cigarette smoking, and death from coronary heart disease. Overall findings and differences by age for 316,099 white men. Multiple Risk Factor Intervention Trial Research Group. *Arch Intern Med*, 1992. 152(1): p. 56-64.

[15] Anderson, K.M., et al., Cardiovascular disease risk profiles. *Am Heart J*, 1991. 121(1 Pt 2): p. 293-8.

[16] Mulrow, C.D., et al., Hypertension in the elderly. Implications and generalizability of randomized trials. *JAMA*, 1994. 272(24): p. 1932-8.

[17] Pocock, S.J., et al., A score for predicting risk of death from cardiovascular disease in adults with raised blood pressure, based on individual patient data from randomised controlled trials. *BMJ*, 2001. 323(7304): p. 75-81.

[18] Major outcomes in high-risk hypertensive patients randomized to angiotensin-converting enzyme inhibitor or calcium channel blocker vs diuretic: The Antihypertensive and Lipid-Lowering Treatment to Prevent Heart Attack Trial (ALLHAT). *JAMA*, 2002. 288(23): p. 2981-97.

[19] Tight blood pressure control and risk of macrovascular and microvascular complications in type 2 diabetes: UKPDS 38. *UK Prospective Diabetes Study Group.BMJ*, 1998. 317(7160): p. 703-13.

[20] Hansson, L., et al., Effects of intensive blood-pressure lowering and low-dose aspirin in patients with hypertension: principal results of the Hypertension Optimal Treatment (HOT) randomised trial. HOT Study Group. *Lancet*, 1998. 351(9118): p. 1755-62.

[21] Barrios, V., et al., Olmesartan medoxomil plus amlodipine increases efficacy in patients with moderate-to-severe hypertension after monotherapy: a randomized, double-blind, parallel-group, multicentre study. *Clin Drug Investig*, 2009. 29(7): p. 427-39.

[22] Schrader, J., et al., BP goal achievement in patients with uncontrolled hypertension : results of the treat-to-target post-marketing survey with irbesartan. *Clin Drug Investig*, 2007. 27(11): p. 783-96.

[23] Kintscher, U., et al., Irbesartan for the treatment of hypertension in patients with the metabolic syndrome: a sub analysis of the Treat to Target post authorization survey. Prospective observational, two armed study in 14,200 patients. *Cardiovasc Diabetol*, 2007. 6: p. 12.

[24] Neldam, S. and C. Edwards, Telmisartan plus HCTZ vs. amlodipine plus HCTZ in older patients with systolic hypertension: results from a large ambulatory blood pressure monitoring study. *Am J Geriatr Cardiol*, 2006. 15(3): p. 151-60.

[25] Pool, J.L., et al., Comparison of valsartan/hydrochlorothiazide combination therapy at doses up to 320/25 mg versus monotherapy: a double-blind, placebo-controlled study followed by long-term combination therapy in hypertensive adults. *Clin Ther*, 2007. 29(1): p. 61-73.

[26] Tuomilehto, J., et al., Combination therapy with valsartan/hydrochlorothiazide at doses up to 320/25 mg improves blood pressure levels in patients with hypertension inadequately controlled by valsartan 320 mg monotherapy. *Blood Press Suppl*, 2008. 1: p. 15-23.

[27] Destro, M., et al., Efficacy and safety of amlodipine/valsartan compared with amlodipine monotherapy in patients with stage 2 hypertension: a randomized, double-blind, multicenter study: the EX-EFFeCTS study. *J Am Soc Hypertens*, 2008. 2: p. 294-302.

[28] Oparil, S., et al., Subgroup Analyses of an Efficacy and Safety Study of Concomitant Administration of Amlodipine Besylate and Olmesartan Medoxomil: Evaluation by Baseline Hypertension Stage and Prior Antihypertensive Medication Use. *J Cardiovasc Pharmacol*.

[29] Destro, M., et al., *Aliskiren, un nuovo inibitore della renina, è ben tollerato e ha un effetto di riduzione pressoria persistente quando somministrato in monoterapia o in associazione a idroclorotiazide nel trattamento a lungo termine dell'ipertensione*

arteriosa., in Poster n. 167, presented at XXIV Congresso Nazionale della Società Italiana dell'Ipertensione Arteriosa, Roma, 4-7 Ottobre 2007. 2007.

[30]   Blumenstein, M., et al., Antihypertensive efficacy and tolerability of aliskiren/hydrochlorothiazide (HCT) single-pill combinations in patients who are non-responsive to HCT 25 mg alone. *Curr Med Res Opin*, 2009. 25(4): p. 903-10.

[31]   Pool, J.L., et al., Aliskiren, an orally effective renin inhibitor, provides antihypertensive efficacy alone and in combination with valsartan. *Am J Hypertens*, 2007. 20(1): p. 11-20.

[32]   Patel, B., et al., Improved persistence and adherence to diuretic fixed-dose combination therapy compared to diuretic monotherapy. *BMC Fam Pract*, 2008. 9: p. 61.

[33]   Jamerson, K., Weber, M. A., Bakris, G. L., et al. Benazepril plus amlodipine or hydrochlorothiazide for hypertension in high-risk patients (2008) *N Engl J Med* 359, 2417-28.

[34]   Devereux, R. B., de Faire, U., Fyhrquist, F.,et al. Blood pressure reduction and antihypertensive medication use in the losartan intervention for endpoint reduction in hypertension (LIFE) study in patients with hypertension and left ventricular hypertrophy (2007) *Curr Med Res Opin* 23, 259-70.

[35]   Bangalore, S., Messerli, F. H., Cohen, J. D., Bacher, P. H., Sleight, P., Mancia, G., Kowey, P., Zhou, Q., Champion, A. and Pepine, C. J. Verapamil-sustained release-based treatment strategy is equivalent to atenolol-based treatment strategy at reducing cardiovascular events in patients with prior myocardial infarction: an INternational VErapamil SR-Trandolapril (INVEST) substudy (2008) *Am Heart J* 156, 241-7.

[36]   Cushman, W. C., Ford, C. E., Cutler, J. A., Margolis, K. L., Davis, B. R., Grimm, R. H., Black, H. R., Hamilton, B. P., Holland, J., Nwachuku, C., Papademetriou, V., Probstfield, J., Wright, J. T., Jr., Alderman, M. H., Weiss, R. J., Piller, L., Bettencourt, J. and Walsh, S. M. Success and predictors of blood pressure control in diverse North American settings: the antihypertensive and lipid-lowering treatment to prevent heart attack trial (ALLHAT) (2002) *J Clin Hypertens* (Greenwich) **4**, 393-404.

[37]   Mancia, G., Brown, M., Castaigne, A., et al. Outcomes with nifedipine GITS or Co-amiloride in hypertensive diabetics and nondiabetics in Intervention as a Goal in Hypertension (INSIGHT) (2003) *Hypertension* 41, 431-6.

[38]   Smith, T. R., Philipp, T., Vaisse, B., Bakris, G. L., Wernsing, M., Yen, J. and Glazer, R. Amlodipine and valsartan combined and as monotherapy in stage 2, elderly, and black hypertensive patients: subgroup analyses of 2 randomized, placebo-controlled studies (2007) *J Clin Hypertens* (Greenwich) 9, 355-64.

[39]   Calhoun, D.A., et al., Triple antihypertensive therapy with amlodipine, valsartan, and hydrochlorothiazide: a randomized clinical trial. *Hypertension*, 2009. 54(1): p. 32-9.

[40]   Destro, M., et al., Triple therapy with amlodipine, valsartan, and HCTZ in Stage 2 hypertensive patients. *International Journal of Clinical Practice*, In press.

[41]   Schrader, J., et al., The combination of amlodipine/valsartan 5/160 mg produces less peripheral oedema than amlodipine 10 mg in hypertensive patients not adequately controlled with amlodipine 5 mg. *Int J Clin Pract*, 2009. 63(2): p. 217-25.

[42]   Kjeldsen SE, A.T., Sierra ADL, et al, Amlodipine and valsartan: calcium channel blockers/angiotensin II receptor blockers combination for hypertension. *Drug Eval*, 2007. 4: p. 31-40.

[43] Smith, T.R., et al., Amlodipine and valsartan combined and as monotherapy in stage 2, elderly, and black hypertensive patients: subgroup analyses of 2 randomized, placebo-controlled studies. *J Clin Hypertens* (Greenwich), 2007. 9(5): p. 355-64.

[44] Chobanian, A. V., Bakris, G. L., Black, et al. The Seventh Report of the Joint National Committee on Prevention, Detection, Evaluation, and Treatment of High Blood Pressure: the JNC 7 report (2003) *Jama* 289, 2560-72.

[45] Mancia, G., De Backer, G., Dominiczak, A.,et al. 2007 Guidelines for the Management of Arterial Hypertension: *The Task Force for the Management of Arterial Hypertension of the European.*

[46] Turnbull, F. Effects of different blood-pressure-lowering regimens on major cardiovascular events: results of prospectively-designed overviews of randomised trials (2003) *Lancet* 362, 1527-35.

[47] Neutel, J. M., Smith, D. H., Silfani, T. N., Lee, Y. and Weber, M. A. Effects of a structured treatment algorithm on blood pressure goal rates in both stage 1 and stage 2 hypertension (2006) *J Hum Hypertens* 20, 255-62.

[48] Arauz-Pacheco, C., M.A. Parrott, and P. Raskin, The treatment of hypertension in adult patients with diabetes. *Diabetes Care*, 2002. 25(1): p. 134-47.

[49] Ong, K.L., et al., Prevalence, awareness, treatment, and control of hypertension among United States adults 1999-2004. *Hypertension*, 2007. 49(1): p. 69-75.

[50] Association, A.D., Standards of medical care in diabetes: 2007. *Diabetes Care,* 2007. 30(Suppl 1): p. S4-S41.

[51] Luft, F., Angiotensin, inflammation, hypertension, and cardiovascular disease. *Curr Hypertens Rep*, 2001. 3: p. 61-67.

[52] Sowers, J.R., et al., Initial combination therapy compared with monotherapy in diabetic hypertensive patients. *J Clin Hypertens* (Greenwich), 2008. 10(9): p. 668-76.

[53] Ridker, P.M., et al., Valsartan, blood pressure reduction, and C-reactive protein: primary report of the Val-MARC trial. *Hypertension*, 2006. 48(1): p. 73-9.

[54] Lacourcière, Y., et al., Antihypertensive efficacy and tolerability of two fixed-dose combinations of valsartan and hydrochlorothiazide compared with valsartan monotherapy in patients with stage 2 or 3 systolic hypertension: an 8-week, randomized, double-blind, parallel-group trial. *Clin Ther*, 2005. 27(7): p. 1013-1021.

[55] Jamerson, K., D. Zappe, and L. Collins, The time to blood pressure (BP) control by initiating antihypertensive therapy with a higher dose of valsartan (160 mg) or valsartan/hydrochlorothiazide compared to low-dose valsartan (80 mg) in the treatment of hypertension: the VELOCITY study *J Clin Hypertens* (Greenwich), 2007. 9(Suppl A): p. A166-A167.

[56] Krairittichai, U. and V. Chaisuvannarat, Effects of dual blockade of renin-angiotensin system in type 2 diabetes mellitus patients with diabetic nephropathy. *Med Assoc Thai*, 2009. 92(5): p. 611-7.

[57] Suzuki, H., et al., Comparison of the effects of angiotensin receptor antagonist, angiotensin converting enzyme inhibitor, and their combination on regression of left ventricular hypertrophy of diabetes type 2 patients on recent onset hemodialysis therapy. *Ther Apher Dial*, 2004. 8(4): p. 320-7.

[58] Solomon, S.D., et al., Effect of the direct Renin inhibitor aliskiren, the Angiotensin receptor blocker losartan, or both on left ventricular mass in patients with hypertension and left ventricular hypertrophy. *Circulation*, 2009. 119(4): p. 530-7.

[59] Zappe, D.H., et al., Metabolic and antihypertensive effects of combined angiotensin receptor blocker and diuretic therapy in prediabetic hypertensive patients with the cardiometabolic syndrome. J Clin Hypertens (Greenwich), 2008. 10(12): p. 894-903.

[60] Furumatsu, Y., et al., Effect of renin-angiotensin-aldosterone system triple blockade on non-diabetic renal disease: addition of an aldosterone blocker, spironolactone, to combination treatment with an angiotensin-converting enzyme inhibitor and angiotensin II receptor blocker. Hypertens Res, 2008. 31(1): p. 59-67.

[61] Abe, M., et al., Renoprotect and blood pressure lowering effect of low-dose hydrochlorothiazide added to intensive renin-angiotensin inhibition in hypertensive patients with chronic kidney disease. Int J Clin Pharmacol Ther, 2009. 47(8): p. 525-32.

[62] McMurray, J.J., et al., Effects of candesartan in patients with chronic heart failure and reduced left-ventricular systolic function taking angiotensin-converting-enzyme inhibitors: the CHARM-Added trial. Lancet, 2003. 362(9386): p. 767-71.

[63] Pfeffer, M., et al., Valsartan, captopril, or both in myocardial infarction complicated by heart failure, left ventricular dysfunction, or both. N Engl J Med 2003. 349(20): p. 1893-906.

[64] Mochizuki, S., et al., Valsartan in a Japanese population with hypertension and other cardiovascular disease (Jikei Heart Study): a randomised, open-label, blinded endpoint morbidity-mortality study. Lancet, 2007. 369: p. 1431-39.

[65] Sawada, T., et al., Effects of valsartan on morbidity and mortality in uncontrolled hypertensive patients with high cardiovascular risks: KYOTO HEART Study. Eur Heart J, 2009. Advance Access published August 31.

[66] Mattace-Raso, F., et al., Arterial stiffness and risk of coronary heart disease and stroke: the Rotterdam Study. Circulation, 2006. 113: p. 657-663.

[67] Hansen, T.W., et al., Prognostic value of aortic pulse wave velocity as index of arterial stiffness in the general population. Circulation, 2006. 113: p. 664-670.

[68] Karalliedde, J., et al., Valsartan improves arterial stiffness in type 2 diabetes independently of blood pressure lowering. Hypertension, 2008. 51(6): p. 1617-23.

[69] Kearney, P., et al., Global burden of hypertension: analysis of worldwide data. Lancet, 2005. 365(9455): p. 217-223.

[70] Chobanian, A., G. Bakris, and H. Black, Seventh Report of the Joint National Committee on Prevention, Detection, Evaluation, and Treatment of High Blood Pressure. Hypertension, 2003. 42(1206-1252).

[71] Committee, G., European Society of Hypertension-European Society of Cardiology guidelines For the management of arterial hypertension. J Hypertens, 2003. 21: p. 1011-1053.

[72] Neutel, J., D. Smith, and M. Weber, Low-dose combination therapy: An important first-line treatment in the management of hypertension. Am J Hypertens, 2001. 14: p. 286-292.

[73] Düsing, R. and F. Sellers, ACE inhibitors, angiotensin receptor blockers and direct renin inhibitors in combination: a review of their role after the ONTARGET trial. Curr Med Res Opin, 2009. 25(9): p. 2287-301.

In: Systolic Blood Pressure
Editor: Robert A. Arfi

ISBN: 978-1-61209-263-8
©2012 Nova Science Publishers, Inc.

Chapter VI

Systolic Blood Pressure: Influences, Associations and Management

Maria Cristina Izar[*]*, Rui M. Póvoa, Henrique A. Fonseca,*
Sílvio A. Barbosa, Henrique T. Bianco and Francisco A. Fonseca
Cardiology Division, Department of Medicine, Federal University of São Paulo,
São Paulo, S.P., Brazil

Abstract

Isolated systolic hypertension (ISH) is defined by the elevation of systolic blood pressure (SBP), with normal levels of diastolic blood pressure (DBP). The condition is recognized as a major cardiovascular risk factor, and current guidelines suggest values of $SBP \geq 140$ mm Hg and $DBP < 90$ mm Hg for the diagnosis and treatment. Age-related changes in large arteries seem to have an important role in the pathogenesis and progression of SBP elevation. Ageing is associated with structural and functional alterations in the intima and media layers, characterized by thickening of large arteries, increased sympathetic activity and decreased sensitivity of beta-receptors, leading to deterioration in arterial compliance. These vessel modifications can determine differences in SBP levels for the same ejected volume. Even in apparently healthy individuals without known cardiovascular disease, SBP tends to increase throughout the life, whereas DBP increases up to 55-60, declining slowly thereafter.

In the elderly, ISH is considered the most common type of hypertension, particularly among very old subjects. For the correct diagnosis of ISH it is necessary to rule out the misdiagnosis of pseudo hypertension, white coat hypertension and to recognize the auscultatory hiatus.

The benefits of hypertension treatment have been fully demonstrated in controlled clinical trials, including those subjects with ISH. Beyond the reduction in major

* Corresponding author: Maria Cristina de Oliveira Izar, MD, PhD, Federal University of São Paulo – São Paulo – SP – Brazil, Rua Pedro de Toledo, 276 – Vila Clementino – São Paulo, S.P., Brazil, ZIPCODE – 04039030, phone/fax: 55-11-50848777, e-mail: mcoizar@terra.com.br

cardiovascular events, treatment of ISH also reduces the incidence of cognitive impairment and dementia.

The treatment goal for blood pressure levels should be below 140/90 mm Hg.

Lifestyle changes have to be encouraged, are less expensive and have proven cardiovascular benefits. Elderly patients with ISH usually present other comorbidities and these conditions should guide the choice of anti-hypertensive agents, preferably with drugs that benefit other preexisting diseases and risk factors, even in borderline or stage I hypertension.

Thiazide diuretics are first-line agents for patients without comorbidities; indapamide, a sulfonamide derivative, seems to have the advantage of not interfering with glucose and lipid levels. When there is renal impairment with glomerular filtration rate < 30 mL/min loop diuretics should be chosen. Dihydropyridine calcium antagonists have been recognized as safe drugs with clear benefits among these patients, but some side effects can be more common in elderly patients. Angiotensin converting enzyme inhibitors are efficacious for treatment of ISH in the elderly, in spite of decreased renin levels. They reduce cardiovascular events, especially in high risk patients. Beta-blockers can be less effective in elderly patients but should be given for those with coronary heart disease or heart failure. Some beta-blockers such as metoprolol and bisoprolol are preferred due to lower risk of central nervous system side effects. Angiotensin receptor blockers (ARBs) are antihypertensives with excellent safety profile, and have proven benefits for ISH in the elderly. Central sympatholytic agents have limited use due to high risk of side effects.

Isolated Systolic Hypertension

The prevalence of hypertension in the United States rises exponentially with age in individuals of both sexes. [1] This effect becomes more pronounced in individuals over 50 years, when isolated systolic hypertension (ISH) is usually detected. The NHANES III study [2] showed that among hypertensive subjects, the ISH was present in 54% of the individuals between the ages 50-59 years and 87% of those aged over 60 years. As a consequence of arterial stiffness, systolic levels continue to rise with age, while diastolic levels tend to reach a plateau during the middle age, declining thereafter. As the population ages, the prevalence of hypertension continues to increase not only in developed, but also in emerging and low-income countries. [3]At the same time, in spite of the widely recognized cardiovascular risk, the disease remains inadequately treated in most patients.[4]Considering the high prevalence of hypertension [5], much more attention should be given, in the early stages of life, to preventive measures, due to its effectiveness and safety.Blood pressure is typically distributed in a log-linear type curve in the population as a whole. In the study "Multiple Risk Factor Intervention Trial" (MRFIT) [6, 7] whose follow-up of approximately 350,000 individuals for 22 years was assessed, the risk of cardiovascular mortality in the long-term correlated to levels of progressive elevation of blood pressure, without any threshold that clearly identifies the potential risk. These data were later confirmed by meta-analysis that measured the relationship between blood pressure and cardiovascular mortality in nearly one million adultsfrom 61 prospective observational studies [8]. Every 20 mm Hg elevation in systolic or 10 mm Hg in diastolic pressure doubles the risk of mortality from coronary heart disease.The first placebo-controlled studies that demonstrate the benefit of antihypertensive treatment in reducing overall and cardiovascular mortality were performed in hypertensive patients with diastolic blood pressure above 115 mmHg, assessing a relatively reduced sample of only 70 patients. However, soon the benefits of antihypertensive treatment where extended to those patients with much lower levels of blood pressure, those more commonly found in community. In the 1970s, the efficacy of antihypertensive treatment in reducing morbidity and mortality was reported in a population of middle-aged adults. One of these pioneering studies in evaluating a representative sample population was the "Veterans Administration Trial" [9], which included mainly middle-aged, hypertensive men. Another important study, "the Hypertension Detection and Follow-up Program" examined a representative cohort of the pyramid population. During the next decade, the emphasis was focused on the so-called mild hypertension, and the most representative study was considered the "Australian Trial of Treatment of Mild Hypertension" [10]. None of these studies, however, was designed specifically to assess the elderly or patients with systolic hypertension, but allowed for analyses of some antihypertensives, mainly diuretics and/or betablockers.In general, these analyses showed similar benefits to those documented in the whole adult population, by reducing morbidity and mortality. However, limited information in the elderly population could be obtained from these initial studies.

In fact, only after the "Systolic Hypertension in the Elderly Program" (SHEP) [11] a double-blind, placebo-controlled, multicenter study, held in the United States, comprising about 4,500 men and women over 60 years, the effects of antihypertensive therapy among old patients was specifically addressed.

Inclusion criteria were SBP between 160 mm Hg and 219 mmHg and DBP below 90 mmHg. Mean blood pressure was 177/70 mm Hg and the mean age was 72 years. Patients were treated with placebo or chlorthalidone (12.5 to 25 mg daily); and atenolol was added to the active treatment when necessary. The mean follow-up was 4-5 years and the active treatment was associated with 37% reduction in fatal and non-fatal stroke, and 27% reduction in the rates of acute myocardial infarction (fatal and nonfatal). This active therapy also reduced in 32% the rates of all cardiovascular events. However, overall mortality was associated with non-significant reduction of 13%. The active treatment produced a reduction of systolic and diastolic pressures in the sitting position of 12 mm Hg and 4 mm Hg, respectively, and the benefits of cardiovascular events compared to the placebo group were justified by these differences in the blood pressure.The "Swedish Trial in Old Patients with Hypertension" (STOP) [12] was a multicenter study conducted in centers of primary health care, and included patients of both sexes ageing 70-84 years. Differently from the SHEP study, patients in the STOP trial should have diastolic blood pressure above 90 mm Hg and SBP between 180 mm Hg and 230 mm Hg. Interestingly, this study included very elderly patients, with large differences between the SBP and DBP (large pulse pressure).

Patients received either placebo or active therapy (hydrochlorothiazide + amiloride or beta blocker). Ironically, due to the acronym of the study, the trial was prematurely stopped after 25 months of follow up, as a result of remarkable benefits in the treated group compared to placebo. For the primary objectives of the study (stroke, myocardial infarction or cardiovascular death) there was a 40% reduction in event rates for the active treatment group. These results were attributed to differences of 20 and 8 mm Hg in SBP and DBP, respectively, between groups. It is of worth to mention that similar to what ocurred in SHEP, the effects of treatment on SBP were more pronounced than those seen on DBP. The STOP-II [13]study was a prospective, randomized study that enrolled 6,614 subjects between 70-84 years with SBP > 180 mm Hg, and/or DBP > 105 mm Hg. During randomization, patients were divided into three classes of drugs as initial therapy: conventional antihypertensive drugs (atenolol, metoprolol, pindolol, or hydrochlorothiazide + amiloride), angiotensin-converting enzyme (ACE) inhibitors (enalapril or lisinopril) or dihydropyridine calcium channel blockers (CCB - felodipine or isradipine). For the achievement of the target blood pressure (BP <160/95 mm Hg), the antihypertensive drugs were progressively added. Study endpoints included fatal stroke, fatal myocardial infarction and fatal cardiovascular disease. There were 719 patients (10.9%) with diabetes at baseline. The results for the primary endpoint of cardiovascular death were similar for all treatment groups. The relative risk of cardiovascular mortality with ACE inhibitors compared to conventional therapy was 1.01 ([95% CI 0.84 to 1.22], P = 0.89). For CCB compared to conventional therapy, the relative risk was 0.97 ([95% CI 0.80 to 1.17], P = 0.97). The relative risk of CV mortality with ACE inhibitors compared with CCB was 1.04 ([95% CI 0.86 to 1.26], P = 0.67). When parameters were considered individually, there was an increased relative risk with CCB compared with ACE inhibitors for myocardial infarction (relative risk = 0.77 [95% CI 0.61 to 0.96], P = 0.018) and congestive heart failure (relative risk = 0.78 [95% CI 0.63 to 0.97], P = 0.025). Similar benefits of the treatment on the primary endpoint of cardiovascular mortality were also observed in 719 patients who had diabetes at baseline. New-onset diabetes was found among 97 patients in the conventional therapy group, 93 patients in the ACE inhibitor group and in 95 patients in the CCB group throughout the study.

High blood pressure is a frequent comorbidity in patients with diabetes, affecting 20% to 60% of patients, depending on the degree of obesity, ethnicity and age. [14] In fact, hypertension substantially increases the risk of the microvascular and macrovascular disease, including coronary artery disease, peripheral vascular disease, retinopathy, nephropathy and possibly neuropathy.[15] In the last years, new data and well-designed randomized clinical trials have demonstrated the effectiveness of aggressive treatment of hypertension in reducing the whole spectrum of diabetes complications [16]. There are substantial evidences showing the effectiveness of antihypertensive therapy in reducing not only cardiovascular events, but microvascular complications such as retinopathy and nephropathy. [17] These results derived from studies using different drug classes, including angiotensin converting enzyme (ACE) inhibitors, angiotensin receptors blockers (ARB), or diuretics as the initial strategies for therapy. However, many patients require three or more drugs to achieve specific target levels. [18].

Overall, there is strong evidence that pharmacologic therapy of hypertension in patients with diabetes substantially affects the rates of cardiovascular disease and microvascular complications [19].

There are data from clinical trials comparing different classes of drugs in patients with diabetes and hypertension. [20] With the use of ACE inhibitors and ARB, there has been spread the concept that cardiovascular effects could be mediated by mechanisms beyond blood pressure reduction. However, many studies of combined regimen of antihypertensive agents have been published, and the superiority of one class over the combination of different therapeutic regimens for diabetes has not been clearly documented.[21] Diuretic agents in combination with adrenergic blockers have been used in United Kingdom Prospective Diabetes Study (UKPDS), SHEP and several trials that include patients with nephropathy.[22] Some studies compared "the old treatments", such as diuretics and beta blockers, with the "new agents", such as ACE inhibitors and CCB, in the (INSIGHT) [23], (NORDIL) [24] and Atherosclerosis Risk in Communities (ARIC) trials.[25] In addition, the

Val-Syst study showed in patients with ISH and high cardiovascular risk, the importance of BP control, which is feasible and can be achieved with a combination of well tolerated antihypertensives.[26]

Pathophysiology

Blood flow in the aorta, coming from the left ventricle, is pulsatile and intermittent. However, the release of blood into the peripheral circulation is continuous. The aorta needs to be compliant expanding during ventricular systole, storing energy to be collected during diastole, and propelling the blood to the microcirculation. The relationship between volume and pressure defines vascular distensibility. [27] The aortic systolic distension triggers a wave that propagates through the aorta and its branches, which is called the pulse wave. The pulse generated in peripheral vessels is a result of this wave pulse and not a direct reflection of blood flow. [28] On reaching the outskirts wave bounces back, forming the so-called reflex wave, which returns to the central circulation, interfering with aortic physiology. Factors affecting the aortic compliance will affect these properties and, therefore, the peripheral circulation and ventricular function. [29]

When compliance is decreased, there is a greater variation in pressure at a given volume ejected. This is the case with aortic stiffening; for the same volume ejected by the left ventricle, there is a greater variation in systolic aortic diameter, which increases by 15% to 35% from 20 to 80 years old. Histologically there is a distortion of the laminar orientation of the fiber wall, fragmentation of elastin and increased collagen content, resulting in decreased elasticity of connective tissue, resulting in increases of both the peripheral vascular resistance and impedance of the aorta [30].

There is strong correlation between normal aging and decreased aortic compliance through various measurement parameters [31]. Elderly subjects with higher physical activity have lower intensity of aortic stiffness [32]. Several factors have been considered possible modulators of progressive development of the ISH. With advancing age, there is an increased production of collagen by smooth muscle cells of aorta determining a larger number of couplings between cells and between cell-matrix extracellular space, regardless of changes in blood pressure but correlated with changes in phenotypes of smooth muscle [33].

Increased sensitivity to sodium found in the elderly and nitric oxide deficiency are related to increased oxidative stress[34].These aspects associated with changes in the phenotype of aortic smooth muscle cells determine vasoconstriction and decreased arterial compliance. These factors acting in combination interfere with the distensibility of the vessels, causing increased systolic blood pressure, large pulse pressure, arterial stiffness and higher pulse wave velocity. The central arterial elasticity is highly dependent of both the content and function of the matrix protein elastin [35].Throughout our lives, fatigue of elastin fibers and the accumulated cyclic stress, as a result of more than 2 billion aortic expansions occurring until the sixth decade of life promotes elastin fractures, and disorders that lead to structural changes of the extracellular matrix, with smooth muscle cell proliferation, collagen and calcium deposition [36]. Figure 1 shows the mechanisms by which changes in the phenotype of endothelial and smooth muscle cells can affect the dynamic of the vessel and thus promote hypertension.

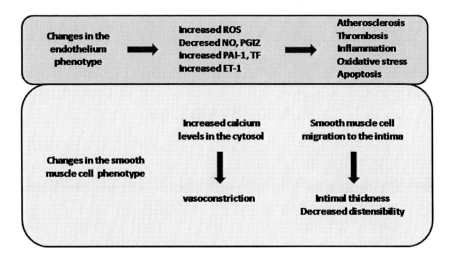

Figure 1. Mechanisms by which changes in the phenotype of endothelial and smooth muscle cells can affect the dynamic of the vessel and thus promote hypertension. ROS – reactive oxygen species; NO – nitric oxide; PGI2 – prostaglandin I2; PAI-1 – plasminogen activator inhibitor factor -1; TF – tissue factor; ET-1 – endothelin-1.

Humoral factors, cytokines and oxidative metabolites can also act as pathogenic mechanisms [37]. This pathological process, classically termed arteriosclerosis, results in increased arterial stiffness of aortic wall independently of blood pressure levels. The vessel diameter is the major determinant of vascular impedance. In subjects with arterial hypertension, the brachial and aortic diameters are increased. The peripheral vascular resistance in hypertension is characteristically high due to changes in the structure and mechanical properties affecting the function of small arteries [38]. The increased vascular resistance is mainly determined by pre-capillary vessels, including arterioles and small arteries. Increased vascular resistance in hypertensive patients is associated with both decreased number of vessels connected in parallel and the narrowing of the lumen of resistance vessels [39].

Besides structural changes, endothelial dysfunction develops over time, triggered by age, hypertension and other comorbidities, contributing functionally to increase arterial stiffness in elderly patients with ISH. The reduced synthesis or secretion of nitric oxide leads to increased thickening of the vessel wall conductance. The fundamental importance of the deficiency of nitric oxide in the ISH is supported by the ability of nitric oxide donors such as nitrates and derivatives, to increase arterial distensibility and compliance and reduce systolic blood pressure without reducing the diastolic pressure [40, 41].

In recent years, considerable attention has been driven to the endothelium apoptosis and its replacement by endothelial progenitor cells (EPC) [42-44].Flow-cytometry assays can estimate the turnover of endothelial cells, and several studies showed an strong association between the higher cardiovascular risk (patients with coronary disease, stroke, diabetes, uncontrolled hypertension, and other classical risk factors), the reduced number of EPC and the increased number of endothelial microparticles (derived from apoptosis of endothelial cells). These interesting findings were also reported in the postmenopause women and in the elderly and can explain the higher number of cardiovascular events occurring in these subjects, particularly in subjects with ISH [45].

Estrogen deficiency, increased salt intake, smoking, increased homocysteine levels and diabetes are factors that decrease central arterial compliance.These factors may alter the endothelium and influence ISH. Increased arterial stiffness also contributes to widening pulse pressure, commonly found in elderly individuals by raising pulse wave velocity to each ejection of blood through the left ventricle. The pressure wave (pulse) generated is propagated from the heart to the peripheral vessels with a finite speed which depends on the elastic properties of conducting arteries. Vessel remodeling can be internal (reduction in lumen diameter) or external (increase in lumen diameter), increasing systolic blood pressure, pulse pressure and afterload, and also decreasing diastolic blood pressure, which can reduce coronary perfusion [46]. The elevation in systolic blood pressure increases cardiac metabolism demand and predisposes to left ventricular hypertrophy (LVH) and heart failure. Angiotensin II is a powerful vasoconstrictor that triggers the secretion of aldosterone, increasing sodium and water retention by the kidneys [47].The system can restore blood pressure in situations of hypotension. However, in pathological conditions, the activation of the cardiac tissue causes vascular inflammation and cardiac and renal fibrosis, besides the development of atherosclerosis in large vessels. The chronic stimulation of the renin angiotensin and aldosterone system (RAAS) leads to proliferation and fibrosis with deleterious effects, including target-organ damage.

In spite of the association of higher birth weight and increased risk of diabetes, a study evaluating 1,543 patients with type 1 diabetes in this population also demonstrated an inverse relationship between low birth weight and systolic blood pressure in adulthood [48, 49].Thus, the contribution of delayed intrauterine growth to increased blood pressure and target-organ damage is currently under investigation.Left ventricular hypertrophy (LVH) is associated with hypertension, although there is debate whether it is caused by increased blood pressure itself or related to the risk factors commonly associated with hypertension [50, 51].

Importantly, regression of LVH during treatment was shown to be associated with a reduction of cardiovascular risk, as demonstrated in the Losartan Intervention for Endpoint Reduction study (LIFE) with 4.8 years of follow-up in patients with baseline LVH [52].

Undoubtedly arterial hypertension results from multiple and complex environmental factors, with many genes interacting to shift the distribution of blood pressure to higher levels [53]. Hypertension is certainly a polygenic disorder involving multiple genes, each of them determining a small role in blood pressure levels [54].

Hypertension is strongly linked to heart disease [55]. Although acute elevations may occur after the onset of ischemic pain, blood pressure may decrease immediately after myocardial infarction, particularly when the ventricular function is compromised. Once the myocardial infarction occurred, the prognosis is affected by the arterial pressure and subsequent consequences [56]. The rate of fatalities at 28 days among 635 men who were affected by an acute myocardial infarction was 24.5% in those with prior SBP below 140 mmHg, 35.6% with prior systolic blood pressure (SBP) between 140-159 mmHg and 48.2% with prior SBP of 160 mmHg or more. If the blood pressure of these individuals remained elevated, the prognosis would be even worse, probably because this would represent an increased work on a diseased myocardium [57]. Systolic hypertension is also a major risk factor for ischemic stroke and brain hemorrhage [58]. Cerebral white matter lesions are relatively common findings on magnetic ressonance imaging, detected of asymptomatic middle-aged subjects [59].

Pathophysiological Consequences of Pulse and Blood Pressure Changes

Aortic wall stiffness increases with ageing and causes augmentation in pulse wave velocity (PWV) [60].In one study, PWV increased by 134% from birth to 90 years, an increase greater than the variation of pressure in the same period.

The increase of PWV is also accompanied by an increase of wave velocity reflex, which returns from the periphery to the central circulation. In young subjects the reflex wave reaches the ascending aorta in early diastole, increasing the initial diastolic pressure. In the elderly, the wave reflex returns to the ascending aorta during systole, contributing to a greater rise in systolic blood pressure. The importance of pulse wave reflection on the systolic pressure increases with age, becoming responsible for more than 20% of central SBP. Increased pulse pressure, frequently present in the elderly [61], has been identified as an important independent cardiovascular risk factor in the elderly.

Thus, the hardening of the aorta contributes greatly to the occurrence of isolated systolic hypertension in the elderly. The increased prevalence of hypertension in the elderly is mainly due to increased frequency of ISH. In the population aged 65 years or more, almost 40% of individuals have ISH, and these represent almost two thirds of all elderly hypertensive [62].

Diastolic Dysfunction

The increase in systolic wall stress elevates left ventricular (LV) pressures, promoting LV hypertrophy. Following the decrease in aortic compliance, left ventricular stiffening can occur even in the absence of hypertrophy. A significant reduction in ventricular relaxation is a frequent cause of heart failure in the elderly, even if they are under normal systolic ventricular function.

Aortic Dissection

It is likely that the degeneration of the middle layer is involved in aortic dissection. The incidence of aortic dissection increases with age and hypertension. The prevention of aortic changes, by decreasing the wall stress (hardening + hypertension + dilatation) could help to prevent degeneration of the middle layer and the dissection. The adequate measurement of blood pressure is a crucial procedure in the evaluation of the cardiovascular system. Despite the assessment of this variable in the clinical setting, by using relatively simple techniques, because of the important prognostic implications of measure, one should examine carefully all factors that can influence blood pressure levels. From the epidemiological point of view, the presence of higher levels of blood pressure alone alters the prognosis of patients in relation to the occurrence of serious cardiovascular events such as myocardial infarction and stroke. Thus, an inappropriate measurement of blood pressure can result in wrong diagnosis, determining, an inappropriate medical treatment, or even treatment of patients with no therapeutic indication.

Measurement of Arterial Blood Pressure

The indirect measurement of blood pressure can be performed, using various techniques, the former being performed with the mercury or aneroid, the most widely used in clinical practice, sphygmomanometer. Especially in the elderly, when ISH is common, incorrect measurement of blood pressure levels can occur and some aspects of its determination should be carefully examined. [63]

Briefly, the sounds or Korotkoff phases can be detected in most individuals if the procedure for the measurement is implemented within the established accuracy for this technique. There are five phases: PhaseI. Corresponds to the onset of the sound, in which the following beats are progressively stronger, of high frequency, and correlate with the level of systolic pressure. Phase II. At this point, the sound begins to diminish and can occur with low frequency sounds, which eventually determine the auscultatory gap. Phase III. The sounds are crisp and intense. Phase IV. Muffling of sounds corresponding to a time close to their disappearance. Phase V. Total disappearance of sounds. Correlates with the diastolic pressure. The evaluation phase of the estimated systolic pressure is important to avoid errors in indirect measurement of blood pressure. Firstly, to estimate the systolic pressure by palpation technique is fundamental, avoiding the most common errors in the BP determination in the elderly. In fact, it avoids errors associated with the phenomenon known as the auscultatory gap. This event takes place for short break in which the Korotkoff sounds are not audible, and may extend for periods up to 40 mm Hg. During the measurement of blood pressure, we can stop inflation eventually within the period of auscultatory gap, and thereby obtain falsely low readings for systolic pressure. This phenomenon usually occurs in elderly patients with hypertension, arteriosclerosis and severe aortic stenosis.

We should avoid repeated inflations and deflations of the cuff, which can cause painful stimuli and variation of blood pressure. It is important to certify that the equipment is calibrated and suitable for that patient. The patient should be resting for 5 minutes, and adviced to avoid ingestion of coffee, tea, alcohol or smoking.

Recent study in the Hospital "Good Samaritan" in Los Angeles evaluated the oscillometric method, now widely used, and compared with the classical auscultary measurement. They found that there were discrepancies between the two techniques, and these differences were significantly higher in individuals over 65 years. They found that the method underestimates the oscillometric blood pressure values at 2.6 mm Hg for SBP and 1.8 mm Hg for DBP[64].

In elderly patients, in view of changes in arterial vessels, the hemodynamic peculiarities of the pulse wave and the processes of deterioration of various functions of the body, the correct measure of the pressure has a number of characteristics.

1. Pressure Variability

There is an increase in pressure variability with age, especially in women. Thus, further steps should be done on these patients prior to determining the presence of hypertension. The measurement of blood pressure follows a Gaussian standard and elderly patients tend to flatter over the curve with a higher standard deviation. Therefore a larger number of measures will lead to greater accuracy of blood pressure level.

2. Auscultatory Gap

During the performance of indirect measurement by auscultation, the bag is inflated above the systolic pressure and thus the flow is interrupted. The auscultatory gap is the interval during which the Korotkoff sounds are audible even when the pressure inside the inflatable bag is high. This interval usually occurs at the end of stage I or II. The cause is not well known but is believed to decrease blood flow to the distal part of the cuff due to increased venous pressure.

This period of silence auscultation may be responsible for incorrect measurements, leading to falsely low SBP.The erroneous assessment of the falsely low SBP due to the auscultatory gap can be avoided by previously using the SBP palpatory technique and the second error can be avoided by getting an eye to the noise until the total deflation of the cuff.

3. Pseudo-Hypertension

Indirect measurements of blood pressure are based on the standpoint of physical collapse in the blood, and restoring blood flow. However the arteries of the elderly may be hardened by fibrosis or atherosclerosis and with that we can have huge discrepancies between indirect measurement and the true pressure value that can only be obtained by arterial catheterization. The pseudo-hypertension, characterized by discrepancies between the real values and the measured blood pressure, greater than 10 mm Hg for SBP or DBP may lead to unnecessary treatment and harm to the elderly. Its prevalence in the elderly varies from 1.5 to 4%. There are no systematic studies that allow an accurate estimate prevalence.In 1985, Messerli et al described a maneuver, named "Osler maneuver" [65] to identify patients with pseudo-hypertension.

It was characterized by the presence of the palpability of the radial artery even after the collapse of the brachial artery induced by the cuff. In that study, patients with positive phenomenon had a significant chance of having pseudo-hypertension. However, the contribution of the technique is uncertain, taking into account various factors, including low levels of the intra-observer reproducibility.

In general pseudo-hypertension is diagnosed clinically. It should be present in the elderly patient that does not respond to antihypertensive treatment, or in those subjects with high SBP without signs of target organ damage.

The suspicion of pseudo-hypertension should also be considered in the presence of symptoms of hypotension in patients that remain with high BP levels detected by indirect measurements despite antihypertensive therapy. The presence of arterial calcifications on the X-Rays reinforces the possibility of pseudo-hypertension.

4. Masked Hypertension

Masked Hypertension (MH) is defined as a clinical situation where the office blood pressure is less than 140/90 mm Hg, but higher levels are observed outside the medical office, such as in home blood pressure measurements (HBPM) or ambulatory blood pressure measurements (ABPM) (> 135/85 mmHg). The term, originally applied to individuals without treatment, can be extended to those patients with controlled office measures of BP. Although little is known about the pathophysiology of MH, some factors were now identified. It is important to consider the circadian rhythm of BP, higher in the morning, and lower later [66]. Assessments at particular times of the day could lead to this misdiagnosis, since MH is much more prevalent in older individuals, and in men with BP at the upper normal limit.Cigarette smoking may also influence MH, as one cigarette raises blood pressure for a period of about 30 minutes. Thus, "heavy-smokers"may raise BP in ABPM [67].Excess of alcohol intake, physical and mental activity would be further exacerbated in those individuals most active during the day or with a high burden of daily stress. The reproducibility of ABPM and HBPM for the diagnosis of MH is good, and prognosis in all studies is very similar to untreated HA, with significant lesions in target organs. Given the impossibility of performing ABPM or HBPM in all patients, MH should be considered in those subjects with normal BP in the office but with damage in target organs, with extension to hypertensive patients that are "controlled" in the office measures with progressive target organ damage.

5. White Coat Hypertension

White-coat hypertension (WCH) is considered when BP measured in the office is $\geq$ 140/90 mmHg, and when measured by HBPM or ABPM during daytime is less than 130/85 mmHg. WCH is very common, especially in the elderly. The condition is still under debate regarding its significance and prognosis.

Verdecchia et al [68]followed patients with WCH and found that the condition is not associated with stroke in the short-term follow-up, but in the long term WCH does not seem to be a benign condition, as it increases the rates of cerebrovascular events.

6. Post-Prandial Hypotension

The age is associated with several changes that may predispose to postural and postprandial hypotension. With the increase of age, a decreased baroreceptor response, autonomic dysfunction, reduced intravascular volume and cardiac output, defects in cerebral auto regulation, and diminished activity of the RAAS predispose to postural hypotension. In the majority of studies performed in the elderly, the BP measurements were done in the sitting position. In 1994, the National High Blood Pressure Education Working Group suggested that blood pressure should also be measured at up-right position to evaluate the effect of antihypertensive drugs in these patients.

During the pilot study of HYVET (Hypertension in the Elderly Trial) which has studied hypertensive patients over 80 years, postural hypertension with treatment was reported in 7.7% of patients [69].

Treatment

Hypertension is a chronic disease, with long asymptomatic course, without immediate consequence of treatment interruption, requiring changes in lifestyle and daily use of medicines. However, among elderly patients, with high frequency of co-morbidities, polypharmacy and the consequent increased risk of drug interactions and adverse effects in the geriatric population, special aspects should be taken into account during the treatment.

At the beginning, the treatment and dosage adjustments are crucial for BP control and adherence. Usually, BP control requires the implementation of frequent outpatient appointments, every 3-4 weeks. The choice of antihypertensive agents should be cautious, paying attention to the number of daily doses, drug interactions and especially for other health problems of the elderly such as heart diseases, urinary incontinence and orthostatic hypotension.

Lifestyle Changes

It was estimated that during human evolution, our ancestors consumed a diet with less than 0.25 grams of salt per day. About 5,000 years ago, the Chinese discovered that salt could be used to preserve food. Then, the salt has become of great economic importance, since it allowed preserving food during the winter and the development of settled communities. More recently, an increased intake of industrialized food products with high salt content, contributed to high salt consume, achieving levels of approximately 9-12 g/day.

Changes in salt intake are a big challenge for the kidneys to excrete these quantities. The consequence is that the intake of salt causes an increase in BP, thereby increasing the risk of cardiovascular disease (strokes, heart attacks and heart failure) and renal diseases.A recent systematic analysis of populationhealth data shows that the increase in blood pressure is a major cause of death and second leading cause of disability. The damage that the elevation in BP does is mainly through its effect on CVD, which is the main cause of death worldwide. High BP accounts for 62% of strokes and 49% of coronary heart disease. Importantly, there is a continuous relationship between BP levels and CVD, beginning at levels above 115/75 mmHg.

Numerous studies in rats, dogs, chickens, rabbits, baboons and chimpanzees have shown that salt intake plays an important role in regulating BP. Moreover, in all forms of experimental hypertension, whatever the animal model, high salt intake seems essential for BP elevation. A study in chimpanzees (98.8% genetic homology with humans) shows that a gradual increase in salt intake of 0.5 g/day up to 10-15 g/day, which is similar to our current salt intake, causes a progressive increase in blood pressure.Epidemiological studies such as the International study of macro-and micro-nutrients and BP and the EPIC-Norfolk (Norfolk cohort of European Prospective Investigation into Cancer) support the important role of salt intake and blood pressure levels in the population[70]. Changes in lifestyle should be encouraged among the elderly, with satisfactory adherence and benefits, as demonstrated by the Trial of Non-pharmacologic Interventions in the Elderly (TONE) [71].In this study, 875 elderly hypertensive subjects receiving antihypertensive monotherapy were randomized to restriction of sodium intake and / or weight reduction in obese, or normal treatment. After the withdrawal of antihypertensive agents, the patients were followed to re-examine blood pressure levels. At 29 months of follow up, 44% of patients in the group of sodium and weight reduction, 37% of the weight reduction group and 34% of the sodium reduction group did not have hypertension or the need for reintroduction of medication, compared to 26% of the control group (p <0.001).

Moderate sodium intake (2.4 g / day) and alcohol (30 ml ethanol / day for men and half for women), consumption of foods rich in potassium, magnesium, calcium and fiber, low content of saturated fat and regular physical activity, associated with weight loss in obese, are important strategies to be achieved in the elderly [72]. With these recommendations, patients can reduce the need of antihypertensive drugs and their cardiovascular risk as well as the quality of life [73]. Despite the widespread notion that it is very difficult to change lifestyle, when the approach is done with good sense, creating healthy alternatives, with clarification of goals and expected results, it is possible to obtain good adherence and treatment effectiveness [74-78].

The maintenance of low levels of blood pressure is closely linked to outcomes such as stroke or myocardial infarction. With this statement, regular exercise becomes a relevant non-pharmacological strategy that contributes for the achievement and maintenance of appropriate blood pressure levels, due to their effectiveness at different levels of hypertension [79]. Brandão-Rondon et al. (2002) found that low intensity exercise in hypertensive subjects with average age of 68 years (blood pressure not exceeding 160/110 mm Hg), promoted reduction in blood pressure during 22 hours and reduced the ventricular end diastolic volume, showing its importance for the treatment of hypertension in elderly subjects [80].

Due to the increased incidence of ISH among older patients, exercise of low intensity and duration of 30-50 minutes can significantly reduce blood pressure values, as reported by reductions of up to 19 mm Hg for SBP and 11 mm Hg for DBP [81]. However, better responses to blood pressure reduction in the ISH are obtained when the practice of physical exercises are conducted before the period of more pronounced changes in the elastic properties of great vessels, a period that comprises betweenfifty and seventy years of life [82]. Following exercise, a post exercise hypotension can occur, which is defined as a reduction in blood pressure after a single block of exercise, achieving BP values below those obtained pre-exercise [83, 84].

The mechanisms that generate the phenomenon of post exercise hypotension are not yet well established, but there may be an alteration in cardiac autonomic function and /or reduction in peripheral vascular resistance, associated with biochemical mediators of vasodilatory actions, such as production of nitric oxide (NO), prostaglandins and histamine [85, 86]. The benefits of reducing BP in relation to physical exercise occur in a dose-dependent manner; even if the reductions in blood pressure are small, they are associated with improvement of endothelial function and benefits on coronary heart disease.

Pharmacological Treatment

The primary goal of treating hypertension is the reduction in the rates of cardiovascular morbidity and mortality. Evidence from studies of clinically relevant outcomes, with relatively short duration, three to four years, demonstrate reduction of morbidity and mortality in studies initially designed to examine the role of diuretics, beta-blocker, ACE inhibitors, ARBs or CCB. However, in the majority of them, the association of antihypertensive drugs was needed.

Clinical trials have identified five classes of drugs that have been used successfully in elderly patients. The benefits were confirmed for diuretics, ACE inhibitors, beta-blockers, ARBs, and CCB.

The seventh report of the Joint National Committee on Prevention, Detection, Evaluation and Treatment of Hypertension (VII JNC) and the European Society of Hypertension (ESH) recommend that therapy with more than one antihypertensive agent should be considered in patients with SBP greater than 20 mm/Hg or DBP greater than 10 mm/Hg above goal and among patients with high cardiovascular risk, as determined by the BP levels and other risk factors. The combination therapy is recommended from the stage 2 of hypertension and seems to be more effective on blood pressure reduction and outcomes than the use of highest doses of a single drug. The VII Joint National Committee recommends diuretics as initial therapy for most patients with hypertension, regardless of age. Thiazides can be administered once a day and are effective at low doses in the elderly [87].

This benefit observed with BP reduction seems not dependent of the class of drugs used. However, recent meta-analysis suggested lower benefit with some beta-blockers in the elderly, particularly atenolol, when compared to other drugs.

Other guidelines (The Joint National Committee, the American Medical Association, American Heart Association, American Society of Hypertension, European Society of Hypertension and European Society of Cardiology) [88] emphasize that the main benefits of therapy are related to blood pressure reduction and its control. Thiazide diuretics and the group of ACE inhibitors seem to be the optimal drugs to safely reduce blood pressure and may provide survival benefits and reduce the risk of stroke or heart failure [89]. The calcium channel blockers may be sequentially added or replaced. As mentioned before, the data suggest that beta-blockers should not be used as primary therapy for hypertension in the elderly.

The RAAS seems to be involved in several complications of hypertension, such as the cardiovascular, cerebral, and renal disease. Its activation is an adaptive mechanism, but it can become overactive, leading to hypertension, heart failure, and impaired glomerular function. Angiotensin II-mediated activation of the angiotensin II type 1 (AT1) receptor has numerous effects, such as vasoconstriction, sodium and water retention, vascular and myocardial fibrosis and hypertrophy, and sympathetic nervous system activation. Thus, the RAAS blockade has been proposed for some subgroups of hypertensive patients with potential advantages.

The ARAMIS trial of 614 patients, who did not necessarily have diabetes, with ISH and albuminuria (2.2 mg/L) showed that the reduction in urinary albumin excretion was greater in the telmisartan (ARB) 20–80 mg group than in the hydrochlorothiazide 12.5 mg group [90].

A recent meta-analysis indicated that the combination of an ACE inhibitor and an ARB reduces proteinuria to a greater extent than does either drug alone. However, the efficacy of this combination in the ONTARGET study failed to demonstrate benefit over the use of ACE inhibitor (ramipril) or the ARB alone. After a follow-up period of 56 months, the primary renal end point (a composite parameter of dialysis, doubling of serum creatinine, and death) was similar for both telmisartan and ramipril, while higher rates for this combined end point were seen with the combination therapy [91]. Currently, the combination of ARB and ACE inhibitors should be prescribed only for patients with heart failure that is not controlled by ACE inhibitors [92, 93].

With respect to stroke prevention, there are important studies reporting huge benefits with antihypertensive treatment. The PROGRESS trial of 6,105 patients showed that a combination of the ACE inhibitor perindopril with the diuretic indapamide reduced the risk of recurrent stroke by 28% compared with placebo after a 4-year follow-up period [94].

In the SCOPE trial, the use of candesartan (ARB) was associated with 42% reduction in the stroke rates in patients with ISH. Early benefits following the use of ARB in the acute phase of stroke were observed as reported in the SCAST trial [95,96].

Clear benefits of antihypertensive therapy, among elderly subjects were confirmed by the results of the HYVET study.Treatment of hypertension is likely to prevent heart failure, reduce stroke and prolong life. Based on the HYVET study, a target blood pressure below 150/80 mm Hg seems both effective and safe.

Current evidence favors the use of diuretics (indapamide or chlorthalidone) as the initial strategy to treat hypertension in the elderly. However, as shown in ALLHAT [97] and HYVET [98], treatment should be effective enough to achieve the target blood pressure independently of the antihypertensive drug class [99].

A number of placebo-controlled studies, including HOPE, EUROPA, IDNT, IRMA2, RENAAL, and TRANSCEND, support the hypothesis that antihypertensive agents may have beneficial effects beyond their blood pressure-lowering effects. A number of other studies, including AMADEO, DETAIL, LIFE, and ONTARGET, which compared active agents in populations that were already receiving other antihypertensive therapies demonstrated effects over and above good blood pressure control [100 - 102].

Important Features of Antihypertensive Agents (97)

1. Be effective orally.
2. Be safe, well tolerated and with relative a good risk - benefit profile for the patient.
3. Allow administration preferably for single daily doses.
4. Be initiated at the lowest effective doses recommended for eachclinical situation and be gradually increased, considering that the higher the dose, the more likely the adverse effect.
5. Be considered in combination for patients with hypertension instages 2 and stage 3 and for patients at high or very high cardiovascular risk
6. Be used for a minimum of four weeks, except when there is need for increasing doses, changes or replacement of monotherapy.

7. Have demonstrated in clinical trials the ability to reduce cardiovascular morbidity and mortality.

Disclosures

The authors report no conflicts of interest in this work.

References

A. Conceptualization and Epidemiology

[1] Burt VL, Whelton P, Roccella EJ, et al.: Prevalence of hypertension in the US adult population. Results from the Third National Health and Nutrition Examination Survey,1988-1991. *Hypertension* 1995;25:305-313.

[2] National Cholesterol Education Program (NCEP) Expert Panel on Detection, Evaluation, and Treatment of High Blood Cholesterol in Adults (Adult Treatment Panel III), Executive Summary of the Third Report of the National Cholesterol Education Program (NCEP) Expert Panel on Detection, Evaluation, and Treatment of High Blood Cholesterol in Adults (Adult Treatment Panel III), *JAMA*2001;285: 2486–2497.

[3] Lloyd-Jones DM, Evans JC, Larson MG, Levy D: Treatment and control of hypertension in the community: A prospective analysis. *Hypertension* 2002;40:640-646.

[4] Mancia G, Grassi G: Systolic and diastolic blood pressure control in antihypertensive drug trails. *J Hypertens*2002;20:1461-1464.

[5] Vassan RS, Beiser A, Seshadri S, et al: Residual lifetime risk for developing hypertension in middle-aged women and men. The Framingham Heart Study. *JAMA* 2002;287:1003-1010.

[6] Neaton JD, Wentworth D. Serum cholesterol, blood pressure, cigarette smoking, and death from coronary heart disease. Overall findings and differences by age for 316,099 white men. Multiple Risk Factor Intervention Trial Research Group. *Arch Intern Med* 1992;152:56-64.

[7] Domanski M, Mitchell G, Pfeffer M, et al: Pulse pressure and cardiovascular disease-related mortality: Follow-up study of the Multiple Risk Factor Intervention Trial (MRFIT). *JAMA* 2002;287:2677-2683.

[8] Lewington S, Clarke R, Qizilbash N, Peto R, Collins R; Prospective Studies Collaboration. Age-specific relevance of usual blood pressure to vascular mortality: A meta-analysis of individual data for one million adults in 61 prospective studies. *Lancet* 2002;360:1903-1913.

[9] Veterans Administration Cooperatives Study Group on Antihypertensive Agents. Effects of treatment on morbidity in hypertension: II. Results in patients with diastolic blood pressure averaging 90 through 114 mm -Hg. *JAMA* 1970;213: 1143-1152.

[10] Reader R. Australian therapeutic trial in mild hypertension. *Med J Aust*1984;140:752-754.

[11] SHEP Cooperative Research Group Prevention of stroke by antihypertensive drug treatment in older persons with isolated systolic hypertension. Final results of the Systolic Hypertension in the Elderly Program. *JAMA*1991; 265: 3255-3264.

[12] Dahlöf B, Hansson L, Lindholm L, Råstam L, Scherstén B, Wester. STOP-hypertension: Swedish trial in old patients with hypertension.*J Hypertens* 1986;4:511-513.

[13] Hansson L, Lindholm LH, Ekbom T, et al.,for the STOP-Hypertension-2 study group. Randomised trial of old and newanti antihypertensive drugs in elderly patients: cardiovascular mortality andmorbidity the Swedish Trial in Old Patients with Hypertension-2 study. *Lancet*1999;354:1751-1756.

[14] Davis TM, Millns H, Stratton IM, Holman RR, Turner RC. Risk factors forstroke in type 2 diabetes mellitus: United Kingdom Prospective Diabetes Study (UKPDS).*Arch Intern Med* 1999;159:1097–1103.

[15] Mogensen CE, Neldam S, Tikkanen I, et al. Randomised controlled trial of dual blockade of renin-angiotensin systemin patients with hypertension, microalbuminuria, and non-insulin dependent diabetes, the candesartan and lisinopril microalbuminuria (CALM)study. *BMJ*2000;321:1440–1444.

[16] Hansson L, Zanchetti, A, Carruthers SG, et al. Effects of intensive blood-pressure lowering and low-dose aspirin in patients with hypertension: principal results of the Hypertension Optimal Treatment (HOT) randomized trial. *Lancet*1998;351:1755–1762.

[17] Zamboli P, De Nicola L, Minutolo R, Bertino V, Catapano F, Conte G. Management of hypertension in chronic kidney disease. *Curr Hypertens Rep* 2006;8:497-501.

[18] Ong KL, Cheung BM, Man YB, Lam KS, Lau CP. Prevalence, awareness, treatment, and control of hypertension among United States adults 1999-2004. *Hypertension.* 2007;49:69–75.

[19] Fogari R, Derosa G, Zoppi A, et al. Effect of telmisartan amlodipine combination at different doses onurinary albumin excretion in hypertensive diabetic patients with microalbuminuria. *Am J Hypertens.* 2007;20:417–422.

[20] Pahor M, Psaty BM, Alderman MH, Applegate WB, Williamson JD, Furberg CD. Therapeutic benefits of ACE inhibitors and other antihypertensive drugs in patients with type 2 diabetes. *Diabetes Care.* 2000;23:888–892.

[21] Weir MR, Bakris GL. Combination therapy with Renin-Angiotensin-aldosterone receptor blockers for hypertension: how far have we come? *J Clin Hypertens (Greenwich)* 2008;10:146–152.

[22] Ishimitsu T, Yagi S, Ebihara A, et al. Long-term evaluation of combinedantihypertensive therapy with lisinopril and a thiazide diuretic in patients with essential hypertension. *Jpn Heart J* 1997;38:831-840.

[23] Brown MJ, Palmer CR, Castaigne A, et al. Morbidity and mortality in patients randomised to double-blind treatment with a long-acting calcium-channel blocker or diuretic in the International Nifedipine GITS study: Intervention as a Goal in Hypertension Treatment (INSIGHT). *Lancet* 2000 Jul 29;356(9227):366-72.

[24] Hansson L, Hedner T, Lund-Johansen P, et al. for the NORDIL Study Group. Randomised trial of effects of calcium antagonists compared with diuretics and blockers on cardiovascular morbidity and mortality in hypertension: the Nordic Diltiazem (NORDIL) study.*Lancet* 2000;356:359-365.

[25] The Atherosclerosis Risk in Communities (ARIC) Study: design and objectives. The ARIC investigators. *Am J Epidemiol* 1989;129:687-702.

[26] Malacco E, Varì N, Capuano V, et al. A randomized, double-blind, active-controlled, parallel-group comparison of valsartan and amlodipine in the treatment of isolated systolic hypertension in elderly patients: the Val-Syst study.*Clin Ther* 2003;25:2765-2780.

B. Pathophysiology

[27] Dart A, Kingwell B. Pulse pressure–a review of mechanisms and clinical relevance. *J Am Coll Cardiol*. 2001;37:975–984.

[28] Wang YX, Fitch RM. Vascular stiffness: measurements, mechanisms and implications. *Curr Vasc Pharmacol*. 2004;2:379 –384.

[29] Nichols W, O'Rourke M. Contours of pressure and flow waves in arteries. In: Nichols W, O'Rourke M, eds. *McDonald's Blood Flow in Arteries. Theoretical, Experimental and Clinical Principles*. London Edward Arnold; 1998.

[30] Wolinsky H, Glagov S. Structural basis for the static mechanical properties of the aortic media. *Circ Res*. 1964;14:400–413.

[31] Vasan RS, Beiser A, Seshadri S, et al. Residual lifetime risk for developinghypertension in middle-aged women and men. *JAMA*. 2002;10:287-288.

[32] Mitchell GF, Parise H, Benjamin EJ, *et al*. Changes in arterial stiffness andwave reflection with advancing age in health men and women. *Hypertension*.2004;43:1239-1245.

[33] Halock P, Benson IC. Studies on the elastic properties of human isolated aorta.*J Clin Invest*. 1937;16:595-602.

[34] Oparil S, Zaman A, Calhoun DA. Pathogenesis of hypertension. *Ann Intern Med*.2003;139:761-766.

[35] Mulvanym J, Baumbach GL, Aalkjaer C, *et al*. Vascular remodeling.*Hypertension*.1996;28:505-506.

[36] Lakatta EG, Levy D. Arterial and cardiac aging: major shareholders incardiovascular disease enterprises: Part I: aging arteries: a "set up" forvascular disease. *Circulation*. 2003;107:139 –146.

[37] Rajagopalan S, Meng XP, Ramasamy S, Harrison DG, Galis ZS.Reactive oxygen species produced by macrophage-derived foam cellsregulate the activity of vascular matrix metalloproteinases in vitro.Implications for atherosclerotic plaque stability. *J Clin Invest*. 1996;98:2572–2579.

[38] Nichols WW, O'Rourke MF. Aortic pulse wave velocity, reflection sitedistance and augmentation index.*Hypertension*. 2008;52:478-483.

[39] Mulvanym J, Baumbach GL, Aalkjaer C, et al. Vascular remodeling.*Hypertension*.1996;28:505-6.

[40] Furchgott, R.F., Zawadzki, J.V. The obligatory role of endothelial cell inthe relaxation of arterial smooth muscle by acetylcholine. *Nature*. 1980;228:373- 376.

[41] Kolpakov, V., Gordon , D. and Thomas , J.K. Nitric oxide-generatingcompoundsinhibit total protein and collagen synthesis in cultured vascularsmooth muscle cells. *Circ. Res*.1995;76:305-309.

[42] Hill JM, et al.Circulating endothelial progenitor cells, vascular function, andcardiovascular risk. *N. Engl. J. Med.*2003;348:593-600.

[43] Bautista LE. Inflammation, endothelial dysfunction, and the risk of highblood pressure:epidemiologic and biological evidence. *J Hum Hypertens.* 2003;17:223-30.

[44] Rajagopalan S, Meng XP, Ramasamy S, Harrison DG, Galis ZS.Reactive oxygen species produced by macrophage-derived foam cellsregulate the activity of vascular matrix metalloproteinases in vitro.Implications for atherosclerotic plaque stability. *J Clin Invest.* 1996;98:2572–2579.

[45] Lewington S, Clarke R, Qizilbash N, Peto R, Collins R. for the ProspectiveStudies Collaboration. Age-specific relevance of usual blood pressure tovascularmortality: a meta-analysis of individual data for one million adultsin 61prospective studies. *Lancet.* 2002;360:1903–1913.

[46] Franklin SS, Khan SA, Wong ND, Larson MG, Levy D. Is pulse pressureuseful inpredicting risk for coronary heart disease? *Circulation.*1999;100:354-360.

[47] Duprez DA. Role of the rennin-angiotensin-aldosterone system in vascularremodeling and inflammation: a clinical review. *J Hypertens.* 2006;24:983-991.

[48] Levitt NS, Steyn K, De Wet T, Morrell C, Edwards R, Ellison GT, Cameron N. An inverse relation between blood pressure and birth weight among 5year old children from Soweto, South Africa. *J Epidemiol Community Health.*1999;53:264–268.

[49] Gennser Gerhard, Rymark Per, Isberg Per Erik. Low birth weight and riskof high blood pressure in adulthood. *Br Med J (Clin Res Ed)* 1988:28;1498–1500.

[50] Gil F. Salles; Roberto Fiszman; Claudia R.L. Cardoso; Elizabeth S.Muxfeldt.Relation of Left Ventricular Hypertrophy With SystemicInflammation and Endothelial Damage in Resistant Hypertension.*Hypertension.* 2007;50:723-728

[51] Baum MA, Underwood DA. Left ventricular hypertrophy: An overlookedcardiovascular risk factor *Cleve Clin J Med.* 2010;77:381-3877.

[52] Dahlof B, et al. LIFE STUDY – Losartan Intervention for Endpoint inHypertension Study. *Lancet.* 2002; 35:9995-1003.

[53] Seventh report of the Joint National Committee on Prevention, Detection,Evaluation, and Treatment of High Blood Pressure. *Hypertension* 2003; 42:1206–1252.

[54] Watanabe Y, Metoki H, Ohkubo T, Katsuya T, Tabara Y, Kikuya M, HiroseT et al.Accumulation of common polymorphisms is associated withdevelopment of hypertension: a 12-year follow-up from the Ohasama studyY.*Hypertens Res.* 2010;33:129-134.

[55] Franklin SS, Pio JR, Wong ND, et al. Predictors of new-onset diastolic andsystolic hypertension. *Circulation.* 2005;111:1121-1127.

[56] Li JJ, Chen JL. Inflammation may be a bridge connecting hypertension andatherosclerosis. *Med Hypotheses.* 2005;64:925-929.

[57] Herlitz J, Bang A, Karlson BW. Five year prognosis after acute myocardialinfarction in relation to a history of hypertension. *Am J Hypertens.*1996;9:70-76.

[58] KaplanNM. Primary hypertension: natural history and evaluation. In:KaplanNM (ed.).*Kaplan's clinical hypertension*. Philadelphia: LippincottWilliams and Wilkins;2006. p.122-60.

[59] Shimada K, Kawamoto A, Matsubayashi K, Ozawa T. Silentcerebrovascular disease in the elderly. Correlation with ambulatory pressure.*Hypertension.* 1990;16:692-699.

[60] Gary F. Mitchell; Paul R. Conlin; Mark E. Dunlap; Yves Lacourcière; J.Malcolm O. Arnold; Richard I. Ogilvie; Joel Neutel; Joseph L. Izzo, Jr; MarcPfeffer Aortic Diameter, Wall Stiffness, and Wave Reflection in SystolicHypertension *Hypertension.* 2008;51:105.

[61] Mitchell GF, Parise H, Benjamin EJ, *et al.* Changes in arterial stiffness andwave reflection with advancing age in health men and women. *Hypertension.*2004;43:1239-1245.

[62] Franklin SS, Jacobs MJ, WongND, L'Italien GJ, Lapuerta P. Predominanceofisolated systolic hypertension among middle-aged and elderly UShypertensives. *Hypertension.* 2001;37:869-874.

[63] Coleman AJ, Steel SD, Ashworth M, Vowler SL, Shennan A. Accuracy of thepressure scale of sphygmomanometers in clinical use within primary care.*Blood Press Monit.* 2005;10:181-238.

[64] Kloner RA, Leor J, Poole WK, Perritt R. Population-bases analysis of the effects of the Northridge Earthquake on cardiac deat in Los AngelesCoutry, California. *J Am Coll Cardiol.* 1997;5:1174-1180.

[65] Messerli FH, Ventura HO, Amodeo C. Osler's maneuver andpeudohypertension. *N Eng J Med.* 1985; 312:1548-1551.

[66] Hoshide S, Ishikawa J, Eguchi K, et al. Masked nocturnal hypertension andtarget organ damage in hypertension and target organ damage inhypertension with well-controlled self-measured home blood pressure.*Hypertens Res.* 2007;30:143-149.

[67] Mann SJ, James GD, Wang RS, Pickering TG. Elevation of ambulatorysystolicblood pressure in hypertensives smokers. A case control. *JAMA*1991; 265:2226- 2228.

[68] Verdecchia P, Reboldi GP, Schwartz JE, et al. Short-and long-term incidenceof stroke in white-coat hypertension. *Hypertension* 2005; 45:203-208.

[69] Beckett NS, Connor M, Sadler JD, et al.Orthostatic fall in blood pressure inthe very-very elderly hypertensive: results from the Hypertension in theElderly Trial pilot (HYVET). *J Hum Hypertens.* 1999; 13:839-840.

C. Treatment

[70] Khaw KT, Bingham S, Welch A, Luben R, O'Brien E, Wareham N, Day N. Blood pressure and urinary sodium inmen and woman: The Norfolk Cohort of the Europe propective Investigation to Cancer (EPIC-Norfolk). *Am J Clin Nutr*2004; 5:1397-1403.

[71] Lawrence J. Appel et al.The Trial of Nonpharmacologic Interventions in theElderly (TONE). *Am Heart J.* 2002;144:625-6299.

[72] Greenberg I, Stampfer MJ, Schwarzfuchs D, Shai I; DIRECT Group. Adherenceand success in long-term weight loss diets: the dietary intervention randomizedcontrolled trial (DIRECT). *Am Coll Nutr.* 2009;28:159-68.

[73] Ebrahim S, Smith GD. Lowering blood pressure: a systematic review of sustainedeffects of non-pharmacological interventions. *J Public Health Med.*1998;20:441- 448.

[74] Mulrow CD, Chiquette E, Angel L, Cornell J, Summerbell C, Anagnostelis B,Grimm R Jr, Brand MB.*Nurs Times.* 2001;97:17-23.

[75] Appel LJ, Moore TJ, Obarzanek E, Vollmer WM, Svetkey LP, Sacks FM *et al.* Aclinical trial of the effects of dietary patterns on blood pressure. DASHCollaborative Research Group. *N Engl J Med.* 1997; 336:1117–1124.

[76] Intersalt Cooperative Research Group. Intersalt: an international study ofelectrolyte excretion and blood pressure. Results for 24 h urinary sodium andpotassium excretion.BMJ 1988; 297: 319–328.

[77] Seventh report of the Joint National Committee on Prevention, Detection,Evaluation, and Treatment of High Blood Pressure. *Hypertension.* 2003; 42:1206–1252.

[78] Seals, D. R., and M. J. Reiling. Effect of regular exercise on 24-hour arterialpressure in older hypertensive humans. *Hypertension.*1991;18:583-592.

[79] Brandão-Rondon MU, Alves MJ, Braga AM, Teixeira OT, Barretto AC, Krieger EM, Negrão CE. Postexercise blood pressure reduction in elderly hypertensivepatients *J Am Coll Cardiol.* 2002;39:676-682.

[80] Lochner J, Rugge B, Judkins D, Saseen J. Clinical inquiries. How effective arelifestyle changes for controlling hypertension? *J Fam Pract.* 2006;55:73-74.

[81] Kingwell BA. Large artery stiffness: implications for exercise capacity andcardiovascular risk. *Clin Exp Pharmacol Physiol.* 2002 ;29:214-217.

[82] Macdonald, JR, Macdougall, JD, and Hogben, CD. The effects of exercisingmuscle mass on post exercise hypotension. *J Hum Hypertens* 2000 ;14: 317–320.

[83] Hagberg, JM, Montain, SJ, Martins, WH. Blood pressure and hemodynamicresponses after exercise in older hypertensives. *Eur J Appl Physiol* 1987;63:270-276.

[84] Rezk, CC, Marrache, RCB, Tinucci, T, Mion, Jr DJ, and Forjaz, CLM. Post-resistance exercise hypotension, hemodynamics, and heart rate variability:influence of exercise intensity. *Eur J Appl Physiol 2006; 98*:105-112.

[85] Bhoola KD, Figueroa CD, Worthy K. Bioregulation of kinins:kallikreins,kininogens, and kininases. *Pharmacol Rev* 1992;44: 1-80.

[86] Cornelissen VA, Fagard RH. Effects of enduranceblood pressure-regulating mechanisms, and cardiovascular risk*Hypertension.* 2005;46:667-675.

[87] Mancia G, Laurent S, Agabiti-Rosei E, et al. Reappraisal ofEuropeanguidelines on hypertension management: a European Society of Hypertensionask force document. *J Hypertens.* 2009;27: 2121-2158. 19.

[88] Mancia G, De BG,Dominiczak A, Cifkova R, Fagard R, Germano G et al. ESH-ESC *Practice Guidelines for the Management of ArterialHypertension*:2007; 25:1751-1762.

[89] Burnier M, Brunner HR. Angiotensin II receptor antagonist. *Lancet.*2000;355:637-645.

[90] Vogt L, Navis G, Köster J, Manolis AJ, Reid JL, de Zeeuw D; for Angiotensin II Receptor Antagonist telmisartan Micardis in Isolated Systolic hypertension (ARAMIS) study group. The angiotensin II receptor antagonist telmisartanreduces urinary albumin excretion in patients with isolated systolic.*J Hypertens.* 2005; 23:2055-2061.

[91] The ongoing telmisartan alone and in combination with ramipril globalendpoint trial program.*Am J Cardiol.* 2003;91:28G-34G.

[92] Cohn JN, Tognoni G; for Valsartan Heart Failure Trial Investigators. Arandomized trial ofthe angiotensin-receptor blocker valsartan in chronicheart failure. *N Engl J Med.* 2001;345:1667-1675

[93] McMurray JJ, Ostergren J, Swedberg K, et al; for CHARM Investigators andCommittees. Effects of candesartan in patients with chronic heart failure

andreducedleft-ventricular systolic function taking angiotensin-converting-enzyme inhibitors: the CHARM-Added trial. *Lancet.* 2003;362:767-771.

[94]   PROGRESS Collaborative Group. Randomised trial of a perindopril- basedblood-pressure-lowering regimen among 6,105 individuals with previousstroke or transient ischaemic attack. *Lancet.* 2001;358:1033-1041.

[95]   Trenkwalder P, Elmfeldt D, Hofman A, Lithell H, Olofsson B, Papademetriou V, Skoog I, Zanchetti A; Study on COgnition and Prognosis in the Elderly (SCOPE). The Study on COgnition and Prognosis in the Elderly (SCOPE) - major CV events and stroke*Blood Press.* 2005;1:31-7.

[96]   Sandset EC, Murray G, Boysen G, Jatuzis D, Kõrv J, Lüders S, Richter PS, Roine RO, Terént A, Thijs V, Berge E; SCAST Study Group. Angiotensin receptor blockade in acute stroke*Int J Stroke.* 2010;5:423-7.

[97]   ALLHAT Officers and Coordinators. Major Outcomes in High- RiskHypertensive Patients Randomized to Angiotensin-Converting EnzymeInhibitoror Calcium Channel Blocker vs Diuretic. *JAMA* 2002;288:2981-97.

[98]   BeckettNS, Peters R, Fletcher AE, *et al.* HYVET Study Group. Treatment ofhypertension in patients 80 years of age or older.*N Engl J Med*8;358:1887-1998.

[99]   VI Brazilian Guidelines of Hypertension.DBH VI *Rev Bras Hipertens* vol.2010;1:5-6.

[100] Yusuf S. From the HOPE to the ONTARGET and the TRANSCEND studies: challenges in improving prognosis. *Am J Cardiol.* 2002;89(2A):18A-25A.

[101] Dahlöf B, Devereux R, de Faire U, Fyhrquist F, Hedner T, Ibsen H, Julius S, Kjeldsen S, Kristianson K, Lederballe-Pedersen O, Lindholm LH, Nieminen MS, Omvik P, Oparil S, Wedel H.The Losartan Intervention For Endpoint reduction (LIFE) in Hypertension study: rationale, design, and methods. The LIFE Study Group.*Am J Hypertens.* 1997;10(7 Pt 1):705-13.

[102] Stojiljkovic L, Behnia R. Role of renin angiotensin system inhibitors in cardiovascular and renal protection: a lesson from clinical trials.*Curr Pharm Des.* 2007;13(13):1335-45.

In: Systolic Blood Pressure   ISBN: 978-1-61209-263-8
Editor: Robert A. Arfi   ©2012 Nova Science Publishers, Inc.

Chapter VII

Systolic Blood Pressure: Implications for Stroke Prevention and Immediate Management

Hebah Hefzy[*1] *and Brian Silver*[2]

[1]Department of Neurology, Allegheny General Hospital, Pittsburgh, PA, US
[2]Department of Neurology, Rhode Island Hospital, Providence, RI, US

Abstract

Hypertension, especially systolic hypertension, is the single most important modifiable risk factor for stroke. A number of recent studies have shown that for primary and secondary stroke prevention, beta blockers should no longer be considered first line agents because of a relatively higher risk of stroke recurrence, mortality (particularly in diabetics) and new onset diabetes compared to other drug classes. First-line choices should include calcium channel blockers, angiotensin converting enzyme inhibitors, angiotensin receptor blockers, and diuretics. Patients with diabetes and chronic kidney disease require specific treatment. Most patients require multiple agents for control. Initial polytherapy may be superior to monotherapy and graduated titration. Acute blood pressure management in stroke is less well defined. The available data suggest that excessive rises and declines in blood pressure may be associated with worse outcomes. Ongoing trials are designed to establish a scientific basis for acute stroke blood pressure management.

Keywords: Stroke, blood pressure, prevention

---

* Correspondence: Hebah Hefzy, MD, Department of Neurology, Allegheny General Hospital, 420 East North Avenue, Suite 206, Pittsburgh, PA 15212, Phone: (412) 359-8850, Fax: (412) 359-8878
Disclosures: Dr. Hefzy has nothing to disclose.Dr. Silver has served as a consultant for Abbott Vascular and as an expert in stroke medical malpractice defense.

Hypertension and Risk of Stroke

Hypertension is the single most important modifiable risk factor for stroke due to its overall prevalence in society and the high relative risk for stroke when present [1-3]. An estimated 72% of stroke survivors have hypertension, with 79% having isolated systolic hypertension (ISH) [4]. An estimated 27% of first ever ischemic strokes among treated hypertensive patients are due to uncontrolled hypertension[5]. Antihypertensive therapy has been shown to reduce stroke recurrence by 25% [6].

Of any blood pressure measure, systolic blood pressure (SBP) alone is the single greatest predictor of stroke risk in men, women, patients with chronic kidney disease, and in the elderly [7-11]. This association remains true for the middle – aged population (aged 45-64) [12] and in stroke patients across all ethnic backgrounds. Myint et. al. reported that in a prospectively followed cohort of British stroke-free patients, risk of stroke increased with age, and a SBP greater than 140 was equal to being 6 years older in regards to risk of stroke [13]. During a mean follow-up period of 11 years, Inoue et. al. found that in a large population of Japanese patients without a history of stroke, the relative hazard of stroke for patients with ISH during 24 hour ambulatory blood pressure monitoring was 2.24 (p=0.002) [14]. In addition to being a known risk factor for stroke throughout Europe and China [15, 16], higher SBP was also found to be an independent risk factor for stroke in a retrospectively studied South Indian population [17].

Maximum SBP, independent of mean SBP, over a range of seven office visits, was found to be a strong predictor of stroke in patients with previous transient ischemic attack (TIA) in the UK-TIA aspirin trial (Hazard Ration [HR] 15.01, p,0.0001) [18]. These results were validated by the same authors in three other TIA cohorts. Using carotid duplex ultrasonography, Lernfelt et. al found that bilateral carotid plaques in an elderly population were independently associated with elevated SBP [19]. Furthermore, men (not women) with bilateral carotid plaques had an increased risk of stroke and mortality during 5-year follow-up.

In addition to increasing the risk of stroke, elevated SBP has been associated with an increased risk of microbleeds as well as white matter hyperintensities on Magnetic Resonance Imaging (MRI) in patients who have previously had a stroke or TIA [20-22]. In patients receiving thrombolytic therapy for acute stroke in the Australian Streptokinase Trial, elevated baseline SBP >165, independent of elevated SBP before therapy, resulted in a > 25% risk of major post-lytic hemorrhage [23].

Further evidence supporting the relationship between elevated SBP and stroke is seen in genetic studies. A genetic predisposition to higher SBP values was seen in a large European population related to the presence of rs17238540 single nucleotide polymorphism on the G allele [24]. These patients had a higher rate of stroke compared to patients who did not carry this trait (p=0.009). Genetic studies in Swedish men have shown that the functional K55R polymorphism of the EPHX2 gene confers a higher risk of hypertension prevalence and increases the risk of incident ischemic stroke in male homozygotes [25].

Many clinicians allow higher SBP's in patients with intracranial arterial stenosis. While this may be an appropriate option for patients with previous stroke or TIA who have bilateral carotid stenosis > or = 70% [26], investigators in the Warfarin-Aspirin Symptomatic Intracranial Disease (WASID) trial found that risk of ischemic stroke and stroke in the territory of the stenotic vessel increased with increasing mean SBP values (p<0.0001); this remained true even after adjustment for all other risk factors [27].

Nocturnal variations in SBP and their effect on risk of ischemic stroke were studied by Kario et. al. They evaluated the ambulatory blood pressure readings (recorded every 30 minutes for 24 hours) of 575 older Japanese patients who were prospectively followed for an average of 41 months and found that patients were at a significantly higher risk of both silent and clinical cerebral infarcts as determined by brain MRI if their nocturnal SBP dipped by > or = to 20% or increased by > or = to 0% (average increase 3.7 +/- 4.5 mm Hg) [28].

Systolic Blood Pressure Target for Stroke Prevention

Treatment of isolated elevated systolic blood pressure reduces stroke incidence and mortality in all age groups, with the greatest effect seen in men and people over the age of 60 [29, 30]. Treatment of SBP to < 160 reduced the incidence of stroke by one-third in the Systolic Hypertension in the Elderly Program (SHEP) [31]. The benefit of antihypertensive medications for stroke risk reduction is only partly explained by their effect on lower SBP; the complete mechanism for stroke risk reduction remains unclear [32]. In fact, some studies have shown antihypertensive medications to be useful in preventing stroke while not significantly lowering SBP [33]. Precise blood pressure targets for secondary stroke prevention are currently being investigated.

Prehypertension (defined as SBP 120-139), though identified as a significant risk factor for coronary heart disease, has not previously been found to increase the risk of stroke [34, 35]. During a 32 year follow-up period, Strandberg et. al. found that the risk of stroke was only increased in patients with SBP > 140 [36]. For ISH > 140, the risk ratio for stroke recurrence after initial stroke has been reported to be 2.2 relative to SBP < 140 [37].

In patients with diabetes mellitus (DM), the risk may be higher with SBP values in the 130-140 range as compared with non-diabetics. Adler et. al. reported that the risk of stroke in patients with type II DM (DM II) is lowest with SBP < 130, and increases significantly with each 10 mm Hg increase in SBP [38]. They found a 19% decrease in the HR of stroke with each decrease in SBP by 10 mm Hg, with the greatest decrease seen in patients who had a SBP < 130. In their model forecasting the risk of first stroke in patients with DM II, Kothari et. al. demonstrate that the chance of a stroke-free survival is higher in patients whose SBP remains < 135 as compared to those whose SBP is > 135 [39]. Investigators on behalf of the Action to Control Cardiovascular Risk in Diabetes (ACCORD) study reported that in 4,733 patients with DM II, intensive reduction of SBP below 120 as compared with moderate reduction (SBP 120-140) decreased the annual risk of stroke from 0.53% to 0.32% (p = 0.01) [40]. However, the investigators found that intensive lowering of SBP to below 120 resulted in an increase in the risk of serious adverse events (e.g. hypotension) by 2% as compared to moderate SBP reduction (p < 0.001).

The hazard of incident stroke in patients with chronic kidney disease (CKD) is elevated beyond that of patients without CKD when the SBP is > or = 140 [41]. In an urban Japanese population, patients with CKD had a significantly lower stroke risk with SBP < 120; this risk increased thereafter with every increase in SBP by 10 mm Hg [42].

The Secondary Prevention of Small Subcortical Strokes (SPS-3) study is a currently ongoing national institutes of health funded trial investigating the efficacy of lowering SBP < 130 in preventing future strokes in patients small subcortical strokes (NINDS: 2 U01 NS38529-04A1).

Recommended Antihypertensive Medications for Stroke Prevention

Many antihypertensive classes have been tested for both primary and secondary stroke prevention. Different patient populations seem to gain the most benefit from different classes of medications. Conflicting data exists regarding the superiority of diuretic therapy in preventing stroke in the elderly population. While some reports indicate that thiazide diuretics appear to confer the greatest reduction in stroke risk in the elderly population [7], others indicate that angiotensin receptor blockers (ARBs) and angiotensin converting enzyme inhibitors (ACE-I) confer a superior stroke risk reduction [33, 43]. Zuliani et. al. reported that ACE-I have been shown to reduce 30 day mortality in patients age 80 and older when given after severe acute ischemic stroke [43]. In patients age 80 and older with a SBP of 160 or more, the diuretic indapamide with or without the ACE-I perindopril has been shown to decrease the risk of fatal or nonfatal stroke by 30% during a follow-up period of 2 years [44]. This combination was found to be effective in reducing the risk of stroke in patients with and without hypertension, irrespective of age in the Perindopril Protection Against Recurrent Stroke Study (PROGRESS) [45]. Perindopril has also been shown to stop or delay the progression of white matter hyperintensities in a population of predominantly male patients (mean age 60) with cerebrovascular disease [21].

Beta blockers are not recommended as first line antihypertensives in patients with uncomplicated hypertension due to their poor ability to prevent future stroke [46, 47]. Atenolol was found in one study to have a 26% higher risk of stroke than other antihypertensives [47]. Not only do beta blockers carry the possibility of increasing future stroke risk, they also have been shown to increase early case fatality [48].

The Antihypertensive and Lipid-Lowering Treatment to Prevent Heart Attack Trial (ALLHAT) established the superiority of diuretic based treatment over alpha-blocker based antihypertensive treatment for the prevention of stroke [49]. There was, however, a greater incidence in new-onset diabetes in diuretic treated patients. Ekbom et. al. report that antihypertensive therapy with beta blockers or diuretics is inferior in stroke prevention to the newer medications (calcium channel blockers [CCBs} and ACE-Is) [50]. In a prospectively followed Japanese population, there was no difference in the 3 year risk of stroke between patients treated with ACE-Is versus CCBs, however, there were significantly more side effects noted with ACE-I therapy [51]. The Losartan Intervention for Endpoint Reduction (LIFE) study group reported that in patients with ISH and evidence of left ventricular hypertrophy on electrocardiographic testing, the incidence of stroke was significantly reduced in patients taking the ARB losartan compared to patients taking atenolol [52]. In addition, there was a lower incidence of new onset diabetes in losartan-treated patients.

CCBs have been found to have a selective benefit in the prevention of stroke, unrelated to the effect on SBP [6, 53-56]. Variability in SBP both in patients on antihypertensive medications as well as those not on medications, separate than the actual SBP value, has been found to be an independent predictor of stroke in patients with previous TIA (HR 6.22, P , 0.0001) [18] as well as those without previous cardiovascular events [57]. Webb, et. al. performed a meta-analysis of all relevant published trials and reported that drug class effects on interindividual blood pressure variation can account for some of the differences in effects of antihypertensives on stroke prevention [58]. They found that compared with placebo, interindividual variation in SBP was reduced the most by calcium-channel blockers (p<0.0001).

Antihypertensive therapy for stroke prevention is tailored differently for diabetic patients as well as those with CKD. Reports indicate that medications interrupting the renin-angiotensin system, such as angiotensin receptor blockers (ARBs) have a particular benefit in stroke reduction in patients with DM [59]. Also supporting the notion that the newer antihypertensive medications have a greater benefit in stroke risk reduction in diabetics with ISH, investigators on behalf of the Systolic Hypertension in Europe Trial (SHET) found that CCB therapy reduced strokes by 73% [60]. In patients with CKD, diuretics alone or in combination with ACE-Is compared with placebo are powerful BP-lowering and stroke preventive agents [61]. Diuretics play a crucial role in treatment of hypertension in CKD patients due to the reduction of volume overload.

Data published over the last decade support the use of the newer antihypertensive agents such as CCBs, ACE-Is, and ARBs as first-line agents for stroke prevention in patients with ISH without CKD. Joint National Committee (JNC) VII recommendations support diuretic use in most antihypertensive patients but this recommendation predates some of the newer studies. [62]. In patients with DM, first-line therapy should include an ACE-I or an ARB [63]. While occasionally ISH is easily treated with one antihypertensive agent, anecdotal experience shows that more often than not, more than one agent is required [64]. The ACCELERATE study found that initiation of dual therapy was more effective than initiation of monotherapy in reducing blood pressure initially and at 24 weeks. [65]

Systolic Blood Pressure Management in Acute Stroke

While lowering systolic blood pressure is important for secondary stroke prevention, the same approach may not be true for the immediate management of systolic blood pressure after acute stroke [31]. Studies have provided conflicting data; some have shown improved outcomes associated with initial hypertension while others have demonstrated the opposite. Interestingly, in a nationally representative population of patients presenting to the emergency room with stroke, higher SBP at presentation was associated with a shorter time to evaluation with patients having SBP > 220 being evaluated in 5 +/- 1 minutes [66]. The American Heart Association recommends that systolic blood pressure not be lowered beyond 220 mm Hg for the first 24 hours after acute stroke [67]. All patients experience a decline in blood pressure within one week after stroke regardless of intervention, with the greatest decline being seen with the highest presenting SBPs [68, 69]. This spontaneous decrease in blood pressure is highest among patients with functional improvement at 6 month follow-up [70].

There is differing data regarding the prognostic significance of elevated SBP at presentation with acute stroke. While some authors have reported that low SBP at ER presentation is associated with high 90 day mortality, others have reported that admission blood pressure is not associated with overall mortality and 6 month outcomes [70-74]. In one study by Oliveira-Filho, et. al, the degree of SBP reduction during the first 24 hours after acute stroke was independently predictive of poor 3 month outcomes [75]. However, after a longer follow-up period (2.5 years), Robinson et. al found that 24 hour SBP > or = 160 after acute stroke was associated with an increased HR of 2.41 (95% confidence intervals: 1.24-4.67) for death compared to a SBP range of 140-159 [76]. Analysis of the data from the International Stroke Trial showed that both high SBP and low SBP were independently associated with poor outcomes both at 2 weeks and 6 months following acute stroke [77]. Early death increased by 18% with each 10 mm Hg decrease in SBP below 150 and by 4% for every increase in SBP above 150, arguing that perhaps, a SBP close to 150 may be the ideal target following acute stroke. There may also be a poor outcome associated with elevations in the weighted-average of SBP and MAP over seven days according to a review of the data collected for the Trial of ORG 10172 in Acute Stroke Treatment (TOAST) [73].

While the influence on overall outcome remains unclear, admission SBP values have been found to be correlated with recanalization rates following treatment with intravenous tissue plasminogen activator (IV tpa). Investigators in the Combined Lysis of Thrombus in Brain ischemia with Transcranial Ultrasound and Systemic TPA (CLOTBUST) trial found that recanalization rates following administration of IV tpa as determined by transcranial Doppler (TCD) sonography were highest among patients with a lower pretreatment SBP (mean SBP 152 +/- 23) [78]. Despite data showing that good outcomes typically mirror recanalization rates [79], in a post-hoc analysis of the National Institute of Neurological Disorders and Stroke (NINDS) r-tPA stroke study group r-tPA trial, Silver et. al. showed a reduced likelihood of good clinical outcomes with each 10 mm Hg reduction in SBP in patients treated with tpa [80]. They do, however, report that patients who received rt-PA had a significantly lower SBP than those who did not, and still had a significantly better overall outcome.

There are several ongoing trials assessing the safety and feasibility of mildly lowering blood pressure in the acute stroke setting with preliminary data showing a trend toward benefit for 3 month mortality [81, 82]. In a retrospective study of 543 patients with acute minor stroke performed by Ogata et. al, SBP of 170 compared with SBP of 160 was significantly associated with clinical deterioration (p = 0.033) which ultimately contributed to a poorer outcome [83]. The ACE-I lisinopril has been shown to lower SBP within 4 hours after first oral dose in patients with acute stroke [84]. In a comprehensive review of literature, CCBs, ACE-Is, ARBs, and glyceroltrinitrate reduced blood pressure when given after acute stroke, however did not alter functional outcome or death [85].

Alternately, several small trials have tested the hypothesis that medically induced hypertension in patients with acute stroke may improve outcomes by increasing blood flow to the ischemic penumbra. These trials have tested various pressor medications, with phenylephrine being the most common, to induce hypertension and looked at patient outcomes. While this therapy appears to be well-tolerated, outcomes remain uncertain and larger trials have yet to be undertaken to test this theory [86, 87].

With the current discord seen in the literature, current practice is tailored to each patient on a case by case basis. If it becomes necessary to medically treat an acute stroke patient with severe hypertension (SBP > 220), the recommended medications include intravenous nicardipine, labetalol, esmolol, and enalaprilat [88].

References

[1] Gorelick PB, Sacco RL, Smith DB, Alberts M, Mustone-Alexander L, Rader D, Ross JL, Raps E, Ozer MN, Brass LM, Malone ME, Goldberg S, Booss J, Hanley DF, Toole JF, Greengold NL, Rhew DC. Prevention of a first stroke: A review of guidelines and a multidisciplinary consensus statement from the national stroke association. *JAMA.* 1999;281:1112-1120

[2] West MJ, White HD, Simes RJ, Kirby A, Watson JD, Anderson NE, Hankey GJ, Wonders S, Hunt D, Tonkin AM, West MJ, White HD, Simes RJ, Kirby A, Watson JD, Anderson NE, Hankey GJ, Wonders S, Hunt D, Tonkin AM. Risk factors for non-haemorrhagic stroke in patients with coronary heart disease and the effect of lipid-modifying therapy with pravastatin. *Journal of Hypertension.* 2002;20:2513-2517

[3] Ruland S, Richardson D, Hung E, Brorson JR, Cruz-Flores S, Felton WL, 3rd, Ford-Lynch G, Helgason C, Hsu C, Kramer J, Mitsias P, Gorelick PB, Investigators A. Predictors of recurrent stroke in african americans. *Neurology.* 2006;67:567-571

[4] Kesarwani M, Perez A, Lopez VA, Wong ND, Franklin SS, Kesarwani M, Perez A, Lopez VA, Wong ND, Franklin SS. Cardiovascular comorbidities and blood pressure control in stroke survivors. *Journal of Hypertension.* 2009;27:1056-1063

[5] Klungel OH, Kaplan RC, Heckbert SR, Smith NL, Lemaitre RN, Longstreth WT, Jr., Leufkens HG, de Boer A, Psaty BM. Control of blood pressure and risk of stroke among pharmacologically treated hypertensive patients. *Stroke.* 2000;31:420-424

[6] Wang JG, Li Y, Wang J-G, Li Y. Primary and secondary prevention of stroke by antihypertensive drug treatment. *Expert Review of Neurotherapeutics.* 2004;4:1023-1031

[7] Nilsson PM, Nilsson PM. Reducing the risk of stroke in elderly patients with hypertension: A critical review of the efficacy of antihypertensive drugs. *Drugs and Aging.* 2005;22:517-524

[8] Bowman TS, Gaziano JM, Kase CS, Sesso HD, Kurth T. Blood pressure measures and risk of total, ischemic, and hemorrhagic stroke in men. *Neurology.* 2006;67:820-823

[9] Tozawa M, Iseki K, Iseki C, Takishita S, Tozawa M, Iseki K, Iseki C, Takishita S. Pulse pressure and risk of total mortality and cardiovascular events in patients on chronic hemodialysis. *Kidney International.* 2002;61:717-726

[10] Brown DW, Giles WH, Greenlund KJ, Brown DW, Giles WH, Greenlund KJ. Blood pressure parameters and risk of fatal stroke, nhanes ii mortality study. *American Journal of Hypertension.* 2007;20:338-341

[11] Psaty BM, Furberg CD, Kuller LH, Cushman M, Savage PJ, Levine D, O'Leary DH, Bryan RN, Anderson M, Lumley T. Association between blood pressure level and the risk of myocardial infarction, stroke, and total mortality: The cardiovascular health study. *Archives of Internal Medicine.* 2001;161:1183-1192

[12] Antikainen RL, Jousilahti P, Vanhanen H, Tuomilehto J. Excess mortality associated with increased pulse pressure among middle-aged men and women is explained by high systolic blood pressure. *Journal of Hypertension.* 2000;18:417-423

[13] Myint PK, Sinha S, Luben RN, Bingham SA, Wareham NJ, Khaw KT, Myint PK, Sinha S, Luben RN, Bingham SA, Wareham NJ, Khaw K-T. Risk factors for first-ever stroke in the epic-norfolk prospective population-based study. *European Journal of Cardiovascular Prevention and Rehabilitation.* 2008;15:663-669

[14] Inoue R, Ohkubo T, Kikuya M, Metoki H, Asayama K, Obara T, Hirose T, Hara A, Hoshi H, Hashimoto J, Totsune K, Satoh H, Kondo Y, Imai Y, Inoue R, Ohkubo T, Kikuya M, Metoki H, Asayama K, Obara T, Hirose T, Hara A, Hoshi H, Hashimoto J, Totsune K, Satoh H, Kondo Y, Imai Y. Stroke risk in systolic and combined systolic and diastolic hypertension determined using ambulatory blood pressure. The ohasama study. *American Journal of Hypertension.* 2007;20:1125-1131

[15] Mazza A, Pessina AC, Pavei A, Scarpa R, Tikhonoff V, Casiglia E. Predictors of stroke mortality in elderly people from the general population. The cardiovascular study in the elderly. *European Journal of Epidemiology.* 2001;17:1097-1104

[16] Fang XH, Longstreth WT, Jr., Li SC, Kronmal RA, Cheng XM, Wang WZ, Wu S, Du XL, Dai XY. Longitudinal study of blood pressure and stroke in over 37,000 people in china. *Cerebrovascular Diseases.* 2001;11:225-229

[17] Lipska K, Sylaja PN, Sarma PS, Thankappan KR, Kutty VR, Vasan RS, Radhakrishnan K. Risk factors for acute ischaemic stroke in young adults in south india. *Journal of Neurology, Neurosurgery and Psychiatry.* 2007;78:959-963

[18] Rothwell PM, Howard SC, Dolan E, O'Brien E, Dobson JE, Dahlof B, Sever PS, Poulter NR, Rothwell PM, Howard SC, Dolan E, O'Brien E, Dobson JE, Dahlof B, Sever PS, Poulter NR. Prognostic significance of visit-to-visit variability, maximum systolic blood pressure, and episodic hypertension. *Lancet.* 2010;375:895-905

[19] Lernfelt B, Forsberg M, Blomstrand C, Mellstrom D, Volkmann R. Cerebral atherosclerosis as predictor of stroke and mortality in representative elderly population. *Stroke.* 2002;33:224-229

[20] Gregoire SM, Brown MM, Kallis C, Jager HR, Yousry TA, Werring DJ, Gregoire SM, Brown MM, Kallis C, Jager HR, Yousry TA, Werring DJ. Mri detection of new microbleeds in patients with ischemic stroke: Five-year cohort follow-up study. *Stroke.* 2010;41:184-186

[21] Dufouil C, Chalmers J, Coskun O, Besancon V, Bousser MG, Guillon P, MacMahon S, Mazoyer B, Neal B, Woodward M, Tzourio-Mazoyer N, Tzourio C, Investigators PMS, Dufouil C, Chalmers J, Coskun O, Besancon V, Bousser M-G, Guillon P, MacMahon S, Mazoyer B, Neal B, Woodward M, Tzourio-Mazoyer N, Tzourio C. Effects of blood pressure lowering on cerebral white matter hyperintensities in patients with stroke: The progress (perindopril protection against recurrent stroke study) magnetic resonance imaging substudy. *Circulation.* 2005;112:1644-1650

[22] van Dijk EJ, Breteler MM, Schmidt R, Berger K, Nilsson LG, Oudkerk M, Pajak A, Sans S, de Ridder M, Dufouil C, Fuhrer R, Giampaoli S, Launer LJ, Hofman A, Consortium C, van Dijk EJ, Breteler MMB, Schmidt R, Berger K, Nilsson L-G, Oudkerk M, Pajak A, Sans S, de Ridder M, Dufouil C, Fuhrer R, Giampaoli S, Launer LJ, Hofman A. The association between blood pressure, hypertension, and cerebral

white matter lesions: Cardiovascular determinants of dementia study. *Hypertension.* 2004;44:625-630

[23] Gilligan AK, Markus R, Read S, Srikanth V, Hirano T, Fitt G, Arends M, Chambers BR, Davis SM, Donnan GA, Australian Streptokinase Trial I. Baseline blood pressure but not early computed tomography changes predicts major hemorrhage after streptokinase in acute ischemic stroke. *Stroke.* 2002;33:2236-2242

[24] Freitas RN, Khaw KT, Wu K, Bowman R, Jeffery H, Luben R, Wareham NJ, Rodwell S, Freitas RN, Khaw K-T, Wu K, Bowman R, Jeffery H, Luben R, Wareham NJ, Rodwell S. Hmgcr gene polymorphism is associated with stroke risk in the epic-norfolk study. *European Journal of Cardiovascular Prevention and Rehabilitation.*17:89-93

[25] Fava C, Montagnana M, Danese E, Almgren P, Hedblad B, Engstrom G, Berglund G, Minuz P, Melander O, Fava C, Montagnana M, Danese E, Almgren P, Hedblad B, Engstrom G, Berglund G, Minuz P, Melander O. Homozygosity for the ephx2 k55r polymorphism increases the long-term risk of ischemic stroke in men: A study in swedes. *Pharmacogenetics and Genomics.* 2010;20:94-103

[26] Rothwell PM, Howard SC, Spence JD, Carotid Endarterectomy Trialists C. Relationship between blood pressure and stroke risk in patients with symptomatic carotid occlusive disease. *Stroke.* 2003;34:2583-2590

[27] Turan TN, Cotsonis G, Lynn MJ, Chaturvedi S, Chimowitz M, Warfarin-Aspirin Symptomatic Intracranial Disease Trial I, Turan TN, Cotsonis G, Lynn MJ, Chaturvedi S, Chimowitz M. Relationship between blood pressure and stroke recurrence in patients with intracranial arterial stenosis. *Circulation.* 2007;115:2969-2975

[28] Kario K, Pickering TG, Matsuo T, Hoshide S, Schwartz JE, Shimada K. Stroke prognosis and abnormal nocturnal blood pressure falls in older hypertensives. *Hypertension.* 2001;38:852-857

[29] Lewington S, Clarke R, Qizilbash N, Peto R, Collins R, Prospective Studies C, Lewington S, Clarke R, Qizilbash N, Peto R, Collins R. Age-specific relevance of usual blood pressure to vascular mortality: A meta-analysis of individual data for one million adults in 61 prospective studies.[erratum appears in lancet. 2003 mar 22;361(9362):1060]. *Lancet.* 2002;360:1903-1913

[30] Staessen JA, Gasowski J, Wang JG, Thijs L, Den Hond E, Boissel JP, Coope J, Ekbom T, Gueyffier F, Liu L, Kerlikowske K, Pocock S, Fagard RH. Risks of untreated and treated isolated systolic hypertension in the elderly: Meta-analysis of outcome trials.[erratum appears in lancet 2001 mar 3;357(9257):724]. *Lancet.* 2000;355:865-872

[31] Perry HM, Jr., Davis BR, Price TR, Applegate WB, Fields WS, Guralnik JM, Kuller L, Pressel S, Stamler J, Probstfield JL. Effect of treating isolated systolic hypertension on the risk of developing various types and subtypes of stroke: The systolic hypertension in the elderly program (shep). *JAMA.* 2000;284:465-471

[32] Boissel JP, Gueyffier F, Boutitie F, Pocock S, Fagard R, Boissel J-P, Gueyffier F, Boutitie F, Pocock S, Fagard R. Apparent effect on blood pressure is only partly responsible for the risk reduction due to antihypertensive treatments. *Fundamental and Clinical Pharmacology.* 2005;19:579-584

[33] Papademetriou V, Farsang C, Elmfeldt D, Hofman A, Lithell H, Olofsson B, Skoog I, Trenkwalder P, Zanchetti A, Study on C, Prognosis in the Elderly study g, Papademetriou V, Farsang C, Elmfeldt D, Hofman A, Lithell H, Olofsson B, Skoog I, Trenkwalder P, Zanchetti A. Stroke prevention with the angiotensin ii type 1-receptor

blocker candesartan in elderly patients with isolated systolic hypertension: The study on cognition and prognosis in the elderly (scope). *Journal of the American College of Cardiology*. 2004;44:1175-1180

[34] Vasan RS, Larson MG, Leip EP, Evans JC, O'Donnell CJ, Kannel WB, Levy D. Impact of high-normal blood pressure on the risk of cardiovascular disease. *New England Journal of Medicine*. 2001;345:1291-1297

[35] Kshirsagar AV, Carpenter M, Bang H, Wyatt SB, Colindres RE, Kshirsagar AV, Carpenter M, Bang H, Wyatt SB, Colindres RE. Blood pressure usually considered normal is associated with an elevated risk of cardiovascular disease. *American Journal of Medicine*. 2006;119:133-141

[36] Strandberg TE, Salomaa VV, Vanhanen HT, Pitkala K. Blood pressure and mortality during an up to 32-year follow-up. *Journal of Hypertension*. 2001;19:35-39

[37] Friday G, Alter M, Lai SM, Friday G, Alter M, Lai S-M. Control of hypertension and risk of stroke recurrence. *Stroke*. 2002;33:2652-2657

[38] Adler AI, Stratton IM, Neil HA, Yudkin JS, Matthews DR, Cull CA, Wright AD, Turner RC, Holman RR. Association of systolic blood pressure with macrovascular and microvascular complications of type 2 diabetes (ukpds 36): Prospective observational study. *BMJ*. 2000;321:412-419

[39] Kothari V, Stevens RJ, Adler AI, Stratton IM, Manley SE, Neil HA, Holman RR, Kothari V, Stevens RJ, Adler AI, Stratton IM, Manley SE, Neil HA, Holman RR. Ukpds 60: Risk of stroke in type 2 diabetes estimated by the uk prospective diabetes study risk engine. *Stroke*. 2002;33:1776-1781

[40] Group AS, Cushman WC, Evans GW, Byington RP, Goff DC, Jr., Grimm RH, Jr., Cutler JA, Simons-Morton DG, Basile JN, Corson MA, Probstfield JL, Katz L, Peterson KA, Friedewald WT, Buse JB, Bigger JT, Gerstein HC, Ismail-Beigi F, Cushman WC, Evans GW, Byington RP, Goff DC, Jr., Grimm RH, Jr., Cutler JA, Simons-Morton DG, Basile JN, Corson MA, Probstfield JL, Katz L, Peterson KA, Friedewald WT, Buse JB, Bigger JT, Gerstein HC, Ismail-Beigi F. Effects of intensive blood-pressure control in type 2 diabetes mellitus. *New England Journal of Medicine*. 2010;362:1575-1585

[41] Khella SL. New insights into stroke in chronic kidney disease. *Advances in Chronic Kidney Disease*. 2008;15:338-346

[42] Kokubo Y, Nakamura S, Okamura T, Yoshimasa Y, Makino H, Watanabe M, Higashiyama A, Kamide K, Kawanishi K, Okayama A, Kawano Y, Kokubo Y, Nakamura S, Okamura T, Yoshimasa Y, Makino H, Watanabe M, Higashiyama A, Kamide K, Kawanishi K, Okayama A, Kawano Y. Relationship between blood pressure category and incidence of stroke and myocardial infarction in an urban japanese population with and without chronic kidney disease: The suita study. *Stroke*. 2009;40:2674-2679

[43] Zuliani G, Cherubini A, Volpato S, Atti AR, Ble A, Vavalle C, Di Todaro F, Benedetti C, Ruggiero C, Senin U, Fellin R, Zuliani G, Cherubini A, Volpato S, Atti AR, Ble A, Vavalle C, Di Todaro F, Benedetti C, Ruggiero C, Senin U, Fellin R. Treatment with angiotensin-converting enzyme inhibitors is associated with a reduction in short-term mortality in older patients with acute ischemic stroke. *Journals of Gerontology Series A-Biological Sciences and Medical Sciences*. 2005;60:463-465

[44] Beckett NS, Peters R, Fletcher AE, Staessen JA, Liu L, Dumitrascu D, Stoyanovsky V, Antikainen RL, Nikitin Y, Anderson C, Belhani A, Forette F, Rajkumar C, Thijs L, Banya W, Bulpitt CJ, Group HS, Beckett NS, Peters R, Fletcher AE, Staessen JA, Liu L, Dumitrascu D, Stoyanovsky V, Antikainen RL, Nikitin Y, Anderson C, Belhani A, Forette F, Rajkumar C, Thijs L, Banya W, Bulpitt CJ. Treatment of hypertension in patients 80 years of age or older. *New England Journal of Medicine.* 2008;358:1887-1898

[45] Chalmers J, Chalmers J. Trials on blood pressure-lowering and secondary stroke prevention. *American Journal of Cardiology.* 2003;91:3G-8G

[46] Rashid P, Leonardi-Bee J, Bath P, Rashid P, Leonardi-Bee J, Bath P. Blood pressure reduction and secondary prevention of stroke and other vascular events: A systematic review. *Stroke.* 2003;34:2741-2748

[47] Wu A, Wu A. Should beta-blockers still be used as initial antihypertensive agents in uncomplicated hypertension? *Annals of the Academy of Medicine, Singapore.* 2007;36:962-964

[48] Blood pressure in Acute Stroke C. Vasoactive drugs for acute stroke. *Cochrane Database of Systematic Reviews.* 2000:CD002839

[49] Antihypertensive, Lipid-Lowering Treatment to Prevent Heart Attack Trial Collaborative Research G. Diuretic versus alpha-blocker as first-step antihypertensive therapy: Final results from the antihypertensive and lipid-lowering treatment to prevent heart attack trial (allhat). *Hypertension.* 2003;42:239-246

[50] Ekbom T, Linjer E, Hedner T, Lanke J, De Faire U, Wester PO, Dahlof B, Schersten B, Ekbom T, Linjer E, Hedner T, Lanke J, De Faire U, Dahlof B, Schersten B. Cardiovascular events in elderly patients with isolated systolic hypertension. A subgroup analysis of treatment strategies in stop-hypertension-2. *Blood Pressure.* 2004;13:137-141

[51] Ogihara T. Practitioner's trial on the efficacy of antihypertensive treatment in the elderly hypertension (the pate-hypertension study) in japan. *American Journal of Hypertension.* 2000;13:461-467

[52] Kjeldsen SE, Dahlof B, Devereux RB, Julius S, Aurup P, Edelman J, Beevers G, de Faire U, Fyhrquist F, Ibsen H, Kristianson K, Lederballe-Pedersen O, Lindholm LH, Nieminen MS, Omvik P, Oparil S, Snapinn S, Wedel H, Group LS, Kjeldsen SE, Dahlof B, Devereux RB, Julius S, Aurup P, Edelman J, Beevers G, de Faire U, Fyhrquist F, Ibsen H, Kristianson K, Lederballe-Pedersen O, Lindholm LH, Nieminen MS, Omvik P, Oparil S, Snapinn S, Wedel H. Effects of losartan on cardiovascular morbidity and mortality in patients with isolated systolic hypertension and left ventricular hypertrophy: A losartan intervention for endpoint reduction (life) substudy. *JAMA.* 2002;288:1491-1498

[53] Verdecchia P, Reboldi G, Angeli F, Gattobigio R, Bentivoglio M, Thijs L, Staessen JA, Porcellati C, Verdecchia P, Reboldi G, Angeli F, Gattobigio R, Bentivoglio M, Thijs L, Staessen JA, Porcellati C. Angiotensin-converting enzyme inhibitors and calcium channel blockers for coronary heart disease and stroke prevention. *Hypertension.* 2005;46:386-392

[54] Staessen JA, Li Y, Thijs L, Wang JG, Staessen JA, Li Y, Thijs L, Wang J-G. Blood pressure reduction and cardiovascular prevention: An update including the 2003-2004

secondary prevention trials. *Hypertension Research - Clinical and Experimental.* 2005;28:385-407

[55]   Kjeldsen SE, Hedner T, Syvertsen JO, Lund-Johansen P, Hansson L, Lanke J, Lindholm LH, De Faire U, Dahlof B, Karlberg BE, Group NS, Kjeldsen SE, Hedner T, Syvertsen JO, Lund-Johansen P, Hansson L, Lanke J, Lindholm LH, De Faire U, Dahlof B, Karlberg BE. Influence of age, sex and blood pressure on the principal endpoints of the nordic diltiazem (nordil) study. *Journal of Hypertension.* 2002;20:1231-1237

[56]   Angeli F, Verdecchia P, Reboldi GP, Gattobigio R, Bentivoglio M, Staessen JA, Porcellati C, Angeli F, Verdecchia P, Reboldi GP, Gattobigio R, Bentivoglio M, Staessen JA, Porcellati C. Calcium channel blockade to prevent stroke in hypertension: A meta-analysis of 13 studies with 103,793 subjects. *American Journal of Hypertension.* 2004;17:817-822

[57]   Pringle E, Phillips C, Thijs L, Davidson C, Staessen JA, de Leeuw PW, Jaaskivi M, Nachev C, Parati G, O'Brien ET, Tuomilehto J, Webster J, Bulpitt CJ, Fagard RH, Syst-Eur i, Pringle E, Phillips C, Thijs L, Davidson C, Staessen JA, de Leeuw PW, Jaaskivi M, Nachev C, Parati G, O'Brien ET, Tuomilehto J, Webster J, Bulpitt CJ, Fagard RH. Systolic blood pressure variability as a risk factor for stroke and cardiovascular mortality in the elderly hypertensive population. *Journal of Hypertension.* 2003;21:2251-2257

[58]   Webb AJ, Fischer U, Mehta Z, Rothwell PM, Webb AJS, Fischer U, Mehta Z, Rothwell PM. Effects of antihypertensive-drug class on interindividual variation in blood pressure and risk of stroke: A systematic review and meta-analysis. *Lancet.* 2010;375:906-915

[59]   Sowers JR, Sowers JR. Treatment of hypertension in patients with diabetes. *Archives of Internal Medicine.* 2004;164:1850-1857

[60]   Tuomilehto J, Rastenyte D, Birkenhager WH, Thijs L, Antikainen R, Bulpitt CJ, Fletcher AE, Forette F, Goldhaber A, Palatini P, Sarti C, Fagard R. Effects of calcium-channel blockade in older patients with diabetes and systolic hypertension. Systolic hypertension in europe trial investigators. *New England Journal of Medicine.* 1999;340:677-684

[61]   Segall L, Oprisiu R, Fournier A, Covic A, Segall L, Oprisiu R, Fournier A, Covic A. Antihypertensive treatment and stroke prevention in patients with and without chronic kidney disease: A review of controlled trials. *Journal of Nephrology.* 2008;21:374-383

[62]   Mancia G, Grassi G. Joint national committee vii and european society of hypertension/european society of cardiology guidelines for evaluating and treating hypertension: A two-way road? *J Am Soc Nephrol.* 2005;16:S74-77

[63]   Whaley-Connell A, Sowers JR, Whaley-Connell A, Sowers JR. Hypertension management in type 2 diabetes mellitus: Recommendations of the joint national committee vii. *Endocrinology and Metabolism Clinics of North America.* 2005;34:63-75

[64]   Waeber B, Waeber B. Trials in isolated systolic hypertension: An update. *Current Hypertension Reports.* 2003;5:329-336

[65]   Brown MJ, McInnes GT, Papst CC, Zhang J, Macdonald TM. Aliskiren and the calcium channel blocker amlodipine combination as an initial treatment strategy for hypertension control (accelerate): A randomised, parallel-group trial. *Lancet.*

[66] Qureshi AI, Ezzeddine MA, Nasar A, Suri MF, Kirmani JF, Hussein HM, Divani AA, Reddi AS, Qureshi AI, Ezzeddine MA, Nasar A, Suri MFK, Kirmani JF, Hussein HM, Divani AA, Reddi AS. Prevalence of elevated blood pressure in 563,704 adult patients with stroke presenting to the ed in the united states. *American Journal of Emergency Medicine*. 2007;25:32-38

[67] Adams HP, Jr., Adams RJ, Brott T, del Zoppo GJ, Furlan A, Goldstein LB, Grubb RL, Higashida R, Kidwell C, Kwiatkowski TG, Marler JR, Hademenos GJ. Guidelines for the early management of patients with ischemic stroke: A scientific statement from the stroke council of the american stroke association. *Stroke*. 2003;34:1056-1083

[68] Semplicini A, Maresca A, Boscolo G, Sartori M, Rocchi R, Giantin V, Forte PL, Pessina AC, Semplicini A, Maresca A, Boscolo G, Sartori M, Rocchi R, Giantin V, Forte PL, Pessina AC. Hypertension in acute ischemic stroke: A compensatory mechanism or an additional damaging factor? *Archives of Internal Medicine*. 2003;163:211-216

[69] Broderick J, Brott T, Barsan W, Haley EC, Levy D, Marler J, Sheppard G, Blum C. Blood pressure during the first minutes of focal cerebral ischemia. *Annals of Emergency Medicine*. 1993;22:1438-1443

[70] Abboud H, Labreuche J, Plouin F, Amarenco P, Investigators G, Abboud H, Labreuche J, Plouin F, Amarenco P. High blood pressure in early acute stroke: A sign of a poor outcome? *Journal of Hypertension*. 2006;24:381-386

[71] Davalos A, Toni D, Iweins F, Lesaffre E, Bastianello S, Castillo J. Neurological deterioration in acute ischemic stroke: Potential predictors and associated factors in the european cooperative acute stroke study (ecass) i. *Stroke*. 1999;30:2631-2636

[72] Stead LG, Gilmore RM, Decker WW, Weaver AL, Brown RD, Jr., Stead LG, Gilmore RM, Decker WW, Weaver AL, Brown RD, Jr. Initial emergency department blood pressure as predictor of survival after acute ischemic stroke. *Neurology*. 2005;65:1179-1183

[73] Jensen MB, Yoo B, Clarke WR, Davis PH, Adams HR, Jr., Jensen MB, Yoo B, Clarke WR, Davis PH, Adams HR, Jr. Blood pressure as an independent prognostic factor in acute ischemic stroke. *Canadian Journal of Neurological Sciences*. 2006;33:34-38

[74] Okumura K, Ohya Y, Maehara A, Wakugami K, Iseki K, Takishita S, Okumura K, Ohya Y, Maehara A, Wakugami K, Iseki K, Takishita S. Effects of blood pressure levels on case fatality after acute stroke. *Journal of Hypertension*. 2005;23:1217-1223

[75] Oliveira-Filho J, Silva SC, Trabuco CC, Pedreira BB, Sousa EU, Bacellar A, Silva SCS. Detrimental effect of blood pressure reduction in the first 24 hours of acute stroke onset. *Neurology*. 2003;61:1047-1051

[76] Robinson TG, Dawson SL, Ahmed U, Manktelow B, Fotherby MD, Potter JF. Twenty-four hour systolic blood pressure predicts long-term mortality following acute stroke. *Journal of Hypertension*. 2001;19:2127-2134

[77] Leonardi-Bee J, Bath PM, Phillips SJ, Sandercock PA, Group ISTC, Leonardi-Bee J, Bath PMW, Phillips SJ, Sandercock PAG. Blood pressure and clinical outcomes in the international stroke trial. *Stroke*. 2002;33:1315-1320

[78] Tsivgoulis G, Saqqur M, Sharma VK, Lao AY, Hill MD, Alexandrov AV, Investigators C, Tsivgoulis G, Saqqur M, Sharma VK, Lao AY, Hill MD, Alexandrov AV. Association of pretreatment blood pressure with tissue plasminogen activator-induced arterial recanalization in acute ischemic stroke. *Stroke*. 2007;38:961-966

[79]   Rha JH, Saver JL, Rha J-H, Saver JL. The impact of recanalization on ischemic stroke
       outcome: A meta-analysis. *Stroke*. 2007;38:967-973

[80]   Silver B, Lu M, Morris DC, Mitsias PD, Lewandowski C, Chopp M, Silver B, Lu M,
       Morris DC, Mitsias PD, Lewandowski C, Chopp M. Blood pressure declines and less
       favorable outcomes in the ninds tpa stroke study. *Journal of the Neurological Sciences*.
       2008;271:61-67

[81]   Potter JF, Robinson TG, Ford GA, Mistri A, James M, Chernova J, Jagger C, Potter JF,
       Robinson TG, Ford GA, Mistri A, James M, Chernova J, Jagger C. Controlling
       hypertension and hypotension immediately post-stroke (chhips): A randomised,
       placebo-controlled, double-blind pilot trial. *Lancet Neurology*. 2009;8:48-56

[82]   Tikhonoff V, Zhang H, Richart T, Staessen JA, Tikhonoff V, Zhang H, Richart T,
       Staessen JA. Blood pressure as a prognostic factor after acute stroke. *Lancet Neurology*.
       2009;8:938-948

[83]   Ogata T, Yasaka M, Wakugawa Y, Ibayashi S, Okada Y, Ogata T, Yasaka M,
       Wakugawa Y, Ibayashi S, Okada Y. Predisposing factors for acute deterioration of
       minor ischemic stroke. *Journal of the Neurological Sciences*. 2009;287:147-150

[84]   Eveson DJ, Robinson TG, Potter JF, Eveson DJ, Robinson TG, Potter JF. Lisinopril for
       the treatment of hypertension within the first 24 hours of acute ischemic stroke and
       follow-up. *American Journal of Hypertension*. 2007;20:270-277

[85]   Geeganage C, Bath PM, Geeganage C, Bath PMW. Interventions for deliberately
       altering blood pressure in acute stroke. *Cochrane Database of Systematic Reviews*.
       2008:CD000039

[86]   Mistri AK, Robinson TG, Potter JF, Mistri AK, Robinson TG, Potter JF. Pressor
       therapy in acute ischemic stroke: Systematic review. *Stroke*. 2006;37:1565-1571

[87]   Marzan AS, Hungerbuhler HJ, Studer A, Baumgartner RW, Georgiadis D. Feasibility
       and safety of norepinephrine-induced arterial hypertension in acute ischemic stroke.
       Neurology. 2004;62:1193-1195

[88]   Heitsch L, Jauch EC, Heitsch L, Jauch EC. Management of hypertension in the setting
       of acute ischemic stroke. *Current Hypertension Reports*. 2007;9:506-511

In: Systolic Blood Pressure
Editor: Robert A. Arfi

ISBN: 978-1-61209-263-8
©2012 Nova Science Publishers, Inc.

Chapter VIII

Computational Fluid Dynamics in Arterial Fluid-Wall Interaction Modelling

M.A. Al-Rawi[1], A.M. Al-Jumaily[1], A. Lowe[2] and J. Lu[3]

[1]Institute of Biomedical Technologies, and
[2]Pulsecor Limited, Auckland New Zealand
[3]Department of Interdisciplinary Studies, AUT University,
Auckland, New Zealand

Abstract

Atherosclerosis and aneurysm occur primarily near areas of disturbed flow such as bifurcations and large curvatures in the arterial tree. Changes to the geometry of these locations are believed to facilitate the development of atherosclerosis lesions and aneurysm ruptures. This fact has been observed *in vivo*, enforcing the importance of studying local hemodynamic conditions in these disease prone arterial sites. Three-dimensional angiographic non-invasive techniques, such as computerized axial tomography (CT) and magnetic resonance imaging (MRI), provide detailed anatomic information. Local hemodynamics can then be studied at patient-specific level using computational fluid-dynamics (CFD) applied to realistic geometric vasculature models. Therefore,it is important to reconstruct geometric models from CT or MR angiographyimages in order to gain accuracy in CFD computations and predictions. The aim of this chapter is to review the use of CFD methods in non-invasivediagnosis or screening of cardiovascular diseases.

Terminologies

1. Vasoregulation: mainly through the production of vasodilator nitric oxide (NO) and vasoconstrictor enothelin-l (ET-1) which bind to receptors on smooth muscle cells.

2. Endothelium:an epithelium of mesoblastic origin composed of a single layer ofthin fl attened cells that lines internal body cavities such as the serouscavities or the interior of the heart.

3. Cardiac catheterisation: the insertion of a catheter into a chamber or vessel of the heart.

4. Poststenotic regions:dilation of an artery, most commonly the pulmonary artery or the aorta.

5. Asynchrony: the quality or state of being asynchronous: absence or lack of concurrence in time.

6. Monolayer: a single, closely packed layer of atoms, molecules, or cells.

7. Antithrombogenic:surfaces or surface coatings which inhibit the formation or development of a thrombus.

8. Ventricles:the pumping chambers of the heart.

Introduction

This literature review focuses on the hemodynamics characteristics of the blood flow and the mechanical properties for the arterial wall when atherosclerosis and aneurysm diseases occur. Thisliterature is based on the hypothesis that the magnitude of stress phase angle between the wall shear stress (WSS) and circumferential strain (CS) can be transformed through pulse wave propagation to develop a non-invasive cardiovascular disease diagnostic methodology.

Since some cardiovascular disease can be identified by the stress phase angle, correlation can be established between this angle and the information carried by the pulse wave analysis.

The aim of this literature survey is to find a validated correlation between WSS and the propagation of waves through the arteries.

For a complete understanding of the field, several related topics will be discussed. Firstly, the physiology and pathophysiology of the cardiovascular diseases are discussed in Section 1. Section 2 covers the current non-invasive clinical cardiovascular diagnostic methods. A major emphasis of this review is on the computational fluid dynamic modelling for the arterial system which will be explained in Section 3. Model outputs from the computational fluid dynamics results are discussed in detail in Section 4. In the last section, future directions and conclusions regarding the use of computational fluid dynamics modelling as a non-invasive diagnostic tool for cardiovascular diseases are listed.

1. Physiology and Pathophysiology of the Cardiovascular System

The wall of large arteries is composed of three layers, the intima, the media and the tunica adventitia(see figure 1). The tunica adventitia comprises the outer layer and is mainly composed of connective tissues, primarily axially oriented collagen fibres. This layer provides mechanical support to the other two layers [1]. The media forms the thickest layer and is composed of smooth muscle cells and connective tissue, mainly collagen and elastin, with both cells and matrix fibres circumferentially oriented. The media layer provides structural integrity while the smooth muscle inside this layer allows for control of artery diameter [2]. The intima layer is composed of a monolayer of endothelial cells on a basement membrane. The intima serves several purposes: it is responsible for the antithrombogenic behaviour of the vascular wall, vasoregulation, control of smooth muscle cell proliferation and control of the transport of water, solutes, macromolecules and cells across the vessel wall [3].

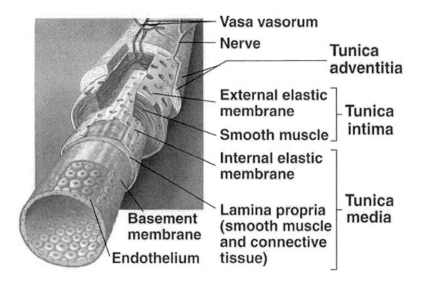

Figure 1. The three artery layers [4].

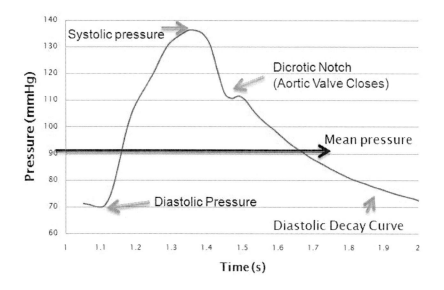

Figure 2. A typical healthy arterial pulse waveform.

When the heart contracts, it generates acontour wave called the arterial pulse wave. This wavetravels along the walls of the arterial tree[5]where it partially reflects at various bifurcations, particularly at the iliac bifurcation[6, 7]. The velocity of the reflected wave is directly dependent on the stiffness of the arteries.Stiff arteries can result in the iliac reflected wave returning to the heart in the systolic phase, which result in pressure increase (see figure 2)[8-10]. It has also been observed that with age both the forward and the reflected wave velocity increase. This can result in the reflected wave coinciding with the forward waveat the heart and a higher total pressure.

Arterial wave reflection propagated along the aorta is a characteristic alteration of the pressure pulse. The magnitude and timing of these waves are important in order to understand their underlying physiology. At any location within the arterial system, the net resultant wave is the superposition of the propagated and reflected waves at that location. A wave returning to the heart during systole would increase the ventricular afterload. If this wave is subtracted from the forward pulse wave, it diminishes the net forward flow. This is disadvantageous to ventricular ejection space [11] and the heart has to overcome it by applying higher pressure and energy [12].

Aneurysms and atherosclerosis are types of cardiovascular diseases affecting both the heart and the circulatory system [13]. The earliest evidence of a developing aneurysm is the local widening of the arterywhichoriginates from a weakness or local absence of the medial layer in the artery wall [14]. The pulse pressure of the circulating blood within the artery stretches the weakened part of the arterial wall,causing the artery to swell. Ultimately, this leads to serious and potentially fatal complications from either the compression of surrounding structures or from rupture of the artery. This may occur in any part of the aorta or major arteriessuch as the ascending aorta, aortic arch, descending aorta and abdominal aorta [15-18].

Atherosclerosis is a condition in which the artery wall is thickened causing a narrowing of the artery and increased resistance to blood flow. Atherosclerosis originates from a small damage to the artery wall due to any possible reason, resulting in a scar tissue and local thickening of the wall. This local thickening in turn, results in a self reinforcing process where progressively more material is deposited, causing the blood passage to become increasingly narrower[19]. The deposited material mostly consists of fats, cholesterol, platelets, cellulose products and calcium. The narrowing of the artery results in a decrease in blood flow and reduction of oxygen supply to the dependent tissues[20].

Both atherosclerosis and aneurysm lead to changes in the diameter of the artery, known as stenosis. Stenosis can cause turbulence inflow resulting in high shear stresses and pressure near the throat of the stenosis. This can activate platelets and thereby induce thrombosis, which can completely block blood flow to the heart or brain[21-24].

2. Non-Invasive Cardiovascular Diagnostic Methods

In this section, devices and techniques used for diagnosing and screening of cardiovascular diseases such as atherosclerosis and aneurysm are discussed. The current non-invasive devices and techniques include, but are not limited to magnetic resonance imaging, blood pressure monitors, pulse wave analysis and central aortic pressure devices. All of these play an important role in the identification and understanding of cardiovascular diseases.Also some of these techniques can be used to extract vascular wall properties for modelling analysis.

2.1. Magnetic Resonance Imaging

MRIis a non-invasive medicalimaging technology for identifying and locating medical conditions [25]. MRI scanning of a disease location gives cross-sectional images that are presented as slices to the radiologist[26]. The procedure of acquiring an MRI scan is as follows:

1. A patient, lying on a table inside the MRI machine, is subjected to a radio frequency wave. The frequency of these waves is selected such that the hydrogen atoms of water molecules are disturbed.
2. A strong magnetic field is applied, which causes these hydrogen atoms to line up in parallel.Subsequently a strong pulse of radio waves is applied to the body, which will knock the nuclei out of their parallel alignment and produce detectable radio signals.
3. These radio signals are converted into grayscale images, with the tone representing the water content at the specific location.

The advantage of using magnetic resonance compared to other imaging techniques (computed tomography(CT) and X-ray) is that it does not use ionizing radiation and provides a much higher contrast between tissue types [27]. MRI allows the physician to accurately determine geometric parameters such as the size of each blood vessel, spatial location, branch position and bifurcation direction [27]. It can also measure velocity components non-invasively with phase contrast techniques, allowing physicians to evaluate various parts of the body and determine the presence of certain diseases that may not be assessed adequately with other imaging methods such as x-ray, ultrasound or CT [28, 29].

2.2. Blood Pressure Monitors

Blood pressure is the force exerted per unit area by the circulating blood on the walls of the blood vessels [30]. From a fluid dynamics point of view, blood pressure is required to generate the flow through the cardiovascular system. The amount of blood pressure needed depends on the resistance of the blood vessels. Small arteries and arterioles provide the largest resistance to flow and hence result in a large pressure drop along the system [31].

The sphygmomanometer is a tool used non-invasivelyto measure the blood pressure from the brachial artery [32, 33]. This device operates by placing a cuff smoothly and snugly around an upper arm. The cuff is inflated until the artery is completely occluded. The pressure in the cuff is slowly released while placing a stethoscope close to the brachial artery at the inner surface of the elbow. When blood flow is detected as a pounding sound from the stethoscope, the pressure is recorded as the systolic pressure.Subsequently, the pressure is further released until the sound disappears, which is then recorded as the diastolic pressure.

Systolic pressure corresponds with contraction of the ventricles, while diastolic pressure occurs when the ventricles are at their maximum blood volume [34]. Systolic and diastolic pressure values in healthy adult males are around 120 and 80 mmHg respectively [35, 36]. Thesevalues vary, not only between subjects but also in time within the same subject. There are many reasons for these variations, ranging from the circadian rhythm to exercise, stress, nutritional factors, drugs or disease [37]. Cardiovascular diseases are often diagnosed based on changes in blood pressure.

The main aim of studying blood pressure measurement from the brachial artery is to assess a relationship for diagnosing cardiovascular diseases between diseases location and brachial site.

2.3 Pulse Wave Analysis Methods

Cardiovascular pulsation is one of the traditional indicators of the human body condition. [38]. From the shape, amplitude and rhythm of pulsation, it is possible to diagnose different cardiovascular diseases. Amplitude and contour are best assessed in the carotid or brachial arteries.

Bickley [32] has shown that the abnormalities of the arterial pulses and pressure waveforms are associated with different diseases and their states (Table 1 and Figure 3). The physiological cause as well as the possible disease conditions indicated by small, weak and large, bounding pulses, bisferiens pulse and pulsus alternans have been explained [32].

The main aim of studying the shape of the pulse wave is to identify and locate different types of cardiovascular diseases from one site to another and determine the correlation between them.

Table 1. Possible diseases which can be diagnosed based on the different types of cardiovascular pulse shapes [32]

Pulse type	Physiological cause	Possible disease
small and weak Pulses	decreased stroke volume	heart failure, hypovolemia, severe aortic stenosis
	increased peripheral resistance	
Large and bounding Pulses	increased stroke volume	fever, anaemia, hyperthyroidism, aortic regurgitation, bradycardia, heart block, atherosclerosis
	decreased peripheral resistance	
	decreased compliance	
Bisferiens Pulse	increased arterial pulse with double systolic peak	aortic regurgitation, aortic stenosis and regurgitation, hypertropic cardiomyopathy
Pulsus Alternans	pulse amplitude varies from peak to peak, rhythm basically regular	left ventricular failure

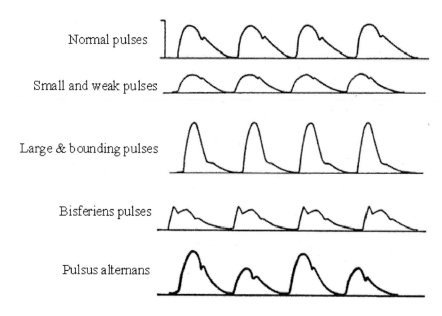

Normal pulses

Small and weak pulses

Large & bounding pulses

Bisferiens pulses

Pulsus alternans

Figure 3. Abnormalities of the Arterial Pulse [32].

2.4. Central Aortic Blood Pressure Methods

Central aortic pressure is the pressure at the root of the heart. It is closely related to the stiffness of the arteries as the stiffness determines the diameter of the arteries, and as such the resistance to flow[39, 40]. In young and healthy people, the systolic pressure is reduced in the brachial artery compared to the central aortic pressure, while the diastolic pressure is increased. Hence the peak to peak amplitude of the pressure waveform is reduced, usually by approximately 30mmHg. However, with age or disease, this reduction can become less as the arteries stiffen [41].

Central blood pressure waveforms are measured invasively through cardiac catheterisation which limits it usability for casual diagnostic analysis [42].To date there is no non-invasive method for aortic blood pressure measurement; however, it can be indirectly determined [43-46]. Current methods of estimating central blood pressure based on non-invasive upper arm blood pressure measurements are not very accurate [47] and they need to be improved in accuracy to make them useful diagnostic tools [48-50].

3. Computational Fluid Dynamics in Arteries

This section discusses available models of blood flow and arterial wall interaction. The defining assumptions for the blood flow models are first introduced. Next modelling of the coupling between the blood flow properties and the arterial wall mechanics using fluid-structure interaction methods is discussed. Finally, the wave propagation and reflection in the cardiovascular system are discussed.

3.1. Assumptions in Modelling Blood Flow

To decide what type of model to use, an understanding of the relevant modelling assumptions is necessary. Figure 4 lists the most commonly used modelling assumptions for blood flow. Itshowsthe different types of models, from the simplest combination of a steady, one dimensional, laminar viscous flow of a Newtonian fluid in a long straight tube of constant cross-section to the most complicated model of an unsteady, 3D non-Newtonian, pulsatile flow in a short, tapered tube with a flexible wall [51, 52]. Each of these assumptions influences the pulsatile flow and the calculated arterial wall characteristics[53]. Early models assumed laminar,continuous, non-pulsatile flow when modelling blood flow [54, 55].However, later studies found that pulsatile flow in arteries tends to be non-laminar, with a flattening velocity profile during systole and a more parabolic velocity profile during diastole[54, 55]. Evidently, changing the modelling assumptions can significantly influence the blood flow parameters, in particular, for diseased arteries. It has been observed that with aneurysms and atherosclerosis, the blood flow profile reacts as transitional or turbulent flow patterns [54, 55].

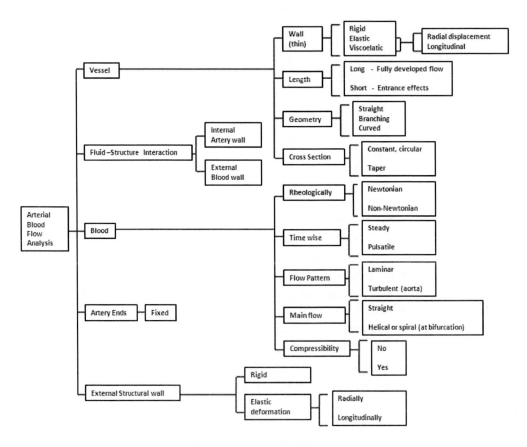

Figure 4. Selection of models for arterial flow analysis (adapted from [24]).

The assumption of either turbulent or laminar flow in diseased arteries, assuming a rigid artery wall, has been used in computer simulation to compare the accuracy with in vivo measurements[56-58]. The turbulence assumption showed better agreement with clinical data with regards to the velocity profile in atherosclerotic arteries [58-61]. It was concluded that the transition from laminar to turbulent flow in arteries occurs at a relatively low Reynolds numbers [61]. On the other hand, Abrahamet al.[15] analyzed a three-dimensional, pulsatile flow model of blood flow in complex tubular geometries using a representation of a plaque-narrowed artery. They found that the removal of the plaque led to a two and a half times increase in the blood flow for both the systole and diastole portions of the cardiac cycle [62].

3.2. Complex Mechanical Interaction

The relatively low stiffness of the artery compared to the viscosity of the blood results in a strong coupling of blood flow and arterial wall mechanics[63]. The pulsatile nature of blood pressure can result in considerable deformations of the artery, which lead to changes in the blood flow characteristics[64]. To address this coupling, a fluid structure interaction method has been developed whichcombines a constitutive model describing the stress distribution in the vessel wall with the computational analysis of blood flow [65, 66]. This method allows for solving the fluid and solid phase coupled problems by accountingfor both the instantaneous fluid mechanical forces on the artery wall such as pressure and wall shear acting, and the effects of wall movement on the fluid motion. Li *et al.*[67]used this approach to investigate the flow and stress field for different diseases, particularly atherosclerosis and aneurysms.They found thatatherosclerosis and aneurysms result in significant wall motion and consequently increasing, blood velocities and decreasing wall shear stress[68].

From a mechanical perspective, changes in arterial geometry represent the clinical manifestations of an induced force exceeding the strength of the artery wall where diseases are located. Wall stress is quantified as either the maximum principal stress or the Von Mises stress resulting from a force exerted along the diseased arterial wall[69].The impinging normal force exerted on the arterial wall is the dominant stress producing the distributed wall deformation. Scotti *et al.*[69]and Leung *et al.*[70] studied the effect of the wall stress and fluid dynamics in an abdominal aortic aneurysm using finite element method. They found that when applying a transient fluid-structure interaction approach, a maximum abdominal aortic aneurysm wall shear stress results, which is higher than that under the assumption of wall stress. Subsequently, in a comparison between models of the aortic arch with and without aneurysm using fluid structure interaction, stresses were found to be much higher at the inflection points in the model with aneurysm [71]. Furthermore, stresses at the media layer are higher for stiffer walls. In a subsequent study, this required the simulation to be performed by considering the artery layer thickness that is modelled as a non-linear hyperelastic material [72]. When modelling the artery wall as individual layers, it was found that stresses in the media layer are the highest, particularly at the outer edge near the adventitia layer[73, 74]. This may explain why tears in the artery wall often originate in the tunica media near the tunica adventitia [74].

3.2.1. Structure of the Arterial Wall

In modelling the arteries, one of the most important decisions to make is what type of artery wall assumptions to be made [75]. The structure of the arterial wall is anisotropic, multilayer and nonlinearly elastic, which makes its material properties highly nonlinear [76, 77].

Previous modellingstudies were carried out under the rigid wall assumption which does not take into account the quantitative influence of the vessel wall motion under pulsatile flow [67, 77]. This has an effect on the flow conditions in both healthy and diseased conditions and on the regions downstream of severe constrictions such as poststenotic regions [78]. This results in a change in the hemodynamics and different wall shear stressvalues [78]. Consequently, to optimize the accuracy and applicability of mathematical models for aneurysms and atherosclerosis, an investigation into the effects of different arterial wall assumptions is required.

3.3. Wave Propagation in Arterial System

Analysis of blood flow and pressure wave propagation in arteries is helpful in exploring the mechanisms associated with the regulation and control of blood circulation in the human body in healthy and diseased cases [79]. With respect to atherosclerosis and aneurysms, the changes in the blood flow patterns around the disease location are of particular interest. As these diseases lead to changes in the arterial wall characteristics, considerable changes in blood flow patterns can be expected [80]. Some studies have analysed the aorta using a simple model of a uniform elastic tube with constant diameter. This simplification seems warranted for sections of the aorta and shows a close agreement with clinical quantities with regards to pulse wave propagation [81]. With progress in computing technologies, more improved modelling using computational fluid dynamics has emerged to investigate the effects of blood flow parameters on the arterial wall[82]. This model measures the pressure gradient using more realistic assumptions, than previous simple assumptions, which assumed the pressure wave propagation velocity is finite [83]. These realistic assumptions introduce some complications in the simulation processes and analysis. Some of these assumptions include, but are not limited to, realistic wall geometry, Newtonian viscous incompressible fluid with non-linear viscoelastic behaviour and the wall tissue with orthotropic material behaviour [84]. These are incorporated by employing the equation of motion for the fluid and using the equation of continuity for the wall, which are then numerically solved to determined the variation of the phase velocities and the transmission coefficients with frequencies for different transmission pressures and initial stress[85, 86]. Thus, mathematical analysis has a potential in understanding the velocity and pressure wave related to the change of the arterial wall properties such as the thickness and diameter that affect the blood flow.

Pulse waves carry a lot of information about the cardiovascular system and if captured in the right context they may help in identifying changes in the dimension and properties of that system [11].

A central parameter in the study of wave reflection is the reflection coefficient which is the ratio of the incoming wave to the reflected wave amplitudes [87].*In vitro* experiments in elastic tubes showed that the reflection coefficient is determined by the mean flow rate and the elastic properties of the proximal unobstructed artery. Consequently, it is strongly influenced by atherosclerosis or aneurysms. In these diseases the reflection coefficient is independent of frequency and pulsatility [88]. However, it has been found that wave reflection properties are weakly dependent on the pulsatility of flow [89]. Because aneurysms and atherosclerosis sites result in wave reflections that are independent of frequency, no phase shift is induced in the reflected waveform [90]. It should be noted that not only the wave reflections, but also the wall stiffness and thickness are affected by atherosclerosis. This results in a change in flow and pressure wave shapes, which is seen primarily as a reduction in pulsatility of distal waves [91]. This reduced pulsatility has an important diagnostic significance in the detection and quantification of peripheral stenosis[91].

4. Model Outputs

4.1. Wall Shear Stress

Wall shear stress (WSS) is the main mechanical regulatory signal that links flow to adaptive changes of the vascular wall and cardiovascular disease lesions[1, 92]. An increased WSS results in remodeling of the vascular wall which is instigated through mechanosensitive pathways in the wall.The calculated WSS values are greatly influenced by the flow condition assumptions. The majority of the literature has assumed that the blood flow is laminar, incompressible, Newtonian and pulsatile, which for the analysis of WSS was found to be quite accurate [20, 93]. Morris et al.[94] and Stroud et al.[95] simulated a 3D model for the human aorta which was obtained from clinical data. The results showed that the maximum wall shear stress occurs along the inner wall of the bend of the aortic arch. The maximum value depends on the assumption, whether steady or pulsatile flow [94-96]. Valenciaet al.[68] found numerically that the pulsatile flow in an artery with atherosclerosis disease is characterized by high wall shear stress and pressure at disease location with recirculation zone. The size of the recirculation zone varies during one cardiac pulse and the recirculation length depends on the degree of disease severity such as stenosis[68].

To contribute to the identification of the earliest stage of cardiovascular diseases, there are some predictions that have significant implications to understanding the local hemodynamic characteristics. In areas of small curvature and high flows assuming a non-Newtonian fluid may be more appropriate. This is due to the fact that the increased red blood cell density on the inside radius of curvature is associated with low WSS [97]. Jung et al.[97] have found that the red blood cell build up is a result of complex recirculation patterns, oscillatory flow with flow reversal, and vessel geometry which result in a prolonged particulate residence time particularly at the end of the diastole cycle. These lead to an increase in the initial plasma viscosity causing lower wall shear stress[97]. These findings are of importance as areas of low WSS have been associated with build up of fatty materials on the artery wall (atherogenesis) [96]. Evidently, theWSS is an important factor in the development or the arrestment of a plaque layer [97]. Hence in a diseased condition, where low WSS occurs in the poststenotic area, which this area represents the narrowing region for the stenosis[98]. A small region of focal low WSS can still be seen as a small irregularity on the inside of the curve of the artery [98]. In addition, the WSS depends strongly on the position of the artery wall, as expected in an arterial geometry with significant primary and secondary curvatures [99-101].

The studies discussed above have indicated that the WSS significantly affects the inner artery wall, which is the main cause of diseases in the artery layers. However, presently there is no clear medical evidence of quantifying the range of WSS changes for different cardiovascular diseases. Also, there is insufficient information on the critical values of this stress for diagnosing atherosclerosis and aneurysm diseases medically.

4.2. Stress Phase Angle

Most *in vitro* studies to date have focused on either WSS or circumferential strain (CS) but not their interaction [102, 103]. WSS and CS and their interaction are believed to play a considerable role in determining artery wall displacementand development of arterial disease [103].

Recently, research has shown that concomitant WSS and CS affect endothelial cellin biochemical responsewhich is modulated by a phase angle called stress phase angle [104]. The stress phase angle is used to characterize the dynamic mechanical stimuli experienced by the endothelial cell monolayer which is expressingthe waveform of stresses. Tada *et al.*[105] found experimentally that these combined forces induce unique endothelial biomolecular responses which were not characterisedas driving forceto modulate an endothelial response[105].An endothelial cell is simultaneously exposed to the mechanical forces of fluidWSS imposed by blood flow and solid circumferential strain induced by the blood vessel's elastic response to the pressure pulse [104].

The stress phase anglehas the possibility to influence vascular remodelling and play a role in the localization of cardiovascular diseases in arteries. This angle is highly radian negative at sites that are prone to atherosclerosis[105-108]. For a better illustration of this angle,a typical transverse arterial cross-section is shown in Figure 5. Pulsatile flow in the axial direction induces pressure and wall shear stress on the endothelium cell lined vascular wall. Pressure imposes a normal radial stress on the wall from the lumen[107].

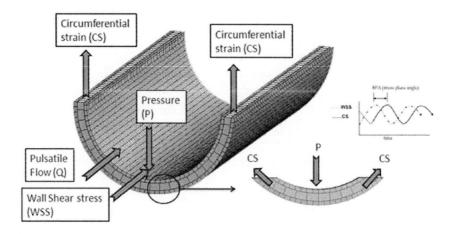

Figure 5. Stress phase angle.

Previous studies have shown how the stress phase angle can be used to indicate disease location. Tada *et al.*[109] simulated 3D, pulsatile flow in carotid bifurcation model with atherosclerosis disease. They found a negative radianstress phase angle on the outer wall of the carotid sinus where diseasewas localized[104]. Torri*et al.*[110]also investigated the effect of changes in flow velocity waveform and arterial wall geometry before and after coronary intervention in the right coronary artery using theCFD method. The results suggested that the stress phase angle measures the degree of asynchrony between pressure and flow waveforms and it is the only parameter that combines WSS and CS (figure 5) [110].

In *in vivo* studies, Dancu*et al.*[111] found that the blood vessel endothelial cellsare subjected to simultaneous pulsatile WSS and CSwhich act approximately in perpendicular directions to each other. In addition, they found that the phase angle between pressure and flow represents the impedance phase angle. They suggested that there is a possible correlation between the stressand the impedance phase angles, which may help in non-invasive screening of cardiovascular diseases [111].

Summary

The above literature indicates the following:

1. Intensive modelling research has been conducted on the cardiovascular system in general and the arteries in particular with an objective of determining the blood flow characteristics. This research has resulted in correlations between these characteristics and the changes in the artery geometry and physical condition caused by various diseases.

2. Intensive research, including that of IBTec [44-46], has been conducted on pulse wave propagation and how the information carried by these waves can be translated in various diagnostic tools.

3. The literature lacks any correlation between the fluid modelling and the wave propagation modelling. It is believed that if such a correlation is established, many of the artery diseases can be identified using pressure wave propagation. This will be one of the main outcomes of this literature survey.

From the above three points, our hypothesisconstitutes the following:

Since some cardiovascular disease can be identified by the stress phase angle, correlation can be established between this angle and the information carried by the pulse wave. It has been shown that the negative values for the phase angle indicate the location of atherosclerosis or aneurysm disease in arteries. It is also believed that there is a correlation between the stress phase angle and impedance phase angle that is generated by the wave reflection. Our research [44-46] has indicated that the hemodynamic characteristics may be predicted from pressure wave signals gathered at the brachial artery. This is anticipated to be a practical approach for diagnosing or screening atherosclerosis and aneurysm diseases from blood pressure measurements at the arm.

The fluid structure interaction method provides realistic results that are possible to validate clinically. Therefore, it is important to include both the dynamics of blood flow as well as the wall motion response associated with the pulsatile nature of the flow to accurately represent an aneurysm or atherosclerosis disease model. However, current models lack the ability to consider the arterial wall thickness and the change in its material properties. Therefore, this research considers the nonlinear arterial wall properties with pulsatile flow. It is anticipated that this model will provide a better validation with the MRI data such as validating the velocity wave form results by simulation with the clinical ones as well for the pressure waveforms.

References

[1]   Wellnhofer, E., et al., Novel non-dimensional approach to comparison of wall shear stress distributions in coronary arteries of different groups of patients. *Atherosclerosis*, 2009. 202 p. 483–490.

[2]   Grigioni, M., et al., A mathematical description of blood spiral flow in vessels: application to a numerical study of flow in arterial bending. *Journal of Biomechanics*, 2005. 38 p. 1375–1386.

[3]   Kagadis, G.C., et al., Computational representation and hemodynamic characterization of in vivo acquired severe stenotic renal artery geometries using turbulence modeling. *Medical Engineering and Physics*, 2008. 30: p. 647–660.

[4]   *http://www.rci.rutgers.edu/~uzwiak/AnatPhys/Blood_Vessels.html.*

[5]   Karamanoglu, M., et al., An analysis of the relationship between central aortic and peripheral upper limb pressure waves in man. *European Heart Journal*, 1993. 14: p. 160-167.

[6]   Hamilton, W.F., The patterns of the arterial pressure pulse. *American Journal of Physiology*, 1944. 141: p. 235-241.

[7]   Kroeker, E.J. and E.H. Wood, Comparison of simultaneously recorded central and peripheral arterial pressure pulses during rest, exercise and tilted position in man. *Circulation Research*, 1955. 3: p. 623-632.

[8]   Ross, R., Atherosclerosis an inflammatory disease. *New England Journal of Medicine*, 1999. 340: p. 115–126.

[9]   Blacher, J., et al., Aortic pulse wave as a marker of cardiovascular risk in hypertensive patients. *Hypertension*, 1999. 33: p. 1111–1117.

[10] Safar, M.E., et al., Recent Advances on large arteries in hypertension. *Hypertension*, 1998. 32: p. 156–161.

[11] Fronek, A., et al., Noninvasivep hysiologicte stsi n the diagnosis and characterization of peripheral arterial occlusive disease. *American Journal of Surgery*, 1973. 126: p. 205-214.

[12] Laurent, S., et al., Aortic stiffness is an independent predictor of all-cause and cardiovascular mortality in hypertensive patients. *Hypertension*, 2001. 37: p. 1236–1245.

[13] Lowe., G.D.O., Different Locations of Atherosclerosis - Different Risk Factors, Different Therapies. *Pathophysiology of Haemostasis and Thrombosis* 2004. 2003/2004; 33: 262-267.

[14] Mitchell, J.R.A. and C.J. Schwarz, Arterial disease. Oxford:Blackwell *Scientific*, 1965.

[15] Abraham, J.P., E.M. Sparrow, and R.D. Lovik, Unsteady, three-dimensional fluid mechanic analysis of blood flow in plaque-narrowed and plaque-freed arteries. *International Journal of Heat and Mass Transfer*, 2008. 51: p. 5633–5641.

[16] Ito, S., et al., Differences in Atherosclerotic Profiles Between Patients With Thoracic and Abdominal Aortic Aneurysms. *The American Journal of Cardiology,* 2008. 101(5): p. 696-699.

[17] Tan, F.P.P., et al., Analysis of flow patterns in a patient-specific thoracic aortic aneurysm model. *Computers and Structures,* 2009. 87(11-12): p. 680-690.

[18] Mantha, A., et al., Hemodynamics in a cerebral Artery before and after the formation of Aneurysm. *American Society of Neuroradiology,* 2006. 27: p. 1113-1118.

[19] Gebbers, J., Atherosclerosis, cholesterol, nutrition, and statins – a critical review. *German medical science,* 2007. 5: p. 1612-3174.

[20] Johnston, B.M., et al., Non-Newtonian blood flow in human right coronary arteries: Transient simulations. *Journal of Biomechanics,* 2006. 39: p. 1116-1128.

[21] Marshall, I., et al., MRI and CFD studies of pulsatile flow in healthy and stenosed carotid bifurcation models. *Journal of Biomechanics,* 2004. 37 p. 679–687.

[22] Lee, B.K., et al., Computed Numerical Analysis of the Biomechanical Effects on Coronary Atherogenesis Using Human Hemodynamic and Dimensional Variables. *Yonsei Medical Journal* 1998. 39(2) p. 166-174.

[23] Deshpande, M.D., et al., Subject-specific blood flow simulation in the human carotid artery bifurcation. *CURRENT SCIENCE,* 2009. 97(9): p. 1303-1312.

[24] Cornelius, T.L., Biomechanical Systems: Biofluid methods in vascular and pulmonary systems. Library of Congress Cataloging-in-Publication Data, 2001.

[25] Bogren, H.G. and M.H. Bounocore, Complex flow patterns in the great vessels: a review. *International Journal of Cardiac Imaging,* 1999. 15: p. 105-113.

[26] Botnar, R.M., et al., Noninvasive coronary vessel wall and plaque imaging with magnetic resonance imaging. *Circulation,* 2000. 102(21): p. 2582-2587.

[27] Laffon, E., et al., Tuning of pulmonary arterial circulation evidenced by MR phase mapping in healthy volunteers. *Journal of Applied Physiology,* 2001. 90: p. 469–474.

[28] Johnson, K., P. Sharma, and J. Oshinski, Coronary artery flow measurement using navigator echo gated phase contrast magnetic resonance velocity mapping at 3.0T. *Journal of Biomechanics,* 2008. 41: p. 595–602.

[29] Kima, D. and J. Park, Internal carotid artery stenosis measurements from 3D reconstructed multi-directional views using phantom data set on MRA image sequence. *European Journal of Radiology,* 2008. 72(1): p. 65-74.

[30] Mirzaee, M.R., et al., Systolic Pressure in Different Percents of Stenosis at Major Arteries. *Proceedings of the World Congress on Engineering and Computer Science* 2008, 2008. WCECS 2008, October 22 - 24, 2008, San Francisco, USA.

[31] Foster, F.K. and D. Turney, Oscillometric Determination of Diastolic, Mean and Systolic Blood Pressure- A Numerical Model. *Journal of Biomechanical Engineering,* 1986. 108: p. 359-364.

[32] Bickley, L.S., *Bates' Guide to Physical Examination and History Taking.* 7th edition J.B. Lippingcott Company, Philadelphia, USA, 1999. Philadelphia, USA.

[33] Wilson, K., MacCallum, H., Wilkinson, I.,B., Hoskins, P., R., Lee, A., J., and Bradbury, A., W, Comparison of Brachial Artery Pressure and Derived Central Pressure in the Measurement of Abdominal Aortic Aneurysm Distensibility. *European Journal of Vascular and Endovascular Surgery,* 2001. Vol. 22(355–360).

[34] Sorvoja, H., *The development of the transducer for the measurement of blood pressure pulse and blood pressure on the wrist.* Licentiate Thesis, 1998. University of Oulu.

[35] Hyman, C., R.L. Paldino, and E. Zimmermann, Local Regulation of Effective Blood Flow in Muscle. *Circulation Research*, 1965. XII.

[36] Hong, H. and M. Fox, Noninvasive detection of cardiovascular pulsations by optical Doppler techniques. *Journal of Biomedical Optics,* 1997. 2: p. 382-385.

[37] Riva, C., B. Ross, and G.B. Benedek, Laser Doppler measurements of blood flow in capillary tubes and retinal arteries. *Investigative Ophthalmology* 1972. 11: p. 91–102.

[38] Pythoud, F., N. Stergiopulos, and J.J. Meister, Modelling of the wave transmission properties of large arteries using nonlinear elastic tube. *Journal of Biomechanics*, 1994. 27: p. 1379–1381.

[39] Hope, S.A., et al., Use of arterial transfer functions for the derivation of central aortic waveform characteristics in subjects with type 2 diabetes and cardiovascular disease: response to Wilkinson and McEniery and Avolio, Cockcroft, and O'Rourke. . *Diabetes Care*, 2004. 27: p. 2565–2567.

[40] Pauca, A.L., M.F. O'Rourke, and N.D. Kon, Prospective evaluation of a method for estimating ascending aortic pressure from the radial artery pressure waveform. *Hypertension*, 2001. 38: p. 932–937.

[41] Roman, M.J., et al., Central Pressure More Strongly Relates to Vascular Disease and Outcome than Does Brachial Pressure. *Hypertension*, 2007. 107.

[42] Stergiopulos, N., B.E. Westerhof, and N. Westerhof, Physical basis of pressure transfer from periphery to aorta: a model-based study. *American Journal of Physiology, Heart and Circulatory Physiology,* 1998. 274: p. H1386–H1392.

[43] Sugimachi, M., et al., A new modelbased method of reconstructing central aortic pressure from peripheral arterial pressure. *The Japanese Journal of Physiology*, 2001. 51: p. 217–222.

[44] Lowe, A., et al., Non-invasive model-based estimation of aortic pulse pressure using suprasystolic brachial pressure waveforms. *Journal of Biomechanics* 2009. 42: p. 2111-2115.

[45] Al-Aklouk, E., A. Al-Jumaily, and A. Lowe, Acoustic Wave Technology as a Diagnostic Tool for Cardiovascular Disease. World *Congress on Medical Physics and Biomedical Engineering*, 2006. 14(1): p. 3386-3389.

[46] Al-Aklouk, E., A. Al-Jumaily, and A. Lowe, Pressure Waves as a Non-Invasive Tool for Artery Stiffness Estimation. *Journal of Medical Devices,* 2008. 2: p. 021001-021008.

[47] Westerhof, B.E., et al., Individualization of transfer function in estimation of central aortic pressure from the peripheral pulse is not required in patients at rest. *Journal of Applied Physiology*, 2008. 105: p. 1858–1863.

[48] Payne, R.A., et al., Similarity between the suprasystolic wideband external pulse wave and the first derivative of the intra-arterial pulse wave. *Br. J. Anaesth.*, 2007. 99: p. 653–661.

[49] McEniery, C.M., et al., On behalf of the anglo-cardiff collaborative trial investigators. Central pressure: variability and impact of cardiovascular risk factors: the anglo-cardiff collaborative trial II. *Hypertension* 2008. 51: p. 1476–1482.

[50] Misra, J.C. and B.K. Sahu, Propagation of Pressure Waves Through Large Blood Vessel:A Mathematical Model of Blood Viscoelasticity. *Mathematical and Computer Modelling*, 1989. 12(3): p. 333-349.

[51] Yilmaz, F., and Gundogdu, M., Y, A critical review on blood flow in large arteries; relevance to blood rheology, viscosity models, and physiologic conditions. *Korea-Australia Rheology Journal,* 2003. Vol. 20, No. 4, December 2008 pp. 197-211.

[52] Womersley, J., Oscillatory motion of a viscous liquid in a thin walled elastic tube: The linear approximation for long waves. *Philosophical Magazine,* 1955. 46(373): p. 199-221.

[53] Peiro, J. and S.J. Sherwin, Automatic reconstruction of a patient-specific high-order surface representation and its application to mesh generation for CFD calculations. *Medical and Biological Engineering and Computing,* 2008. 46: p. 1069–1083.

[54] Sulaiman, A., et al., In vitro non-rigid life-size model of aortic arch aneurysm for endovascular prosthesis assessment. *European Journal of Cardio-thoracic Surgery,* 2008. 33: p. 53-57.

[55] Pontrelli, G., Blood Flow Through an Axisymmetric Stenosis *Journal of Engineering in Medicine,* 2001. 215(1): p. 1-10.

[56] Lee, D. and J.J. Chiu, Intimal thickening under shear in a carotid bifurcation--A numerical study. *Journal of Biomechanics,* 1996. 29(1): p. 1-11.

[57] Ku, D.N. and D.P. Giddens, Laser Doppler anemometer measurements of pulsatile flow in a model carotid bifurcation. *Journal of Biomechanics,* 1987. 20(4): p. 407-421.

[58] Varghese, S.S., S.H. Frankel, and P.F. fischer, Direct numerical simulation of stenotic flows, Part 2: Pulsatile flow. *Journal of Fluid Mechanics,* 2007. 582: p. 281-318.

[59] Giddens, D.P., C.K. Zarins, and S. Glagov, The role of fluid mechanics in the localisation and detection of atherosclerosis. *Journal of Biomechanical Engineering,* 1993. 115(4): p. 588–594.

[60] Ojha, M., et al., Pulsatile flow through constricted tubes: an experimental investigation using photochromic tracer methods. *Journal of Fluid Mechanics* 1989. 203: p. 173–197.

[61] Cebral, J.R., M.A. Castro, and C.M. Putman, Numerical simulation of flow alterations after carotid artery stenting from multi-modality image data. Computational Fluid and Solid Mechanics, 2005. *Third MIT Conference on Computational Fluid and Solid Mechanics:* p. 607-611.

[62] Zhao, S.Z., et al., Blood flow and vessel mechanics in a physiologically realistic model of a human carotid arterial bifurcation. *Journal of Biomechanics,* 2000. 33 p. 975-984.

[63] Ivankovic, A., et al., Towards Early Diagnosis of Atherosclerosis: The Finite Volume Method for Fluid-Structure Interaction. *Biorheology,* 2002. 39: p. 401-411.

[64] Bathe, M. and R.D. Kamm, A fluid-Strcture Interaction Finite Element Analysis of Pulsatile Blood Flow Through a Compliant Stenotic Artery. *Journal of Biomechanical Engineering,* 1999. 121: p. 361-369.

[65] Tang, D., et al., Steady Flow and Wall Compression in Stenotic Arteries: A Three-Dimensional Thick-Wall Model With Fluid–Wall Interactions. *Journal of Biomechanical Engineering,* 2001. 123: p. 548-557.

[66] Vito, R.P. and S.A. Dixon, Blood Vessel Constitutive. *Annual Review of Biomedical Engineering,* 2003. 5: p. 413-439.

[67] Li, H.J., J.H. Haga, and S. Chien, Molecular basis of the effects of shear stress on vascular endothelial cells. *Journal of Biomechanics,* 2005. 38(10): p. 1949-1971.

[68] Valencia, A. and F. Baeza, Numerical simulation of fluid–structure interaction in stenotic arteries considering two layer nonlinear anisotropic structural model. *International Communications in Heat and Mass Transfer,* 2009. 36 p. 137–142.

[69] Scotti, C.M., et al., Wall stress and flow dynamics in abdominal aortic aneurysms: finite element analysis vs. fluid–structure interaction. *Computer Methods in Biomechanics and Biomedical Engineering*, 2008. 11(3): p. 301–322.

[70] Leung, J.H., et al., Fluid structure interaction of patient specific abdominal aortic aneurysms: a comparison with solid stress models. *BioMedical Engineering OnLine*, 2006. 5(33)(1-15).

[71] Gao, F., et al., Fluid-structure Interaction within a Layered Aortic Arch Model. *Journal of Biological Physics*, 2006. 32: p. 435–454.

[72] Kim, Y., et al., Blood Flow in a Compliant Vessel by the Immersed Boundary Method. *Annals of Biomedical Engineering*, 2009. 37(5): p. 927–942.

[73] Gao, F., O. Ohta, and T. Matsuzawa, Fluid structure interaction in layered aortic arch aneurysm model assessing the combined influence of arch aneurysm wall stiffness. *Australsian Physical and Engineering Sciences in Medicine*, 2008. 31: p. 32-41.

[74] Demiray, H. and R.P. Vito, On large periodic motions of arteries. *Journal of Biomechanics*, 1983. 16(8): p. 643-648.

[75] Steinman, D.A., et al., Reconstruction of carotid bifurcation hemodynamices and wall thickness using computational fluid dynamics and MRI. *Magnetic Resonance in Medicine*, 2002. 47(1): p. 149–159.

[76] Weydahl, E.S. and J.E. Moore, Dynamic curvature strongly affects wall shear rates in a coronary artery bifurcation model. *Journal of Biomechanics*, 2001. 34(9): p. 1189-1196.

[77] Chandran, K.B. and T.L. Yearwood, Experimental Study of Physiologcial Pulsatile Flow in a Curved Tube. *Journal of Fluid Mechanics*, 1981. 111: p. 59–85.

[78] Perktold, K., D. Hilbert, and . Numerical simulation of pulsatile flow in a carotid bifurcation model. *Journal of Biomedical Engineering*, 1986. 8: p. 193–199.

[79] Cox , R.H., Comparison of linearized wave propagation models for arterial blood flow analysis. *Journal of Biomechanics*, 1969. 2: p. 251–265.

[80] Atabek, H.B., Wave propagation through a viscous liquid contained in a tethered, initially stressed, orthotropic elastic tube. . *Biophysical Journal*, 1968. 8: p. 626–649.

[81] Avolio, A.P., M.F. O'roukre, and M.E.D. Webster, Pulse-Wave Propagation in the Arterial System of the Diamond Python Morelia Spilotes. AJP - *Regulatory, Integrative and Comparative Physiology*, 1983. 245: p. 831-836.

[82] Thurston, G.B., Effect of viscoelasticity of blood on wave propagation in the circulation. *Journal Biomechanics*, 1976. 9: p. 13–20.

[83] Cox, R.H., Wave propagation through a Newtonian fluid contained within a thick-walled viscoelastic tube: the influence of wall compressibility. *Journal of Biomechanics*, 1970. 3: p. 317–335.

[84] Misra, J.C. and K. Roychoudhuri, Effect of initial stresses on the wave propagation in arteries. *Journal of Mathematical Biology*, 1983. 18: p. 53–67.

[85] Atabek, H.B. and H.S. Lew, Wave propagation through a viscous incompressible fluid contained in an initially stressed elastic tube. *Biophysical Journal*, 1966. 6: p. 481–503.

[86] Chow, J.C. and J.T. Apter, Wave propagation in a viscous incompressible fluid contained in flexible viscoelastic tubes. *Journal of the Acoustical Society of America*, 1968. 44: p. 437–443.

[87] Freudenburg, H. and P.R. Lichtlen, The normal wall segment in coronary stenosis-a postmortem study. *Kardiologie*, 1981. 70: p. 863-869.

[88] Stergiopulos, N., et al., On The Wave Transmission and Reflection Properties of Stenoses. *Journal of Biomechanics*, 1996. 29: p. 31- 38.

[89] Olufsen, M.S., Structured tree outflow condition for blood flow in larger systemic arteries. *American Physiological Society*, 1999. 276: p. H257-H268.

[90] Liu, B., *Computer simulations of flow in curved tubes with stenosis, in COMSOL Multiphysics User's Conference.* 2005: Boston.

[91] Liu, B., Flow patterns in curved atherosclerotic arteries. Far *East Journal of Applied Mathematics*, 2004. 14(2): p. 157-177.

[92] Soulis, J.V., et al., Non-Newtonian models for molecular viscosity and wall shear stress in a 3D reconstructed human left coronary artery. *Medical Engineering and Physics*, 2008. 30 p. 9–19.

[93] Lee, S.E., et al., Direct numerical simulation of transitional flow in a stenosed carotid bifurcation. *Journal of Biomechanics* 2008. 41: p. 2551-2561.

[94] Morris, L., et al., 3-D Numerical Simulation of Blood Flow Through Models of the Human Aorta. *Journal of Biomechanical Engineering*, 2005. 127: p. 767-775.

[95] Stroud, J.S., B.A. A, and D. Saloner, Numerical Analysis of Flow Through a Severely Stenotic Carotid Artery Bifurcation. *Journal of Biomechanical Engineering*, 2002. 124: p. 9-20.

[96] Zeng, D., et al., Effects of Cardiac Motion on Right Coronary Artery Hemodynamics. *Annals of Biomedical Engineering*, 2003. 31: p. 420-429.

[97] Jung, J., et al., Multiphase hemodynamic simulation of pulsatile flow in a coronary artery. *Journal of Biomechanics*, 2006. 39(11): p. 2064-2073.

[98] Nguyena, K.T., et al., Carotid geometry effects on blood flow and on risk for vascular disease. *Journal of Biomechanics*, 2008. 41p. 11–19.

[99] Kenjereš, S., Numerical analysis of blood flow in realistic arteries subjected to strong non-uniform magnetic fields. International *Journal of Heat and Fluid Flow*, 2008. 29: p. 752–764.

[100] Torii, R., et al., A CFD Study on Coronary Artery Hamodynamics With Dynamic VEssel Motion Based on MR Images *Journal of Biomechanics* (Abstracts of the 16th Congress, European Society of Biomechanics), 2008. 41: p. S212.

[101] Fayad, Z.A. and V. Fuster, The human high-risk plaque and its detection by magnetic resonance imaging. *American Journal of Cardiology*, 2001. 88(2A): p. 42E–45E.

[102] Chen, J. and X. Lu, Numerical investigation of the non-Newtonian blood flow in a bifurcation model with a non-planar branch. *Journal of Biomechanics*, 2004. 37 p. 1899–1911.

[103] Qui, Y. and J.M. Tarbell, Interaction between Wall Shear Stress and Circumferential Strain Affects Endothelial Cell Biochemical Production. *Journal of Vascular Surgery*, 1999. 37: p. 147-157.

[104] Lee, B.K., et al., Hemodynamic Effects on Atherosclerosis-Prone Coronary Artery: Wall Shear Stress/ Rate Distribution and Impedance Phase Angle in Coronary and Aortic Circulation. *Yonsei Medical Journal*, 2001. 42: p. 375-383.

[105] Tada, S. and J.M. Tarbell, A Computational Study of Flow in a Compliant Carotid Bifurcation–Stress Phase Angle Correlation with Shear Stress. *Annals of Biomedical Engineering*, 2005. 33 (9): p. 1202-1212.

[106] Dancu, M.B. and J.M. Tarbell, Large Negative Stress Phase Angle (SPA) attenuates nitric oxide production in bovine aortic endothelial cells. *Journal of Biomechanical Engineering,* 2006. 128(3): p. 329-34.

[107] Wang, D.M. and J.M. Tarbell, Nonlinear analysis of flow in an elastic tube (artery): steady streaming effects. *The Journal of Fluid Mechanics,* 1992. 239: p. 341-358.

[108] Urbina, E.M., et al., Impact of multiple coronary risk factors on the intima-media thickness of different segments of carotid artery in healthy young adults (The Bogalusa Heart Study). *American Journal of Cardiology,* 2002. 90: p. 953–958.

[109] Tada, S., Dong, C., and Tarbell, J., M, Effect of the Stress Phase Angle on the Strain Energy Density of the Endothelial Plasma Membrane. *Biophysical Journal,* 2007. Volume 93: p. 3026–3033.

[110] Torii, R., et al., Stress phase angle depicts differences in coronary artery hemodynamics due to changes in flow and geometry after percutaneous coronary intervention. *Am J Physiol Heart Circ Physiol,* 2009. 296: p. H765–H776.

[111] Dancu, M.B., et al., Asynchronous Shear Stress and Circumferential Strain Reduces Endothelial NO Synthase and Cyclooxygenase-2 but Induces Endothelin-1 Gene Expression in Endothelial Cells. *Arteriosclerosis, Thrombosis, and Vascular Biology,* 2004. 24(11): p. 2088-2094.

In: Systolic Blood Pressure
Editor: Robert A. Arfi

ISBN: 978-1-61209-263-8
©2012 Nova Science Publishers, Inc.

Chapter IX

Measures of Coupling Strength and Synchronization in Non Linear Interaction of Heart Rate and Systolic Blood Pressure in the Cardiovascular Control System[*]

Elio Conte, Antonio Federici[†], Mauro Minervini,
Annamaria Papagni and Joseph P. Zbilut

Department of Pharmacology and Human Physiology and TIRES-Center
for Innovative Technologies for Signal Detection and Processing,
University of Bari, Policlinico, I-70124, Bari, Italy
Department of Physiology, Rush Medical College,
Rush University, Chicago, Illinois, 60612, US

Abstract

Beat-to-Beat R-R intervals and systolic blood pressure (SBP) variability signals were used for a quantitative study of coupling strength and synchronization in non linear interaction of heart rate and systolic blood pressure during spontaneous and controlled breathing. In addition to linear analysis that was based on spectral and cross-spectral analysis, we applied the independence of complexity test, the recurrence and the cross recurrence quantification analysis in order to estimate the values of coupling and synchronization in the two conditions of experimentation. The results indicate that the

---

[*] A version of this chapter also appears in *Chaos and Complexity Research Progress*, edited by Franco F. Orsucci, published by Nova Science Publishers, Inc. It was submitted for appropriate modifications in an effort to encourage wider dissemination of research.

[†] Address for correspondence: Antonio Federici, M.D. Dipartimento di Farmacologia e Fisiologia Umana Policlinico, Piazza Giulio Cesare 11, I-70124, Bari, Italia, Tel.: ++39 80 5478 414, Fax : ++39 80 5478 417 E-mail address: fisio2@fisiol.uniba.it

non linear R-R:SBP interaction is influenced at a high degree by the respiratory component because coupling strength and synchronization resulted strongly reduced during controlled respect to spontaneous respiration. In particular, the recurrence quantification analysis enabled us to confirm that a non deterministic dynamics, mathematically supported by the so called relaxation of Lipschitz conditions, is at the basis in cardiovascular control system.

1. Introduction

Heart rate (HR) and blood pressure variability (BPV) reflect the function of the cardiovascular control system. Periodic fluctuations were observed for the first time in arterial blood pressure (BP) in 1773 by Stephen Hales (Hales, 1773). He did not consider the possibility of relating these variations to respiration. Some years later, in 1778, Albrecht von Haller (Haller, 1778) recognized that fluctuations exist in heart rate (HR), and that these fluctuations are in synchrony with respiration. In 1847 Carl Ludwig (Ludwig, 1847) noted fluctuations in BP connected to respiration from observations of physiological signals recorded from dogs and horses.

Although fluctuations in blood pressure and heart rate were identified over 100 years ago, they continue to be a subject of considerable interest relative to the idea that their fluctuations are indicative of sympathetic or parasympathetic control of the cardiovascular system (Akselrod et al., 1981). The initial effort was to consider that the presence of non linear mechanisms would be reflected mainly in the long-term recordings of variability while instead, during short-term stationary recordings in stable conditions, the signals were assumed to behave according to a linear small-signal model with non linearity being negligible. Consequently, linear methods such as spectral analysis and linear parametric modeling were employed in the analysis of short-term variability. More recently, instead, a growing importance arose in the assessment of HR and BP short term variability with non-linear methods. Starting with the measurements of Mayer (Mayer, 1877) and of Guyton and Harris (Guyton and Harris, 1951) in 1951, research on cardiovascular variability was centered on questions to ascertain if baroreceptors and sympathetic outflow are determinants in regulating the oscillations. A great variety of animal and human studies have suggested some important results, the first being that at least two frequency bands are present in heart rate and blood pressure with autonomic involvement. One band of oscillation is associated with respiration and another at a slower frequency in the order of 0.1 Hertz in humans.

The analysis of short term cardiovascular control using non linear methods has indicated that very complex mechanisms are involved in cardiovascular regulation and that they interact with each other in a non linear way. Still, the relevant role of random variations in cardiovascular system has been also considered in detail. Spontaneous fluctuations are common in physiological systems, and such variations in blood pressure may be regarded as noise. Three major noise sources may be identified in the system as systemic resistance noise, random baromodulation and vagal noise. A vagal noise source is present since afferent systems from heart, lungs and other organs excite or inhibit cardiac vagal efferent activity. It has been shown that the low frequency variations in heart rate below 0.1 Hz have a 1/f power spectrum in a range of approximately 0.025-0.04 Hz (Butler et al.,1993-1994). 1/f characteristics have been also found in heart rate in the frequency range 0.01-0.4 Hz (Lipsitz et al., 1990).

A movement to change the dominant paradigm of literature regarding heart rate variability and centered around the concept of modulation by feedback, has also been repeatedly promulgated (Zbilut et al., 1988). In this framework, studies aimed to decide whether the particular behaviors of the observed R-R time series are due to autonomic control or must be conceived as a basic characteristic of cardiac rhythm independent of control (Giuliani et al.,1996). A number of studies were performed on the problem of intrinsic beat mechanism of heart devoid of external influences. In 1993 Wilders and Jongsma (Wilders and Jongsma, 1993) showed that individual and cell clusters of heart beat stochastically. Certainly this result has not resolved still the problem of coupling to the atrium. However, all such results suggest that the random walk paradigm could be more appropriate in the analysis of control dynamics in the cardiovascular system. It was repeatedly outlined (Zbilut et al., 1988) that the noise level and non stationarity characterizing cardiovascular signals severely prohibit the uncritical application of some linear and non linear methods of signal processing. At the same time it was evidenced that strong conceptual problems remain in the same manner to conceive classically the control dynamics of the system. Chaotic systems are fully determined by initial conditions and they are unpredictable only because our lack of precision. Living organisms are adaptive throughout a range of time scales. Instead, the rigidity of an adopted mechanism of deterministic or chaotic-deterministic nature forces the dynamics of a system into some narrow predetermined behavior rendering it incapable of responding to the continuous adjustments that instead are required in consequence of its interaction with its environment. Still, given the tremendous amounts of noise in biological systems and the extreme sensitivity to initial conditions of chaotic systems, the energy expended to run adaptive controllers would be considerable. Certainly the stability of such systems would come into question since infinitesimal differences in control parameters should result in enormously different effects.

In conclusion, in analysing cardiovascular system, the problem does not seem to be the adoption of non linear dynamics per se but the adoption of uniqueness criteria (Lipschitz conditions) that, from its starting of classical physics, were required for the solution of differential equations. If such conditions are relaxed (Zbilut et al., 1988), the dynamics becomes more tractable from a general view point and with respect to noise. It becomes a non deterministic dynamics. A new class of phenomena arises which cannot be represented by chaos directly. It delineates a discrete events dynamics where randomness appears as point events since there is a sequence of random occurrences at fixed or random times but there is no additional component of uncertainty between these times. The system dynamics becomes more adaptive since the presence of singular points in the mathematical treatment can be considered to be part of a larger chain of oscillators which become self–organizing. In previous studies experiments were conducted (Giuliani et al., 1996) on normal and anesthetized rats. From the analysis emerged a picture of autonomic control as constraining the probabilistic fluctuations of the R-R intervals around the last achieved state. The control did not try to level the system to the most probable, ground state, rather it only constrained the size of the oscillations. When the system escaped the constraint of one state, it was adjusted to the new state reached. When the autonomic control was off (anesthesia of the rats), the R-R dynamics resulted in a simple random walk between states. Thus the before mentioned non Lipschitz model was more appropriate with non deterministic dynamics governed by noise in a central manner in the cardiovascular system.

The present paper moves in the framework previously delineated. The purpose is to give a contribution to the comprehension of the specific problems regarding the degree of involvement of the different cardiovascular control systems in the appearance of the non linear components of R-R interval variability and systolic blood pressure (SBP). Our aim is to give detailed results concerning the non linear interaction acting between R-R behavior and systolic blood pressure (SBP) and to assess the degree of linear and non linear coupling between these two cardiovascular variables during baseline and condition of controlled respiration for cardiovascular system.

2. Materials and Methods

2.1. Experimental Protocol and Data Acquisition

The interference between spontaneous fluctuations in R-R intervals and systolic blood pressure (SBP) has been studied in two different conditions of respiratory activity, in 6 healthy female subjects whose age ranged from 26 to 30 years. Subjects were studied while resting in supine position in a quiet but not acoustically isolated environment. All the experimental sessions took place between 9.00 and 11.00 in the morning.

The following parameters were recorded: II lead electrocardiogram by an analogic electrocardiograph; thoracic respiratory movements, by an estensimetric belt; arterial sphygmogram by a photopletysmographic device (Finapres, Ohmeda) applied at a finger of the left hand. Data were digitally converted (sampling rate: 500 Hz; resolution: 16 bit) by an A/D interface (MP 100, Biopac Systems) and stored on the hard disk of a PC.

The subjects were equilibrated to the environment and resting for about 15 min before of recording. In fact, as previously said, biological signals, in addition to being non linear, tend to be non stationary, noisy and then high dimensional. Therefore, a satisfactory compromise was reached not to exceed 10 min for each stage of acquisition of data. The protocol consisted of two different steps, the first one with the subject spontaneously breathing lying supine at the rest, and the second one with the subject controlled to breath at a frequency of about 0.2 Hz, driven by experimenter's commands.

Signal preprocessing included the detection of QRS complexes in electrocardiogram and systolic peaks in arterial blood pressure with a software calculating times between peaks for R-R and values of SBP.

2.2. Preprocessing Data. Testing for Non Stationarity and Non Linearity

Statistical drift was employed to evaluate non stationarity of data. Statistical indexes were used as mean, S.D., median, variance and RMS. Figure 1, as example, evidences non stationarity for R-R intervals and SBP values as they were obtained by mean values with a window of 20 in the case of subject 2. No different results were obtained in the case of the data examined for the other subjects in the different conditions of experimentation.

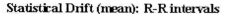

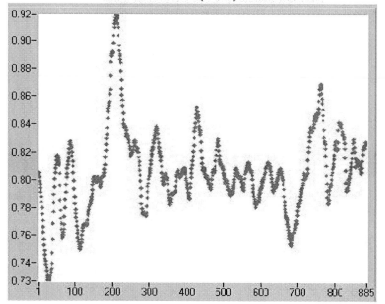

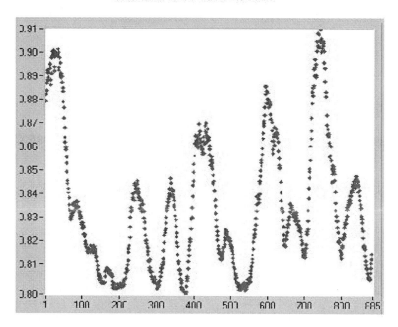

Figure 1. Non Stationarity of Data.

Figure 2 evidences the trend in the same case of R-R intervals and SBP values for subject 2. Also in this case no substantial differences in the results were obtained for the other subjects and in the two conditions of experimentation. The results highly confirmed non stationary and noise behavior of the data.

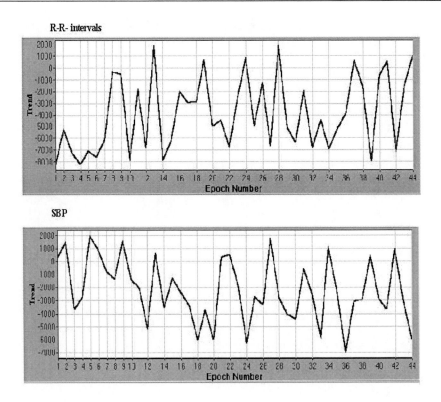

Figure 2. Non Stationarity of Data.

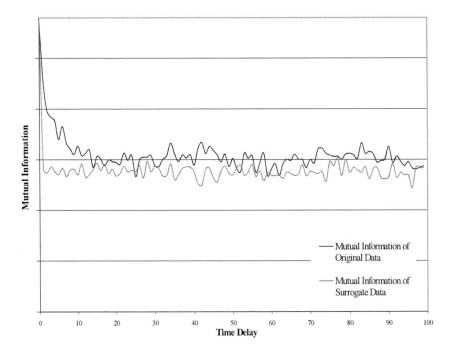

Figure 3. Mutual Information of Original and Surrogate Data. R-R Time Series.

Testing for non linearity. Surrogate Data. Surrogate data were generated through Amplitude Adjusted Fourier Transform (AAFT). In this case surrogate series has the same distribution of amplitudes as the original one but it does not have the same power spectrum. Mutual Information (MI) and autocorrelation function (Acf) were used as discriminant statistics (Baselli et al., 2002). Acf is a linear operator.

If Acf values of original and surrogate series do not differ significantly, this is indication of a correct surrogating process since it retains linearities. Instead, MI is a non linear operator and thus large differences are expected between original and surrogate as non linear relations in the time series have been not destroyed. In this case one may discard the null hypothesis of linear process. Figure 3 evidences high non linearity for time series regarding R-R intervals for subject 3 with values of time delays $\tau = 1$ and $\tau = 6$ that were obtained as first minimum of MI in the case of surrogate and original data respectively. The same significant results were obtained using SBP values as well as in the case of the other subjects under investigation.

On the basis of the previous results it was possible to conclude that all the recorded signals exhibited an highly non stationary and non linear structure.

3. Analysis of the Data

3.1. Estimate of Coupling between R-R Intervals and SBP

A preliminary analysis for testing linear coupling between R-R and SBP was performed. The cross correlation function (CCF) was used to detect the linear relationship. The behaviors are reported in figures 4 and 5 for subject n1 but substantially equivalent results were obtained also in the other investigated cases.

It is well known that spontaneous oscillations of R-R and SBP were repeatedly analyzed in the past by Fourier mathematical tools with the aim to extract the main related frequency information. Such linear analysis confirmed, as just we outlined in the introduction, that these signals exhibit some approximate periodicities. Studies identified three bands of spectral activity in adults healthy subjects, a very low frequency, approximately 0.05 Hertz, possibly related to thermoregulation, a slightly higher frequency, approximating 0.1 Hertz, associated with baroreceptor activity of control and a region between 0.12-0.5 Hertz corresponding to the respiratory frequency (R.I. Kitney and O. Rompelman, The Study of Heart-Rate Variability, Oxford U.P.,Oxford,1980). It is important to outline here that such periodicities are not constant for each subject but fluctuate often or also disappear or still may be entrained to each other as it is the case of subjects with respiratory periodicity approaching baroreceptor frequency .We also performed spectral and cross spectral analysis for R-R and SBP data. In this case a rough estimation of R-R : SBP linear coupling may be obtained by calculation of the α - BRS index (BaroReceptorSensitivity), calculated as square rooted ratio of R-R and SBP powers in given frequency bands and for values of coherence greater of 0.5.LF and HF peaks were detected and evaluated by us for the subjects in normal and controlled breathing conditions The values of coherence were also accounted at LF (0.1 Hertz) and HF (0.25 Hertz) for subjects in normal conditions of spontaneous respiration with LF (0.1Hertz) and HF (0.2 Hertz) in the case instead of controlled respiration. Also phase shifts were estimated between R-R and SBP at the same LF and HF ranges in the two previously indicated conditions of experimentation.

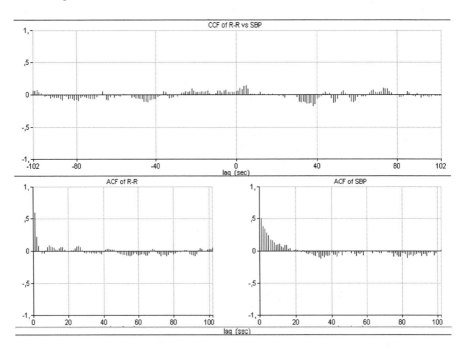

Figure 4. R-R vs SBP: Spontaneous Respiration.

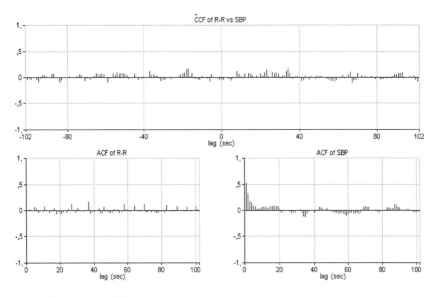

Figure 5. R-R vs SBP: Controlled Respiration.

The non linear coupling between R-R and SBP was estimated using the text of independence of complexity, C_{RR-SBP}, that was introduced by D. Hoyer et al. in 1998 (Hoyer et al., 1998). It is the ratio of the sum of the absolute values of the differences between the joint correlation dimension and each individual correlation dimension over the sum of the individual correlation dimensions according to the following formulas

$$C_{RR-SBP} = \frac{|CD_{RR-SBP} - CD_{RR}| + |CD_{RR-SBP} - CD_{SBP}|}{CD_{RR} + CD_{SBP}}$$

where CD_{RR-SBP} is the correlation dimension of the jointly embedded series R-R and SBP while CD_{RR} and CD_{SBP} are the correlation dimension of the individual series of R-R and SBP respectively. The coupling strength results to be

$$C_\gamma = \frac{1}{C_{RR-SBP}}$$

and it has its maximum value when the two series are strongly coupled ($CD_{RR-SBP} = CD_{RR} = CD_{SBP}$), and its minimum value ($C_\gamma = 1$) for completely independent series ($CD_{RR-SBP} = CD_{RR} + CD_{SBP}$).

The aim of the analysis was to estimate the coupling strength C_γ between R-R and SBP in the two conditions of experimentation, the spontaneous and controlled respiration, respectively. According to Takens' theorem (Tackens, 1980), the dynamics of the systems (R-R or SBP) were reconstructed by using time-delays values of the single observed time series as state variables while the joint system dynamics of the two coupled subsystems, (RR-SBP), was reconstructed by an analogous delay vector using the values of the two interacting subsystems

$$p(t) = [x_{RR}(t), x_{RR}(t-\tau), ..., x_{RR}(t-m\tau), x_{SBP}(t), x_{SBP}(t-\tau), ..., x_{SBP}(t-n\tau)]$$

with embedding dimension m and n for R-R and SBP respectively, and joint embedded system with dimension m+n. False Nearest Neighbours technique (Fraser and Swinney, 1986) was used to estimate embedding dimensions while correlation dimensions were calculated according to Grasberger-Procaccia's method (Grasberger and Procaccia, 1993).

3.2. Recurrence Quantification Analysis and Cross Recurrence Quantification Analysis

Another non linear analysis of the data was started by means of recurrence quantification analysis (RQA) and cross recurrence quantification analysis (KRQA). The recurrence plot technique (RP) was introduce by Eckmann et al. (Eckmann et al, 1987) in 1987 for analysis of dynamical systems. Zbilut and Webber introduced instead RQA and KRQA starting with 1994 (Webber and Zbilut, 1994). The RQA analysis was conceived to investigate the dynamics of a system in presence of non linearity, non stationarity and noise by identification of time correlations of single embedded time series. The recurrence plot looks for repeated sequences in the data in the half of an $n \times n$ matrix where data are considered to be recurrent when their distance results to be less than a small prefixed value. The diagonal lines result to be of particular interest in such plots. In fact, given a series of n points, let p the number of the recurrence points. The percentage of recurrences will result to be % Rec = 100 p/m being m the number of points in the half of the $n \times n$ matrix with exclusion of the principal diagonal. In order to estimate trajectories that at similar levels remain parallel, a given Length is fixed and the number d of recurrent points in diagonal lines of a given Length L, is calculated. In this manner the percentage of determinism results to be %Det = 100 d/p. Other variables of interest may be also calculated in RQA (see (Webber and Zbilut, 1994) for details). To analyze R-R intervals and SBP we embedded R-R and, respectively, SBP data in a m-dimensional (n-dimensional) Euclidean space using mutual information for time delay reconstruction and False Nearest Neighbours technique for detecting dimension at 5% false nearest neighbours (Fraser and Swinney, 1986). A distance R about 80 was obtained following the strategy that was indicated in (Zbilut et al., 2002). %Rec was calculated for several increasing values of r, the results were plotted on a log-log plot to detect a satisfactory scaling region in consideration of the non stationarity of the data. Finally, a Length measure of 2 was selected for the analysis and dimension d=10. This is the procedure that was employed to provide qualitative and quantitative information about the non linear dynamical structure of only one, R-R or SBP, single time series in the two conditions of experimentation, respectively of spontaneous and controlled breathing.

Some studies appeared (Porta et al., 1996; Shockley et al., 2002; Censi et al., 2002) ascertaining that RQA may be applied also to analyze whether repetitive patterns may be used to investigate the interaction between two given time series. The derived method is called KRQA. In this method two time series $x_1(t)$ and $x_2(t)$ are given and RP results to be a representation of the normalized distances between points $[x_1(i), x_2(i)]$ and $[x_1(j), x_2(j)]$ in time domain. Plots are obtained on the basis of a normalized distance. In this condition, a recurrent point in (i,j) means that the interaction between the signals in the instant i is almost the same as in the instant j and this is to say that the interaction between the two signals is happening. An occasional recurrence point indicates an isolated recurrence of the phase relationship between the signals happening by chance or noise or actual interaction. Line segments parallel to the main diagonal will indicate instead the presence of points close to each other forward in time according to (i,j), $(i+t_1,j+t_1)$, $(i+t_2,j+t_2)$,........., $(i+T,j+T)$ $(T>......>t_2>t_1$). A recurrent diagonal will indicate a stable recurrence of the phase relationship for a time interval corresponding to the length of the diagonal (T) and the time interval separating diagonals will be the recurrence period. Also in this case some variables may be introduced and precisely %Rec expressing the percent ratio between the number of recurrence points and the total number of points, the %Det defining the percent ratio between the number of recurrence points forming diagonal lines and the total number of recurrence points. Still, a given threshold Length will be fixed, and, finally, a third variable will be defined, the entropy E that will be the Shannon entropy of the diagonal length distribution. According still to references (Censi et al., 2002, Porta et al., 1996), the more periodic the signal dynamics is, the higher will result the %Rec value. %Det will contain instead information about the duration of a stable interaction so that the longer will be the interactions and higher will result %Det values. Finally, E will result an index of the deterministic structure of the dynamics as measured in bits of information. The more deterministic is the structure of the recurrence plot, the smaller will be the number of bits required to represent such structure. In conclusion, for increasing coupling and synchronization, one will have increasing values of %Rec and %Det but decreasing values of E. We applied such KRQA method in order to analyze coupling and synchronization between R-R and SBP time series in the two conditions of controlled respect to spontaneous respiration.

Results and Conclusion

As expected, our preliminary tentative to detect any linear relationship of coupling between R-R and SBP by CCF did not give relevant results (i.e. see also, Suder et al. 1998). With 95% significance, values of 0.09 and 0.11 were obtained by CCF analysis in the two cases of spontaneous and controlled respiration, respectively.

Regarding instead the test of independence of complexity that we used to evaluate non linear coupling strength in R-R: SBP in the two conditions of experimentation, we have to state first a fundamental specification.

As we know, the last decade witnessed the original hope that chaos theory would help elucidating the complexities of the biological processes. Initially, it was retained in fact that the calculation of chaotic invariants would capture subtle non linear aspects of dynamics of biological systems.

However, more investigations have cleared that chaotic specific measures as Lyapunov exponents and correlation dimensions may be utilized on the basis of some specific requisites and limitations that must be rigorously respected in order chaos analysis to have a sense. An important recognition in this respect is that biological signals, in addition to being non linear, tend to be non stationary, noisy and high dimensional and such complex of features lead many doubts on the correct applicability of chaos measures in the analysis of biological signals. In the course of the present analysis we just utilized the test of independence of complexity whose computation requires in particular the calculation of correlation dimensions as it was explained in detail in the previous section. Thus, we applied such test in the case of non stationary, noisy and high dimensional signals. Therefore the obtained results should be taken with care considering the present calculation more as a phenomenological tentative to evaluate non linear coupling strengths rather than an accurate and definitive estimate. The results are reported in Figure 6.

It is seen that the coupling strength between R-R and SBP results to be $C_\gamma = 15.08 \pm 6.60$ in the case of R-R: SBP coupling in condition of spontaneous respiration while instead it results $C_\gamma = 8.81 \pm 3.01$ in the case of R-R: SBP coupling during controlled respiration. We identified a reduction of about 41% in the value of the non linear coupling strength between R-R and SBP in passing from spontaneous to controlled respiration. Thus, one first result seems to be phenomenologically reached. Respiratory component appears to be strongly involved in non linear R-R:SBP interaction since R-R:SBP coupling strength results profoundly reduced during controlled respect to spontaneous respiration.

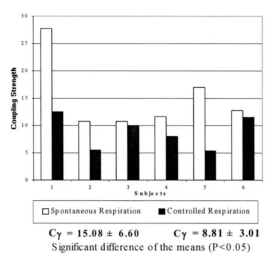

$C\gamma = 15.08 \pm 6.60$ $C\gamma = 8.81 \pm 3.01$

Significant difference of the means (P<0.05)

Figure 6. Values of Coupling Strength in non Linear Interaction R-R : SBP During Spontaneous and Controlled Respiration.

In order to confirm these novel results, we employed this time RQA and KRQA methods which are uniquely suited to the case of analysis with non linear, non stationary, noisy and high dimensional signals. To confirm a decreasing of coupling strength in R-R:SBP non linear interaction in the case of controlled versus spontaneous respiration, we expected to obtain decreasing values of %Rec and of %Det but increasing values of E by KRQA in the condition of controlled versus spontaneous respiration on the basis of the arguments of the previous section. The results are reported in Figure 7. KRQA confirmed substantially the results previously obtained by the test of independence of complexity. For R-R:SBP we had %Rec = 20.29±1.18 , %Det =31.93±8.27, and E=2.60±0.50 in the case of spontaneous respiration, and %Rec = 11.25 ± 5.01, %Det = 13.50 ± 8.49, and E=3.58±0.48 in the case of controlled respiration.

Such results characterized non linear interaction and thus R-R: SBP coupling strength and synchronization in the case of spontaneous respiration and of controlled respiration. They confirmed and indeed established in rigorous quantitative terms that a fall of coupling strength and synchronization happens during R-R:SBP non linear interaction in controlled versus spontaneous respiration. Significant differences were found by using two-way analysis of variance (P<0.05).

A conclusion may be than fixed. During controlled respiration we have a reduction of RR:SBP non linear interaction with regard to its periodicity (%Rec.) and to the duration (%Det.) of such stable interaction respect to the condition of spontaneous respiration.

However, it was of course the RQA analysis that furnished the most interesting results. We calculated %Rec, %Det, and Max Line. While both %Rec and %Det may be considered to be indicative of the regularity of the signal over the time, L_{max} is inversely related to the Lyapunov exponent and gives a measure of the sensibility of the system to the initial conditions in the case of a chaotic deterministic system while, generally considering, it is a measure of system divergence for a system subjected to transients and singularities, as it is as example the case of a system relaxing Lipschitz conditions. We expected to find substantial differences for the values of %Rec, of %Det and of L_{max} variables for R-R intervals and for SBP in spontaneous respect to controlled respiration. The results are reported in Figure 8.

and, as seen, no substantial differences were found in the mean values of the variables in the two conditions of experimentation as well as no results of significant difference were obtained by using two-way analysis of variance. The important result, however, is that for R-R intervals a very large standard deviation was calculated for %Rec and %Det in controlled versus spontaneous respiration (see Figure 8 for the details).

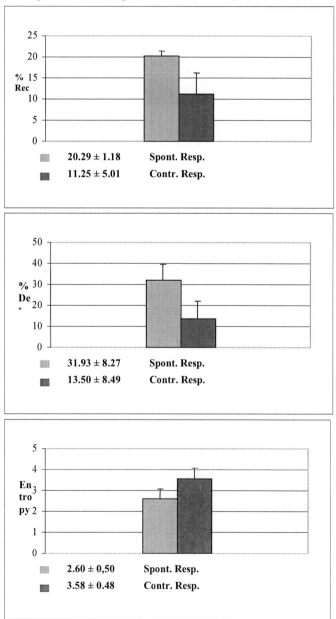

Figure 7. Cross Recurrence Quantification Analysis: Mean Values and Standard Deviation of %REC, %DET and Entropy During R-R: SBP non linear interaction.

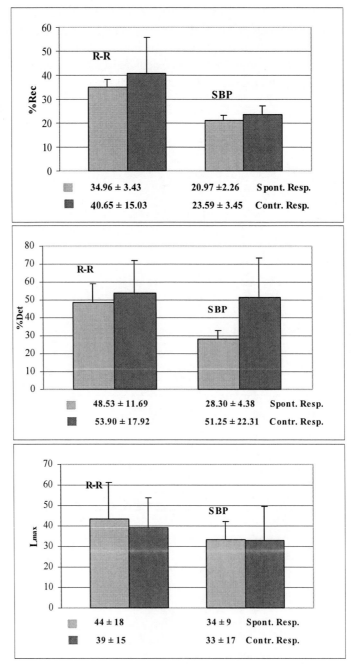

Figure 8. Recurrence Quantification Analysis: Mean Values and Standard Deviation of %REC, %DET and Max Line.

Since we ascertained by the previous analysis (C_γ and KRQA analysis, respectively) that we had a fall in non linear coupling strength as well as in dynamical modalities (synchronization) of non linear R-R:SBP interaction during controlled respect to spontaneous breathing, it had a sense to examine the results obtained by RQA analysis for each subject comparing RQA results of controlled respiration with those obtained by spectral and cross spectral analysis. Table 1 gives the results of our spectral analysis in frequency-domain. We give the values of power expressed in ms^2 and mmHg^2 for R-R and SBP respectively.

Table 1. Frequency domain results analysis. Power values of heart period (R-R) and systolic blood pressure (SBP) in low (LF) and high (SF) frequency range in six subjects during spontaneous and controlled respiration

Subjects	Spontaneous Respiration				Controlled Respiration			
	R-R		SBP		R-R		SBP	
	LF (power ms^2) (0.10 Hz)	HF (power ms^2) (0.25 Hz)	LF (power mmHg^2) (0.10 Hz)	HF (power mmHg^2) (0.25 Hz)	LF (power ms^2) (0.10 Hz)	HF (power ms^2) (0.20 Hz)	LF (power mmHg^2) (0.10 Hz)	HF (power mmHg^2) (0.20 Hz)
n. 1	751	82	2.03	5.37	1309	397	15.40	15.34
n. 2	377	14	2.86	1.70	631	57	1.85	0.59
n. 4	775	103	2.94	6.00	509	383	0.98	2.39
n. 5	381	653	1.92	3.64	363	27	5.87	0.73
n. 7	419	398	1.58	1.34	621	300	2.68	1.51
n. 11	296	112	2.30	1.60	402	183	3.20	2.15

Table 2 gives results of our cross-spectral analysis, and we express the considered values for frequency, coherence and phase shift in degree. The calculated values of α-BRS, the index of baroreflex sensitivity, were also obtained by square rooted ratio of R-R and SBP powers at the given frequency of 0.1 Hz. In table 6 the results may be compared with those of RQA analysis for %Rec. and %Det. as they were obtained for each subject. It is seen that for subjects n. 1, 7, and 11 increasing values of %Rec and %Det in condition of controlled respect to spontaneous breathing, corresponded to increasing values of the powers calculated for LF at 0.1 Hertz. In such cases we also observed maintenance of the LF value peaked at 0.1 Hz during spontaneous as well as controlled respiration. This result suggests that such frequency value was preserved in the two conditions of experimentation during the linear action of baroflex control mechanism on heart rate. The increasing values of %Rec. and %Det just confirmed that the non linear mechanism of control slowed down during R-R:SBP interaction in condition of controlled respect to spontaneous respiration with greater support of the linear R-R:SBP interaction leading the system to a more deterministic and periodic behavior. It is important to outline also that we had increasing values of the coherence in condition of controlled respect to spontaneous respiration as well also the phase shift remained constant at 0.1 Hz around the value of about -90 degrees. The negative phase shift in LF indicates that R-R oscillations lag behind SBP oscillations with a delay of about 1 beat for heart.

The conclusion is thus that in such cases, under controlled respiration, we had an R-R:SBP interaction that is quite mutilated in its non linear component with consequent enhancement of the linear component of the interaction leading the system to a more periodic and deterministic behavior. In subject n.2 we had rather similar behavior but with some important modifications. With respect to R-R we had again increased determinism in condition of controlled respiration but periodicity tended to remain the same in the two conditions of experimentation. In spectral analysis the peak at 0.1 Hz remained unchanged. Instead in SBP we had again increased periodicity and determinism of the oscillations in controlled respect to spontaneous respiration but the basic features of the interaction changed in the sense that the peak of LF changed respect to the value of 0.1 Hz of about 20%.

Table 2. Example of spectral and cross-spectral analysis in spontaneous respiration of a subject

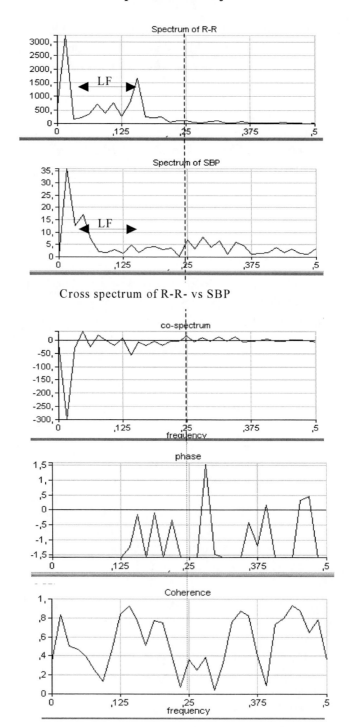

Table 2. Results of spectral and cross-spectral analysis (Continued)

Subject	1	2	4	5	7	11
Spont. Resp.						
HF (0.25 Hz)						
Coherence	0.174	0.117	0.362	0.706	0.204	0.410
Phase	*	*	*	*	*	*
LF (0.1 Hz)						
Coherence	0.009	0.015	0.448	0.213	0.019	0.527
Phase	*	*	*	*	*	*
α-BRS	19.20	11.48	16.20	14.00	16.28	11.30
Contr. Resp.						
HF (0.20 Hz)						
Coherence	0.922	0.252	0.190	0.242	0.851	0.780
Phase	-90°	76.9°	8.1°	-51.8°	-90°	-90°
LF (0.1 Hz)						
Coherence	0.964	0.309	0.985	0.009	0.856	0.817
Phase	-90°	48.2°	32.5°	-58°	-90°	-90°
α-BRS	9.20	18.46	22.70	7.86	15.32	11.20

(*) rather constant value of – 90°.

This is to say that the system was forced to rearrange itself about new values of frequency in LF.

The same thing happened for subject n.4 for R-R and for SBP. A rearrangement of the values for frequencies happened for subject n.5 and this time the R-R:SBP interaction determining also a reduction of periodicity and determinism but only for R-R .in order to reach its periodicity and determinism. As it may be seen from Table 2 the values of coherence resulted largely increased in subjects n.1, 7, 11 with a constant value of phase shift while instead coherence and phase shifts resulted profoundly and differently modified when a rearrangement of frequencies happened. Still, the values of baroreflex sensitivity decreased in subjects n.1, 7, and 11 in condition of controlled respect to spontaneous respiration, while instead they assumed the tendency to increase (subjects n.2, and 4) or still to decrease (subject n.5) when the mechanism of the R-R:SBP interaction was subjected to a rearrangement of its frequencies in LF band.

In conclusion, in such cases, provided that the non linear R-R:SBP interaction slowed down owing to the imposed condition of controlled respiration, the system followed the way to rearrange itself about a new dynamics selecting new possible peaked values of frequencies and phases for its basic oscillations and reorganizing itself about new values of determinism and periodicity.

In this manner, we have arrived on one hand to clear the essential role of the non linear component of R-R:SBP interaction evidencing that, through its slow down, the system may run about the values of periodicity and determinism that do not pertain to it naturally (that is, in condition of spontaneous respiration) or, instead, the system may attempt also to rearrange and to reorganize itself about new patterns. In brief, the cardiovascular system configures itself as a kind of adaptive system able to modify its characteristics and its control mechanisms by a fine tuning in order to respond to the conditions imposed from the outside. It delineates itself as a large chain of oscillators that become self-organizing owing to the presence of singularities having in relaxation of Lipschitz condition the mathematical counterpart.

As it was outlined in a previous paper (Giuliani et al., 1996) by a study conducted on anesthetized rats, the emerging picture of autonomic control seems to be that one of constraining the probabilistic fluctuations of the R-R intervals around the last achieved state. The control does not try to level the system to the most probable, ground state. It, instead, functions as a fine tuning constraining the size of the oscillations.

We have interpreted the results of the present paper accounting obviously for the central role of respiration in the cardiovascular system. One way, in fact, has been to consider the relevant role of the respiratory oscillation in blood pressure that may be ascribed to the cyclic variation in intrathoracic pressure with breathing perturbing mechanically venous return, cardiac output, and thus blood pressure.

In this condition it is currently accepted that such changes are detected by baroreceptors that cause changes in autonomic activity to the heart and thus fine tuning changes in heart rate. Another confirmation of this paper is that heart rate does not inherently contain a respiratory related oscillation without it being also present in blood pressure, suggesting it as a function of the baroreflex.

We may sketch a brief model to this regard. Baroreceptor activity B_a is marked mainly by the presence of noise.

We have effects of baroreflex activity to the instantaneous value of phase of respiration φ but baroreflex activity determines the efferent sympathetic activity B_{as} and vagal or parasympathetic activity B_{ap} by the fine tuning acted by the respiratory influence R_i that is depending from B_a through its dependence from the instantaneous value of the phase of respiration φ. We may express roughly φ -B_a dependence in the following manner

$$\frac{d\varphi}{dt} = v_{resp.} - k_{coupling}(B_a - B_{threshold})$$

where $1/v_{resp}$ is the constant period of respiration. R-R results quite non linearly decoupled to SBP during controlled respiration since, during controlled respiration, the phase φ ceases to depend directly from B_a, $k_{coupling} \rightarrow 0$. Of course, this equation could enter in the general model that we (Conte et al., 2003) discussed recently as possible biological mechanism of control and exhibiting non-deterministic chaotic behavior.

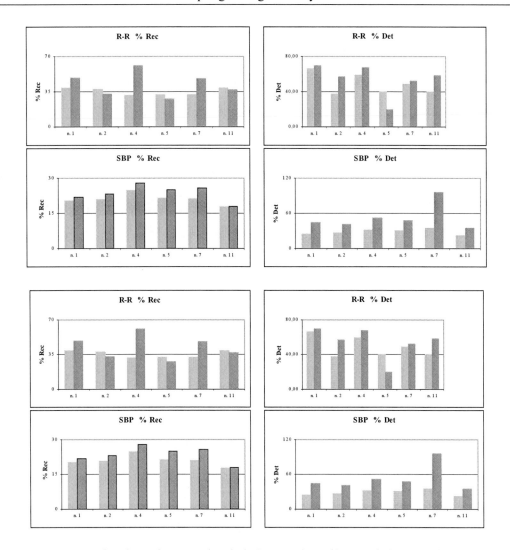

Figure 9. Frequency-domain results: spactral analysis. Power values of heart period (R-R) and systolic blood pressure (SBP) in low (LF) and high (HF) frequency range in six subjects during spontaneous ( ) and controlled ( ) respiration.

Acknowledgments

This research was supported by TIRES and University of Bari grants (Fondi di Ateneo 2003).

References

Akselrod S., Gordon D., Ubel F.A., Shannon D.C., Barger A.C., Cohen R.J., (1981) Power Spectrum Analysis of Heart Rate Fluctuations: a Quantitative Probe of Beat-to Beat Cardiovascular Control, *Science*, 213, 220-222, and references therein.

Baselli G., Cerutti S., Porta A., Signorini M.G., (2002) Short and Long Term non Linear Analysis of RR variability Series, *Medical Engineering and Physics*.24, 21-32.

Censi F., Calcagnini G., Cerutti S., (2002) Coupling Patterns between Spontaneous Rhythms and Respiration in Cardiovascular Variability Signals, *Computer Methods and Programs in Biomedicine*, 68, 32-47.

Conte E, , Federici A. , Zbilut J.P. , (2003) On a Simple Case of Possible non-Deterministic Chaotic Behavior in Compartment Theory of Biological Observables, *Chaos ,Solitons and Fractals,*22, 277-284.

Eckmann J.P., Kamphorst S.O., Ruelle D., (1987) Recurrence Plot of Dynamical Systems, *Europhys. Letters*, 4, 973-977.

Fraser A. M., Swinney H.L., (1986) Independent Coordinates for Strange Attractors from Mutual Information, *Phys. Rev.* A33, 1134-1141.

Giuliani A., Lo Giudice P., Mancini A.M., Quatrini G., Pacifici L., Webber C.L., Zbilut J.P, (1996) A Markovian Formalization of Heart Dynamics Evinces a Quantum-Like Hypothesis, *Biolog. Cybern.*74, 181-187.

Grassberger P., ProcacciaI., (1993) Estimation of Kolmogorov Entropy from a Chaotic Signal, *Phys. Review A*, 28, 2591-2593.

Guyton A.C., Harris J.W.,(1951) Pressoreceptor-Autonomic Oscillation: a Probable Cause of Wavemotor Waves, *Am. J. Physiol.* 165,158-166.

Hales S. (1733) *Statistical Essays: containing haemastatics; or an account of some hydraulik and hydrosstatical experiemnts made on the blood and blood-vessels of animals*, Innys W., Manby R., Woodward T., London, United Kingdom.

Von Haller A., (1788) *De partium corporis humani praecipuarum fabrica et functionibus,*Bern, Prelis Societarum Typographicarum.

Hoyer D., Bauner R., Walter B., U. Zwiener, Estimation of Nonlinear Couplings on the Basis of Complexity and Predictability – A New Method Applied to Cardiorespiratory Coordination,IEEE Transactions on Biomedical Engineering, 45,545-552,1998.

Ludwig C.,(1847) Beitrage zur kennuthiss des einflusses der respirations be wgungen auf den blutlauf im aortensysteme, Muller's Arch. Anat. *Physiol. Med.* 242-302.

Mayer S., (1877) Studien zur Physiologie des Herzens und der Blutgefasse uber Spontane Blutdruschwankungth, Sitzungsberichte Kaiserlich Akad Wissenschaft *Mathemat-Natwrwissenschaften Classe*74, 281-307.

Porta A., Baselli G., Montano N., Gnecchi-Ruscone T., Lombardi F., Malliani A., Cerutti S., (1996) Classification of Coupling Patterns among Spontaneous Rhythms and Ventilation in the Sympathetic Discharge of Decerebrated Cats, *Biol. Cybern.* 75, 163-172.

Shockley K., Butwill M., Zbilut J.P., Webber C.L., (2002) Cross Recurrence Quantification of Coupled Oscillators, *Physics Letters A*, 305, 59-69.

Suder K. Drepper F.M.R. , Schiek M. , Abel H. H. , (1998) One-dimensional , non Linear Determinism Characterizes Heart Rate Patterns during Paced Respiration , *Am. J. Physiol.* 275, H1092-H1102

Tackens F., (1980*) Detecting Strange Attractors in Turbulence, in Dynamical Systems in Turbulence*, D. Rand and L.S. Young Eds. Springer Verlag, 366-381.

Webber C.L., Zbilut J.P., (1994) Dynamical Assessment of Physiological Systems and States Using Recurrence Plot Strategies, *J. Appl. Physiol.*76, 965-973.

Wilders R., Jongsma H.J., (1993) Beating Irregularity of Single Pacemaker Cells Isolated from the Rabbit Sinotrial Node, *Biophysical Journal*, 65, 2601-2613.

Zak M., (1997) Dynamical Simulation of Probabilities, *Chaos, Solitons and Fractals*, 8, 793-804 and references therein.

Zbilut J.P, Gottfried G., Geist K., (1988) Dimensional Analysis of Heart Rate Variability in Heart Transplant Recipients, *Math. Biosciences*, 90, 49-70.

Zbilut J.P., Webber C.L., Zak M., (1986) *Quantification of Heart Rate Variability Using Methods Derived from Non Linear Analysis, Assessment and Analysis of Cardiovascular Function*, New York, Springer Verlag 114-122, (Editors G. Drzewiecki, JK-I Li);

Zbilut J.P, Zak M., Webber C.L., (1995) Physiological Singularities in Respiratory and Cardiac Dynamics, *Chaos, Solitons and Fractals*, 5, 1509-1516, and references therein.

Zbilut J.P, Huber A., Webber C.L., (1996) *Physiological Singularities Modeled by Non deterministic Equations of Motion and the Effect of Noise, Fluctuations and Order, The New Synthesis*, New York, Springer Verlag, 397-417, (editor M. Millonas).

Zbilut J.P, Zinghong H., Giuliani A., Webber C.L., (2000) *Singularities of Heart Beat as Demonstrated by RQA*, Proceedings of the World Congress of Medical Physics, Chicago

Zbilut J.P., Thomasson N., Webber C.L., (2002) Recurrence Quantification Analysis as a Tool for nonlinear Exploration of Nonstationary Cardiac Signals, *Med. Engineering and Physics*, 24, 53-60.

In: Systolic Blood Pressure
Editor: Robert A. Arfi

ISBN: 978-1-61209-263-8
©2012 Nova Science Publishers, Inc.

Chapter X

Angiotensin-Converting Enzyme Inhibitors in Coronary Artery Disease and Preserved Left Ventricular Systolic Function[*]

Fadi Alqaisi and Mouaz H. Al-Mallah[†]
Henry Ford Heart and Vascular Institute, Detroit, MI, US

Abstract

Angiotensin converting enzyme inhibitors (ACEI) have been shown to be beneficial in patients with hypertension, recent myocardial infarction (MI), patients undergoing percutaneous coronary intervention (PCI) and/or left ventricular (LV) dysfunction. However, the evidence for routine administration of ACEI has been conflicting in patients with coronary artery disease (CAD) with preserved LV systolic function.In this chapter, we will review the potential anti-atherosclerotic mechanisms of ACEI.In addition, we will summarize the randomized clinical trials supporting the potential benefitsof ACEI in patient with CAD and preserved LV function. The potential differences in the study design, patient population, individual ACEI pharmacokinetic and pharmacodynamic characteristics and therapeutic blood pressure differences between the trials will be addressed. In addition, we will also present an updated meta-analysis of the above trials.In summary, we believe that the current evidence supports that routine treatment with ACEIin patients with CAD who have preserved LV function.

---

[*] A version of this chapter also appears in *Angiotensin Converting Enzyme Inhibitors*, edited by Anne N. DeBrue, published by Nova Science Publishers, Inc. It was submitted for appropriate modifications in an effort to encourage wider dissemination of research.

[†] Send Correspondence to:Mouaz Al-Mallah, MD, Henry Ford Heart and Vascular Institute2799 West Grand Blvd., K 14, Detroit, MI48202, Tel: 313 916 2721, Fax: 313 916 4531, Email: malmall1@hfhs.org.

Abbreviations

ACEI	Angiotensin converting enzyme inhibitors
echo	echocardiography
MPI	myocardial perfusion imaging
LV	left ventricle
CHF	congestive heart failure
EF	ejection fraction
CP	Chest pain;
MI	myocardial infarction
SE	Stress echocardiography
CVA	cerebrovascular accident
CV	cardiovascular
IMAGINE	Ischemia, Management with Accupril post-bypass Graft via Inhibition of the converting Enzyme
PCI	percutaneous intervention
QCA	Quantitative Coronary Angiography
CABG	coronary artery bypass surgery
SCATT	The Simvastatin/Enalapril Coronary Atherosclerosis Trial
SD	Standard deviation; SBP: systolic blood pressure
DBP	Diastolic blood pressure
NA	Not available

*Median Follow-Up

† CAD equivalent patients had stroke, peripheral vascular disease, or diabetes plus at leastone other cardiovascular risk factor (hypertension, elevatedtotal cholesterol levels, low high-density lipoprotein cholesterollevels, cigarette smoking, or documented microalbuminuria)

‡ At 4 years

§ 68% had CAD

Since the early 1980's, the incidence of coronary artery disease (CAD) in the united states has been decreasing mostly because of a reduction in cigarette smoking and low-density lipoprotein (LDL) cholesterol levels. According the American heart association statistics, the decrease in the incidence of CAD is not paralleled by a decrease in the mortality rate in patients with CAD despite the fact that most patients with CAD have normal left (LV) ventricular function.[1] Multiple therapies have been tested to assess their impact on survival in patients with CAD. In this chapter, we will review the effect of Angiotensin converting enzyme inhibitors (ACEI) in patients with CAD and preserved LV function.

Potential Mechanisms of ACEI Beneficial Activity in Patients with CAD

The role of ACE in the development of CAD is not well identified. Although ACE may be isolated from plasma, it primarily exists within tissues located on the endothelium of all blood vessels as well as in the parenchyma of the heart, kidneys, brain, and adrenal glands[2]. Substantial experimental evidence has established that injury to the heart results in a marked ACE induction. This was demonstrated in pressure overloaded, hypertrophied hearts, in volume overloaded hearts, myocardial infraction, and heart failure.[3-8]ACE is also linked to the development of cardiac hypertrophy where it has been shown to enhance protein synthesis independent of load in both the intact heart and in the isolated myocyte[9]. In addition, locally produced Angiotensin II (AII) is among the most important substances that may affect endothelial function. In healthy individuals, AII maintains a balance between vasoconstrictors and vasodilators that results in minimal vasomotor tone. Endothelial ACE, however, may be unregulated in response to injury (e.g., hypercholesterolemia, smoking, hypertension, aging, diabetes), thus mediating the formation of excess local AII. AII adversely affects the redox state of the endothelium and consequently, by increasing the activity of reduced nicotinamide-adenine dinucleotide-dependent oxidase, produces superoxide anion and hydrogen peroxide that can inactivate NO.[10] Oxidative stress also activates the transcription of factor NF-κB that induces the expression of genes controlling cytokine formation and leukocyte adhesion to the vessel wall. [11,12] In addition, ACE degrades and inactivates bradykinin, a vasoactive peptide that promotes the generation of nitric oxide (NO) and other endothelial derived vasodilators. [13,14] NO also inhibits vascular smooth muscle cell VSMC growth and migration, and the expression of pro-inflammatory molecules, such as vascular cell adhesion molecule-1 and monocyte chemoattractant protein-1 [13,14]; therefore, reductions in NO result in not only vasoconstriction, but also an increased propensity for inflammation. AII also stimulates the production of endothelin-1 (a very potent vasoconstrictor) and plasminogen activator inhibitor-1 (PAI-1). [15]

Bradykinin can stimulate the synthesis of plasminogen activator. Thus, by synthesizing AII and degrading bradykinin, ACE regulates vascular fibrinolytic balance in favor of thrombosis. Reductions in AII and increases in bradykinin may contribute to the vasculoprotective effects of ACEI by way of tilting the vascular fibrinolytic balance in favor of fibrinolysis [16].

Clinical Uses of ACEIin Cardiovascular Diseases

All the above potential injuries suggested by ACE made it reasonable to use ACEI and AII receptor blocker in coronary artery disease and left ventricular dysfunction. ACEI have been shown to be beneficial in patients with hypertension, recent myocardial infarction (MI), patients undergoing percutaneous coronary intervention (PCI) and/or left ventricular (LV) dysfunction. [17-29].There are multiple mechanisms that couldexplain the benefit of ACEIpost MI includingnumber of modalities may be beneficial in the management of the patient with acute myocardial infarction (MI), including reduction in ventricular remodeling and infarct size, interference with ischemic preconditioning, improvement in the oxygen supply/demand ratio of the myocardium by reversing angiotensin II-induced vasoconstriction and inotropic activity,improvement in endothelial, improvement in the hypercoagulable state after an MI by reducing plasma plasminogen activator inhibitor-1 (PAI-1, inhibition of the activation and accumulation of macrophages and monocytes by diminishing the levels of monocyte chemoattractant protein-1 and potentially reducing exercise-induced ischemia[30,31].Similar mechanisms may be beneficial in patients with ischemic or non ischemic cardiomyopathy,

Thus, the current AmericanCollege of Cardiology and American HeartAssociation guidelines for the management of ST segment elevation myocardial infarction recommend that an ACEI should be prescribed at discharge to all patients with ST segment elevation myocardial infarction (Class I). [32].

On the other hand, Post hoc analyses of patients from the Studies of Left Ventricular Dysfunction (SOLVD) [27]and the and the Survival and Ventricular Enlargement (SAVE) [26] trials showed a reduction in the rate of acute MI in patients who were treated with ACE-I.

However, the routine administration of ACEI in patients with CAD and preserved LV systolic function remains controversial. Multiple trials have addressed this question and are discussed below. These trials are summarized in table 1.

Randomized Clinical Trials Examining the Use of ACEI in Patients with CAD and Preserved LV Systolic Function

Heart Outcomes Prevention Evaluation Study (Hope)

The HOPE trial [33,34] was the first trial to address this Question. The trial randomized 9297 high risk patientswith normalLV ejection fraction (LVEF) and followed them up between 1994 and 2000.

The mean age was 66 ± 7 years and 80.4% had CAD, defined as previous myocardial infarction (MI), previous revascularization or history of chronic stable angina. Only 46.8% had hypertension and 38.5% had DM, At the end of the five year follow up, 14% in the Ramipril group died of cardiovascular causes or had a myocardial infarction or stroke, as compared to 17.8% in the placebo group (relative risk, 0.78; 95% confidence interval, 0.70 to 0.86; P<0.001) (figure 1).

The benefit was consistent in a subgroup analysis that included only patients with CAD. Ramipril also decreased rates of revascularization, cardiac arrest, worsening angina, heart failure and new diagnosis of DM. If is important to note that the effect of Ramipril on systemic blood pressure was modest in this study. At baseline, both groups had BP of 139/79. At the end of the study, the Ramipril group BP was 136/76 as compared to 139/77 in the placebo group.

The benefit in outcome seen between the two groups can be partially attributed to the reduction in blood pressure, but protective effects against atherosclerosis may have contributed to the benefit. Based on number to treat analysis, treating 1000 patients with Ramipril for four years might prevent about 150 events in approximately 70 patients.

Table 1. Characteristics of the Trial Evaluating the Effects of ACEI in patients with CAD and Normal LV Function (adapted with Permission from (43))

	HOPE(33)	EUROPA (39)	PEACE (41)	QUIET (36)	PART-2 (35)	CAMELOT (40)	IMAGINE (42)
Enrollment Period	12/93 – 7/95	10/97 – 6/00	11/96 - 6/00	91 - 96		4/99 – 3/04	11/1999- 9/2004
Publication Year	2000	2003	2004	2001	2000	2004	2008
Enrolling Sites	US, Europe, South America, Mexico	Europe	US, Canada,Italy	US, Canada,Europe	New Zeeland	US, Canada,Europe	Canada,Belgium,France, Netherland
ACEI	Ramipril	Perindopril	Trandolapril	Quinapril	Ramipril	Enalapril	Quinapril
Preserved LV definition	EF>40% or clinical absence of CHF	Clinical absence of CHF	Echo, MPI preserved EF>40%	Angiography, Echo EF>40%	Absence of Clinical CHF	EF>40%	EF>40%
CAD definition	Documented CAD or "CAD equivalent " †	Angiography, SE (in men with CP)	MI, Angiography	Angiography	MI, SE, CVA§	Angiography	Post CABG patients
Primary Endpoint	CV death, MI, Stroke	CV death, MI, Cardiac arrest	CV death, MI, Revascularization	CV death, CV arrest, non fatal MI, Revascularization or hospitalization	Carotid Intimal Thickening	CV death, CV arrest, non fatal MI, Revascularization, CVA, PVOD or CV hospitalization	CV death, CV arrest, non fatal MI, Revascularization, UA ± hospitalization, CVA, stroke or CHF hospitalization
Sample Size	9297	12218	8290	1750	617	1997	2553
Mean Follow Up (yr)	4.5	4.2	4.8 yr *	2	4	2	4
Age (year ± SD)	66 ± 7	60 ± 9	64 ± 8	58	61	58	61
Females (%)	25	15	18	18	18	28	13
Prior MI (%)	53	65	55	49	42 §	39	39
Prior PCI (%)	18	29	42	100	NA	29	18
Prior CABG (%)	26	29	39	NA	NA	7	3
Hyper-tension (%)	47	27	46	47	Excluded	60	47
Diabetes (%)	38	12	17	16	8	18	10

Table 1. (Continued)

	HOPE(33)	EUROPA (39)	PEACE (41)	QUIET (36)	PART-2 (35)	CAMELOT (40)	IMAGINE (42)
Anti platelets (%)	76	92	90	73	81	95	95
Beta Blockers (%)	40	62	60	26	43	77	63
Lipid Lowering Therapy (%)	29	58	70	0.1	29	83	85
Beta Blockers (%)	40	62	60	26	43	77	79
Calcium Channel blockers (%)	47	31	36	0	25	9	37
Diuretics (%)	15	9	13	NA	NA	30	NA
SBP/DBP lowering (mm Hg)	3/2	5/2	3/1	NA	6/4	5/2	4/2
% On Study Drug at 3 years	71	81	75	76	74% ‡	Unknown	81

(PART-2) Trial: Randomized, Placebo-Controlled Trial of the Angiotensin-Converting Enzyme Inhibitor, Ramipril, in Patients with Coronary or Other Occlusive Arterial Disease

In the same year of 2000, the PART-2 trial[35] challenged the concept of protective effects of ACEI against atherosclerosis. This trial evaluated the effect of daily 5-10mg of Ramipril on carotid sclerosis, as assessed by B-modeUS recordings, and LVH, as assessed by M-mode echocardiogram. A total of 617 patients with previous MI, angina with documented CAD, transient ischemic attacks, or intermittent claudication were randomized to Ramipril or placebo and were followed between 1994 and 1999. All patients did not have clinical congestive heart failure or hypertension. At baseline, both groups had BP of 133/79. At the end of the study, the Ramipril group BP was 127/74 as compared to 132/78 in the placebo group. And so, there was 6/4 reduction in the BP (both p<0.0001). Despite a significant reduction in blood pressure (more than the HOPE trial), there were no significant differences in the change in common carotid far wall thickness or carotid plaque score from baseline to follow up. At the end of follow up, there was a significant reduction in the LV mass index in the Ramipril group and a small, yet significant, increase in LV end diastolic dimension in the placebo group. Although this study was not powered to look at clinical outcomes, it is important to note that there was a non significant trend towards improved survival on Ramipril (7.1% in the Ramipril group died of cardiovascular causes or had a myocardial infarction, as compared to 10.7% in the placebo group; relative risk, 0.66; 95% confidence interval, 0.39 to 1.14).

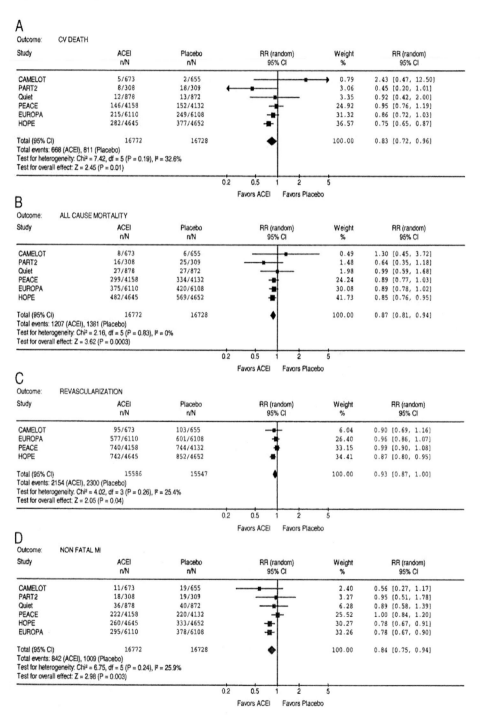

Figure 1. Kaplan–Meier Estimates of the Composite Outcome of Myocardial Infarction, Stroke, or Death from Cardiovascular Causes in the Ramipril Group and the Placebo Group in the HOPE trial.[33] The relative risk of the composite outcome in the ramipril group as compared with the placebo group was 0.78 (95 percent confidence interval, 0.70 to 0.86).(adapted with permission from [33]).

This trial showed that there was no significant protective effect of ACE-I on atherosclerosis. This trial that reduced BP and LV mass among patients treated with ACE-I may be more relevant that initially thought. The authors acknowledged that the trial with 617 patients, as compared to 9297 patients in the HOPE trial, was underpowered to detect significant differences in the clinical outcomes between the two groups, though trends of favorable outcome in the Ramipril group were evident. This trial also emphasized the ongoing discussion about the use of surrogate endpoint versus clinical outcomes as endpoints.

The Quinapril Ischemic Event Trial (QUIET)

One year later, in 2001, the QUIET trial(36) studied the effect of daily 20mg of quinapril on ischemic events (cardiac death, resuscitated cardiac arrest, nonfatal MI, coronary artery bypass graft surgery, coronary angioplasty, or hospitalization for angina pectoris) in 1750 patients who had undergone successful coronary angioplasty or atherectomy at baseline and had at least 1 coronary artery that had not been subjected to mechanical revascularization. All patients had a documented LV ejection fraction of $\geq$40%. Patients were followed for a total of three years for incident ischemic events. At the end of followup duration, 37.7% in the quinapril group had an ischemic event as compared to 38.5% in the placebo group; (relative risk, 1.04; 95% confidence interval, 0.89 to 1.22; P=0.6). In addition, there was no significant difference in any of the individual events between the two groups. In a sub-study [37] evaluating the progression of atherosclerosis in coronary arteries as assessed by coronary angiography, there was no difference between the active therapy and placebo. This trial showed that quinapril had no beneficial effect on ischemic events. Multiple limitations could have resulted in such results including sample size (1750 patients as compared to 9297 patients in the HOPE trial) and short duration of follow up (3 years as compared to 4.5 years in the HOPE trail) as well as low dose of quinapril (20 mg as compared to 40 mg in the TREND trial [38] which showed improvement of coronary artery endothelial reactivity with quinapril).

European Trial on Reduction of Cardiac Events with Perindopril in Stable Coronary Artery (EUROPA Trial)

This landmark trial was published in 2003. The EUROPA trial [39] evaluated the beneficial effect of daily 4-8 mg ofPerindopril on clinical outcomes of cardiovascular death, MI and cardiac arrest in 12218 Patients with evidence of CAD and no previous CHF were followed up between 1997 and 2000. In contrast to the HOPE study, all patients had CAD, defined as previous MI, previous revascularization or angiographic evidence of $\geq$70% narrowing of one or more major coronary arteries. At the end of the follow-up duration, 18% of the patient in the Perindopril group died of cardiovascular causes or had a MI or cardiac arrest, as compared to 9.9% in the placebo group(relative risk, 0.80; 95% confidence interval, 0.71 to 0.91; P<0.001). Perindopril also significantly reduced hospital admissions for heart failure (1% vs. 1.7%; relative risk, 0.61; 95% confidence interval, 0.44 to 0.83; P=0.002). Although the relative risk reduction in the EUROPA trial (0.8) was similar to the HOPE trial

(0.78), treating 50 patients with perindopril for four years would prevent one major cardiovascular event. The rate of cardiac events in the HOPE trial was higher. This is despite the fact that patients enrolled in the EUROPA lower risk patients in the trial. Patients in the HOPE trial were older, more females, more hypertensive and diabetic and used less antiplatelets, BB and lipid lowering agents. The reduction of BP achieved in the Perindopril group (mean of 5/2) by the end of the study couldn't explain the treatment effect since the outcome benefits exceeded what is expected from this BP reduction. And so, the antiatherosclerotic effects of ACE-I could not be neglected.

Effect of Antihypertensive Agents on Cardiovascular Events in Patients with Coronary Disease and Normal Blood Pressure Study: (CAMELOT) Study

The CAMELOT study [40] compared the effects of 10-20 mg of Enalapril, 5-10 mg of Amlodipine and placebo on cardiovascular events (cardiovascular death, nonfatal myocardial infarction, resuscitated cardiac arrest, coronary revascularization, hospitalization for angina pectoris, hospitalization for congestive heart failure, fatal or nonfatal stroke or transient ischemic attack (TIA), and any new diagnosis of peripheral vascular disease)in patients with CAD, controlled BP (with or without antihypertensive medications) and no CHF. A total of 1991 patients were followed between 1999 and 2004. The study population was similar to patients in other trials although all of them had angiographic evidence of coronary atherosclerosis. At the conclusion of follow-up, 20.2% in the Enalapril group had an event, as compared to 23.1% in the placebo group; (relative risk, 0.85; 95% confidence interval, 0.67 to 1.07; P=.16) Individual components of the primary end point and secondary end points generally showed fewer events with Enalapril treatment, but none of the comparisons reached statistical significance, though, in this trial, Enalapril decreased BP significantly by 4.9/2.9 mmHg (p<0.11 vs. placebo).

In a sub study of the CAMELOT study, 274 patients (13.8%) underwent evaluation of the antiatherosclerotic effects of the study medications using intravascular ultrasound. Both, Enalapril and Amlodipine showed statistically insignificant trends of favorable antiatherosclerotic effect on coronary arteriesas assessed by IVUS. Although this trial was not powered to assess event reduction by ACEI, it provided an in-vivo evidence that ACEI could result in a reduction in the atherosclerotic burden assessed invasively.

Angiotensin-Converting-Enzyme Inhibition in Stable Coronary Artery Disease. The PEACE Trial

The goal of the Prevention of Events with Angiotensin Converting Enzyme Inhibition (PEACE) Trial[41] was to test whether ACE-inhibitor therapy, when added to modern conventional therapy, would reduce the rate of nonfatal myocardial infarction, death from cardiovascular causes, or revascularization in low-risk patients with stable coronary artery disease and normal or slightly reduced left ventricular function. The study enrolled 8290 patients with CAD (defined as previous myocardial infarction, previous revascularization or angiographic evidence of ≥50% narrowing of one or more major coronary arteries) and normal left ventricular ejection fraction (LVEF) who were followed between 1996 and 2003. This cohort had a lower risk compared to the HOPE and EUROPA trials and was more evidence based therapies for CAD including beta blockers, aspirin and lipid-lowering agents.At the end of the follow-up duration, 21.9% in the trandolapril group died of cardiovascular causes or had a myocardial infarction or coronary revascularization, as compared to 21.9% in the placebo group; relative risk, 0.96; 95% confidence interval, 0.88 to 1.06; P=0.43. Individual components of the primary or secondary endpoints were similar in both groups. Subgroup analysis did not show benefit in terms of primary end point in any of the subgroups. In this trial, trandolapril lowered the BP significantly by 4.4/3.6mmHg which could have impacted the primary endpoint.

Ischemia Management with Accupril Post Bypass Graft via Inhibition of Angiotensin Converting Enzyme (IMAGINE) Trial

Recently, the IMAGINE trial[42] which was a double-blind, placebo-controlled study of 2553 post bypass patients who were randomly assigned to quinapril, target dose 40 mg/d, or placebo, who were followed up to a maximum of 43 months. These patients were relatively at low risk of cardiovascular events given the recent revascularization.

Although in this trial, quinapril lowered the BP significantly by 3.9/2.1mmHg, 13.7% in the quinapril group had a new ischemic event, as compared to 13.7% in the placebo group; relative risk, 1.15; 95% confidence interval, 0.92 to 1.42; P=0.212.

Individual components of the primary or secondary endpoints were similar in both groups. What was new in this study is that the incidence of adverse events, particularly early after CABG was increased on the ACEI group. This study suggests that early after CABG, initiation of angiotensin-converting enzyme inhibitor therapy should be individualized and continually reassessed over time according to risk.

Meta Analysis of the Effects of ACEI in Patients with Normal LV Function and CAD

We performed a Meta analysis [43] to assess the effect of ACEI in patients with normal LV function and CAD.In the pooled analysis, ACEI therapy resulted in a mean of 3.9 mmHg drop in the systolic blood pressure and 1.8mmHg drop in the diastolic blood pressure. Patients enrolled in the HOPE and EUROPA trails had a more significant drop in systolic (4.1 mmHg vs. 3.5 mmHg) and diastolic (2.0 mmHg vs. 1.4 mmHg) blood pressure which may explain part of the therapeutic benefits. Figure 2 shows that pooled effect of ACEI therapy on outcomes. ACEI therapy was associated with a decrease in cardiovascular mortality (RR 0.83, 95% CI 0.72 – 0.96, p=0.01), non-fatal MI (RR 0.84, 95% CI 0.75 – 0.94, p=0.003), all cause mortality (RR 0.87, 95% CI 0.81 – 0.94, p=0.0003) and revascularization rates (RR 0.93, 95% CI 0.87 – 1.00, p=0.04). The number needed to treat with ACEI to prevent either of the adverse outcomes (one cardiovascular death or any death, or non-fatal MI, or revascularization) is 100. There were no differences in the effect among the studies as evident by I^2 estimates for different outcomes. In addition, we did not detect any evidence of publication bias.

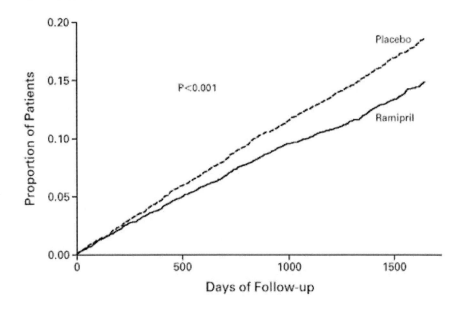

Figure 2. Pooled data of the above trials. The angiotensin-converting enzyme inhibitor (ACEI) therapy was associated with a decrease in cardiovascular (CV) death(A), all-cause mortality(B), revascularization(C), and nonfatal myocardial infarction (MI) (D). CAMELOT = Effect of Antihypertensive Agents on Cardiovascular Events in Patients With Coronary Disease and Normal Blood Pressure Trial; EUROPA = European Trial on Reduction of Cardiac Events With Perindopril in Stable Coronary Arteries trial; HOPE = Heart Outcomes Prevention Evaluation trial; PART-2 = Prevention of Atherosclerosis With Ramipril Trial; PEACE = Angiotensin-Converting Enzyme Inhibition in Stable Coronary Artery Disease; QUIET = Quinapril Ischemic Event Trial; RR = relative risk. (adapted with permission from [43])

Putting it Together

As discussed above, not all the individual trials showed a statistically significant benefit of ACEI in patients with CAD and normalLV function. The meta analysis discussed above have demonstrated a favorable response. Multiple reasons could explain the differences between the trials

- First, except for the CAMELOT trial, all trials showed a reduction in all cause mortality in patients receiving ACEIs as evidence by the individual RR from each study. However, this reduction did not reach statistical significance in some because of a small sample size and lack of statistical power. A meta-analysis can overcome this limitation and detect smaller changes in outcome.

- Second, differences in the risk profile and baseline therapies of patients enrolled among different trials have impacted the final results by reducing event ratio. The baseline characteristics of the patients and adjunctive co-therapies in the trials were consistently different. Patients in the HOPE trials had the highest risk of cardiac event (older, higher prevalence of female gender and diabetes). On the other hand, patients enrolled in the PEACE trial were more often on proven adjunctive therapies for coronary artery disease and had better risk factor modification.

- Third, the follow up duration was not the same among different trials. The QUIET and CAMELOT trials, for example, followed patients for only two years compared to HOPE, EUROPA and PEACE in which follow up was four years or more. The beneficial effects of therapy started after one year in EUROPA and two years in the HOPE trial. We did not find a statistically significant interaction between follow up duration and effect size.

- Fourth, the pharmacokinetic and pharmacodynamic characteristics of different ACEIs might have impacted the final trial results. We do not believe this is an important factor in this Meta analysis as the majority of the patients received a tissue specific ACEI.

- Fifth, the dose of the ACEI used might have been small in certain trials. In the QUIET trial, 20 mg of quanipril did not affect the overall progression of coronary atherosclerosis. This dose is less than "the standard" 40mg dose most often used.

- Sixth, differences in blood pressure drop might account for difference in efficacy estimates. Numerous experimental studies and clinical trials support the emerging realization that ACEI's restore endothelial function or prevent endothelial dysfunction more than what is expected from blood pressure reduction aloneThe HOPE and PEACE trials were associated with the same degree of blood pressure drop, yet the impact of ACEI treatment on the primary endpoint of both trials have been different. Thus, difference in the magnitude of blood pressure drop is not the only reason for inconsistency among these two trials. In addition, Subgroup analysis from HOPE and EUROPA indicates that the benefits of ACEI were universal in normotensive as well as hypertensive patients

- Seventh, there was a difference in the rate of statin use between the different trials. ACEI and statins inhibit superoxide production in the cell, thus they may have similar anti-inflammatory effects. Thus, a high statin use rate may mask the anti-atherosclerotic benefit of an ACEI.

In conclusion, treatment with ACE-I, when added to conventional therapy, reduces all cause morality, cardiovascular mortality, non-fatal myocardial infarction, and subsequent revascularization in patients with coronary artery disease who have preserved left ventricular function.

References

[1]   Rosamond W, Flegal K, Furie K, et al. Heart disease and stroke statistics--2008 update: a report from the American Heart Association Statistics Committee and Stroke Statistics Subcommittee. *Circulation* 2008;117:e25-146.

[2]   Nash DT. Comparative properties of angiotensin-converting enzyme inhibitors: relations with inhibition of tissue angiotensin-converting enzyme and potential clinical implications. *Am. J. Cardiol.* 1992;69:26C-32C.

[3]   Fabris B, Jackson B, Kohzuki M, Perich R, Johnston CI. Increased cardiac angiotensin-converting enzyme in rats with chronic heart failure. *Clin. Exp. Pharmacol. Physiol.* 1990;17:309-14.

[4]   Hirsch AT, Talsness CE, Schunkert H, Paul M, Dzau VJ. Tissue-specific activation of cardiac angiotensin converting enzyme in experimental heart failure. *Circ. Res.* 1991;69:475-82.

[5]   Hokimoto S, Yasue H, Fujimoto K, et al. Expression of angiotensin-converting enzyme in remaining viable myocytes of human ventricles after myocardial infarction. *Circulation* 1996;94:1513-8.

[6]   Pieruzzi F, Abassi ZA, Keiser HR. Expression of renin-angiotensin system components in the heart, kidneys, and lungs of rats with experimental heart failure. *Circulation* 1995;92:3105-12.

[7]   Ruzicka M, Skarda V, Leenen FH. Effects of ACE inhibitors on circulating versus cardiac angiotensin II in volume overload-induced cardiac hypertrophy in rats. *Circulation* 1995;92:3568-73.

[8]   Schunkert H, Dzau VJ, Tang SS, Hirsch AT, Apstein CS, Lorell BH. Increased rat cardiac angiotensin converting enzyme activity and mRNA expression in pressure overload left ventricular hypertrophy. Effects on coronary resistance, contractility, and relaxation. *J. Clin. Invest.* 1990;86:1913-20.

[9]   Baker KM, Aceto JF. Angiotensin II stimulation of protein synthesis and cell growth in chick heart cells. *Am. J. Physiol.* 1990;259:H610-8.

[10]   Rajagopalan S, Kurz S, Munzel T, et al. Angiotensin II-mediated hypertension in the rat increases vascular superoxide production via membrane NADH/NADPH oxidase activation. Contribution to alterations of vasomotor tone. *J. Clin. Invest.* 1996;97:1916-23.

[11]   Collins T, Read MA, NeishAS, Whitley MZ, Thanos D, Maniatis T. Transcriptional regulation of endothelial cell adhesion molecules: NF-kappa B and cytokine-inducible enhancers. *FASEB J.* 1995;9:899-909.

[12]   Marui N, Offermann MK, Swerlick R, et al. Vascular cell adhesion molecule-1 (VCAM-1) gene transcription and expression are regulated through an antioxidant-sensitive mechanism in human vascular endothelial cells. *J. Clin. Invest.* 1993;92:1866-74.

[13]   Britten MB, Zeiher AM, Schachinger V. Clinical importance of coronary endothelial vasodilator dysfunction and therapeutic options. J Intern Med 1999;245:315-27.

[14]   Drexler H, Hornig B. Endothelial dysfunction in human disease. *J. Mol. Cell Cardiol.* 1999;31:51-60.

[15] Vaughan DE, Lazos SA, Tong K. Angiotensin II regulates the expression of plasminogen activator inhibitor-1 in cultured endothelial cells. A potential link between the renin-angiotensin system and thrombosis. *J. Clin. Invest* .1995;95:995-1001.

[16] VaughanDE, Rouleau JL, Ridker PM, Arnold JM, Menapace FJ, Pfeffer MA. Effects of ramipril on plasma fibrinolytic balance in patients with acute anterior myocardial infarction. HEART Study Investigators. *Circulation* 1997;96:442-7.

[17] Effects of enalapril on mortality in severe congestive heart failure. Results of the Cooperative North Scandinavian Enalapril Survival Study (CONSENSUS). The CONSENSUS Trial Study Group. *N. Engl. J. Med.* 1987;316:1429-35.

[18] Effect of ramipril on mortality and morbidity of survivors of acute myocardial infarction with clinical evidence of heart failure. The Acute Infarction Ramipril Efficacy (AIRE) Study Investigators. *Lancet* 1993;342:821-8.

[19] GISSI-3: effects of lisinopril and transdermal glyceryl trinitrate singly and together on 6-week mortality and ventricular function after acute myocardial infarction. Gruppo Italiano per lo Studio della Sopravvivenza nell'infarto Miocardico. *Lancet* 1994;343:1115-22.

[20] ISIS-4: a randomised factorial trial assessing early oral captopril, oral mononitrate, and intravenous magnesium sulphate in 58,050 patients with suspected acute myocardial infarction. ISIS-4 (Fourth International Study of Infarct Survival) Collaborative Group. *Lancet* 1995;345:669-85.

[21] Ambrosioni E, Borghi C, Magnani B. The effect of the angiotensin-converting-enzyme inhibitor zofenopril on mortality and morbidity after anterior myocardial infarction. The Survival of Myocardial Infarction Long-Term Evaluation (SMILE) Study Investigators. *N. Engl. J. Med.* 1995;332:80-5.

[22] Flather MD, Yusuf S, Kober L, et al. Long-term ACE-inhibitor therapy in patients with heart failure or left-ventricular dysfunction: a systematic overview of data from individual patients. ACE-Inhibitor Myocardial Infarction Collaborative Group. *Lancet* 2000;355:1575-81.

[23] Kober L, Torp-Pedersen C, Carlsen JE, et al. A clinical trial of the angiotensin-converting-enzyme inhibitor trandolapril in patients with left ventricular dysfunction after myocardial infarction. Trandolapril Cardiac Evaluation (TRACE) Study Group. *N. Engl. J. Med.* 1995;333:1670-6.

[24] Neal B, MacMahon S, Chapman N. Effects of ACE inhibitors, calcium antagonists, and other blood-pressure-lowering drugs: results of prospectively designed overviews of randomised trials. Blood Pressure Lowering Treatment Trialists' Collaboration. *Lancet* 2000;356:1955-64.

[25] Otsuka M, Yamamoto H, Okimoto T, et al. Long-term effects of quinapril with high affinity for tissue angiotensin-converting enzyme after coronary intervention in Japanese. *Am. Heart J.* 2004;147:662-8.

[26] Pfeffer MA, Braunwald E, Moye LA, et al. Effect of captopril on mortality and morbidity in patients with left ventricular dysfunction after myocardial infarction. Results of the survival and ventricular enlargement trial. The SAVE Investigators. *N. Engl. J. Med.* 1992;327:669-77.

[27] Pfeffer MA, Greaves SC, Arnold JM, et al. Early versus delayed angiotensin-converting enzyme inhibition therapy in acute myocardial infarction. The healing and early afterload reducing therapy trial. *Circulation* 1997;95:2643-51.

[28] Staessen JA, Wang JG, Thijs L. Cardiovascular protection and blood pressure reduction: a meta-analysis. *Lancet* 2001;358:1305-15.

[29] Turnbull F. Effects of different blood-pressure-lowering regimens on major cardiovascular events: results of prospectively-designed overviews of randomised trials. *Lancet* 2003;362:1527-35.

[30] Pfeffer MA, Lamas GA, Vaughan DE, Parisi AF, Braunwald E. Effect of captopril on progressive ventricular dilatation after anterior myocardial infarction. *N. Engl. J. Med.* 1988;319:80-6.

[31] Pretorius M, Rosenbaum D, VaughanDE, BrownNJ. Angiotensin-converting enzyme inhibition increases human vascular tissue-type plasminogen activator release through endogenous bradykinin. *Circulation* 2003;107:579-85.

[32] Antman EM, Anbe DT, Armstrong PW, et al. ACC/AHA guidelines for the management of patients with ST-elevation myocardial infarction--executive summary: a report of the American College of Cardiology/American Heart Association Task Force on Practice Guidelines (Writing Committee to Revise the 1999 Guidelines for the Management of Patients With Acute Myocardial Infarction). *Circulation* 2004;110:588-636.

[33] Yusuf S, Sleight P, Pogue J, Bosch J, Davies R, Dagenais G. Effects of an angiotensin-converting-enzyme inhibitor, ramipril, on cardiovascular events in high-risk patients. The Heart Outcomes Prevention Evaluation Study Investigators. *N. Engl. J. Med.* 2000;342:145-53.

[34] Dagenais GR, Yusuf S, Bourassa MG, et al. Effects of ramipril on coronary events in high-risk persons: results of the Heart Outcomes Prevention Evaluation Study. *Circulation* 2001;104:522-6.

[35] MacMahon S, Sharpe N, Gamble G, et al. Randomized, placebo-controlled trial of the angiotensin-converting enzyme inhibitor, ramipril, in patients with coronary or other occlusive arterial disease. PART-2 Collaborative Research Group. Prevention of Atherosclerosis with Ramipril. *J. Am. Coll. Cardiol.* 2000;36:438-43.

[36] Pitt B, O'Neill B, Feldman R, et al. The QUinapril Ischemic Event Trial (QUIET): evaluation of chronic ACE inhibitor therapy in patients with ischemic heart disease and preserved left ventricular function. *Am. J. Cardiol.* 2001;87:1058-63.

[37] Cashin-Hemphill L, Holmvang G, Chan RC, Pitt B, Dinsmore RE, Lees RS. Angiotensin-converting enzyme inhibition as antiatherosclerotic therapy: no answer yet. QUIET Investigators. QUinapril Ischemic Event Trial. *Am. J. Cardiol.* 1999;83:43-7.

[38] Mancini GB, Henry GC, Macaya C, et al. Angiotensin-converting enzyme inhibition with quinapril improves endothelial vasomotor dysfunction in patients with coronary artery disease. The TREND (Trial on Reversing ENdothelial Dysfunction) Study. *Circulation* 1996;94:258-65.

[39] Fox KM. Efficacy of perindopril in reduction of cardiovascular events among patients with stable coronary artery disease: randomised, double-blind, placebo-controlled, multicentre trial (the EUROPA study). *Lancet* 2003;362:782-8.

[40] Nissen SE, Tuzcu EM, Libby P, et al. Effect of antihypertensive agents on cardiovascular events in patients with coronary disease and normal blood pressure: the CAMELOT study: a randomized controlled trial. *JAMA* 2004;292:2217-25.

[41] Braunwald E, Domanski MJ, Fowler SE, et al. Angiotensin-converting-enzyme inhibition in stable coronary artery disease. *N. Engl. J. Med.* 2004;351:2058-68.

[42] Rouleau JL, Warnica WJ, Baillot R, et al. Effects of angiotensin-converting enzyme inhibition in low-risk patients early after coronary artery bypass surgery. *Circulation* 2008;117:24-31.

[43] Al-Mallah MH, Tleyjeh IM, Abdel-Latif AA, Weaver WD. Angiotensin-converting enzyme inhibitors in coronary artery disease and preserved left ventricular systolic function: a systematic review and meta-analysis of randomized controlled trials. *J. Am. Coll. Cardiol* 2006;47:1576-83.

Index

E

I

O

N

T